Health, Social Problems and Well-Being of Patients with Chronic Diseases, Quality of Life, and the Need for Emotional and Social Support

Health, Social Problems and Well-Being of Patients with Chronic Diseases, Quality of Life, and the Need for Emotional and Social Support

Guest Editors

Grażyna Bączyk
Dorota Formanowicz

MDPI

Basel • Beijing • Wuhan • Barcelona • Belgrade • Novi Sad • Cluj • Manchester

Guest Editors
Grażyna Bączyk
Department of Nursing
Poznan University of
Medical Sciences
Poznan
Poland

Dorota Formanowicz
Department of Medical Chemistry
and Laboratory Medicine Poznan
University of Medical Sciences
Poznan
Poland

Editorial Office
MDPI AG
Grosspeteranlage 5
4052 Basel, Switzerland

This is a reprint of the Special Issue, published open access by the journal *Healthcare* (ISSN 2227-9032), freely accessible at: https://www.mdpi.com/journal/healthcare/special_issues/N6MY5Z43CV.

For citation purposes, cite each article independently as indicated on the article page online and as indicated below:

Lastname, A.A.; Lastname, B.B. Article Title. *Journal Name* **Year**, *Volume Number*, Page Range.

ISBN 978-3-7258-6358-7 (Hbk)
ISBN 978-3-7258-6359-4 (PDF)
https://doi.org/10.3390/books978-3-7258-6359-4

Contents

About the Editors vii

Preface ix

Saja H. Almazrou, Shiekha S. Alaujan and Nouf F. AlSaad
Assessing the Roles and Responsibilities of Informal Caregivers from the Perspective of Adult Patients in Saudi Arabia: A Cross-Sectional Study
Reprinted from: *Healthcare* **2025**, *13*, 1038, https://doi.org/10.3390/healthcare13091038 1

Cristina Flores Mata and Carmina Castellano-Tejedor
Relationship Between Instagram, Body Satisfaction, and Self-Esteem in Early Adulthood
Reprinted from: *Healthcare* **2024**, *12*, 2153, https://doi.org/10.3390/healthcare12212153 11

Chiu-Hsiang Lee, Yu-An Chen, Chiu-Ming Yang, Kuang-Hua Huang, Tung-Han Tsai, Yuanmay Chang and Shwn-Huey Shieh
Risk Factors Associated with Unplanned Hospitalization Among Long-Term Care Facility Residents: A Retrospective Study in Central Taiwan
Reprinted from: *Healthcare* **2024**, *12*, 2069, https://doi.org/10.3390/healthcare12202069 28

Jessi Hanson-DeFusco, Decontee Davis, Meghana Bommareddy and Zainab Olayemi Olaniyan
Understanding Ethical Concerns Involving Vulnerable Human Participant Populations in Medical Research: Mixed-Method Analysis of Liberian Ebola Survivors' Experiences in PREVAIL I–VII
Reprinted from: *Healthcare* **2024**, *12*, 1989, https://doi.org/10.3390/healthcare12191989 37

Leona Yuen-Ling Leung, Hon-Lon Tam, Isaac Sze-Him Leung, Alex Siu-Wing Chan, Yueheng Yin, Xiubin Zhang, et al.
Perceived Well-Being among Adults with Diabetes and Hypertension: A National Study
Reprinted from: *Healthcare* **2024**, *12*, 844, https://doi.org/10.3390/healthcare12080844 59

Katarzyna Krefft-Trzciniecka, Hanna Cisoń, Alicja Pakiet, Danuta Nowicka and Jacek C. Szepietowski
Enhancing Quality of Life and Sexual Functioning in Female Androgenetic Alopecia: Therapeutic Potential of Hair Follicle-Derived Stem Cells
Reprinted from: *Healthcare* **2024**, *12*, 608, https://doi.org/10.3390/healthcare12060608 71

Izolde Bouloukaki, Antonios Christodoulakis, Katerina Margetaki, Antonia Aravantinou Karlatou and Ioanna Tsiligianni
Exploring the Link between Social Support and Patient-Reported Outcomes in Chronic Obstructive Pulmonary Disease Patients: A Cross-Sectional Study in Primary Care
Reprinted from: *Healthcare* **2024**, *12*, 544, https://doi.org/10.3390/healthcare12050544 82

Philippos Klonizakis, Noémi Roy, Ioanna Papatsouma, Maria Mainou, Ioanna Christodoulou, Despina Pantelidou, et al.
A Cross-Sectional, Multicentric, Disease-Specific, Health-Related Quality of Life Study in Greek Transfusion Dependent Thalassemia Patients
Reprinted from: *Healthcare* **2024**, *12*, 524, https://doi.org/10.3390/healthcare12050524 100

Patricia Solís García, María Souto Serrano, Mª Ángeles Alcedo Rodríguez, Elsa Peña Suárez, Ignacio Pedrosa and Antonio León Aguado Diaz
Ageing with Parkinson's: Identification of Personal Needs in the Northern Spanish Context
Reprinted from: *Healthcare* **2024**, *12*, 498, https://doi.org/10.3390/healthcare12040498 115

Grażyna Bączyk, Anna Pleszewa, Dorota Formanowicz and Katarzyna A. Kozłowska
Quality of Life for Polish Women with Ovarian Cancer during First-Line Chemotherapy
Reprinted from: *Healthcare* **2023**, *11*, 2596, https://doi.org/10.3390/healthcare11182596 . . . . . **126**

Enrica Cogodi, Jessica Ranieri, Alessandra Martelli and Dina Di Giacomo
Emotional Dysregulation in Anorexia Nervosa: Scoping Review of Psychological Treatments
Reprinted from: *Healthcare* **2024**, *12*, 1388, https://doi.org/10.3390/healthcare12141388 . . . . . **144**

Marcin Kuryłło and Ewa Mojs
Do Atopic Dermatitis and Psoriasis Have an Impact on Cognitive Decline—Latest Research Review
Reprinted from: *Healthcare* **2024**, *12*, 1170, https://doi.org/10.3390/healthcare12121170 . . . . . **157**

About the Editors

Grażyna Bączyk

Grażyna Bączyk is an Associate Professor and Head of the Department of Nursing Practice, Faculty of Health Sciences, Poznan University of Medical Sciences, and is also an Associate Professor at the Academy of Applied Sciences in Gniezno. She specializes in surgical nursing, and her research interests closely reflect her clinical and teaching expertise. She focuses on the care and functioning of patients with chronic diseases—including autoimmune disorders, connective tissue diseases, and inflammatory bowel diseases—as well as patients requiring surgical treatment. Her main research areas include the assessment of the quality of nursing care in postoperative pain management and the evaluation of quality of life in patients with chronic diseases and those undergoing surgical procedures. From 2018 to 2021, she participated in the international InovSafeCare project, which aimed to educate students on innovative methods of infection prevention and control in healthcare facilities. A key outcome of this initiative was the development of an e-book for students on the prevention and control of healthcare-associated infections (HAI). She is currently involved in the InfPrev4frica project, a continuation of InovSafeCare. Assoc. Prof. Bączyk has completed several internships at international centers and is an active member of the Polish Nursing Association. She is the author of more than 200 scientific articles and several textbook chapters and serves as an editor of student textbooks. Additionally, she is an active reviewer of nursing articles for several scientific journals.

Dorota Formanowicz

Dorota Formanowicz is a Professor and Head of the Department of Medical Chemistry and Laboratory Medicine at the Poznan University of Medical Sciences, where she also leads the Laboratory of Biology and Systems Medicine. Her research focuses on systems medicine, atherosclerosis, and the molecular and systemic mechanisms underlying chronic diseases, including diabetes, chronic kidney disease, and cardiovascular disorders. She is particularly interested in biomarker discovery, oxidative stress, and the complexity of disease networks. She earned her medical degree in 2001, completed her Ph.D. in 2005, habilitation in 2015, and was awarded the title of Professor in 2021. She specializes in internal medicine and actively supervises Ph.D. candidates. Prof. Formanowicz has authored more than 200 scientific articles, reviews, and book chapters, with a cumulative Impact Factor of approximately 300, an h-index of 22, and nearly 1830 citations. She was recognized among MDPI's Top 1000 Reviewers in 2024 and received the Outstanding Reviewer Award 2024 in *Biomedicines*. She is also a recipient of the Silver Cross of Merit for her contributions to medical science. Additionally, she has received numerous scientific and teaching awards from the Rector of the Poznan University of Medical Sciences. Her professional activities include editorial roles in scientific journals, participation in international research collaborations, and a strong commitment to advancing evidence-based medicine, systems biology, and innovative approaches in laboratory diagnostics.

Preface

This Special Issue aims to explore health, social, and emotional issues, assess quality of life, and assess the need for social and emotional support in people with chronic illnesses. Research on these aspects allows us to obtain valuable information from patients. This includes not only disease symptoms and treatment side effects, but also assessment of psychological (well-being), social, and spiritual dimensions. Research findings on these specific issues occurring in people with chronic illnesses will help guide treatment and patient care through evidence-based medicine (EBM) and evidence-based nursing practice (EBNP).

This Reprint addresses the complex health, social, and emotional challenges faced by individuals living with chronic diseases. Its scope includes research on quality of life, psychosocial well-being, and the need for social and emotional support. The aim is to provide evidence-based insights that guide clinical practice and nursing care. We were motivated by the growing importance of holistic approaches in managing chronic diseases. This Reprint is intended for healthcare professionals, researchers, and policy makers seeking to improve patient-centered care. We sincerely thank all contributing authors and reviewers for their valuable efforts in making this collection possible.

Grażyna Bączyk and Dorota Formanowicz
Guest Editors

healthcare

MDPI

Article

Assessing the Roles and Responsibilities of Informal Caregivers from the Perspective of Adult Patients in Saudi Arabia: A Cross-Sectional Study

Saja H. Almazrou [1,*], Shiekha S. Alaujan [1] and Nouf F. AlSaad [2]

[1] Clinical Pharmacy Department, College of Pharmacy, King Saud University, Riyadh 11362, Saudi Arabia; salaujan@ksu.edu.sa

[2] Royal Commission Hospital, Jubail 31961, Saudi Arabia; noof.f.alsaad@gmail.com

* Correspondence: salmazrou@ksu.edu.sa

Abstract: Objectives: This study aim to determine the characteristics, roles, responsibilities, and challenges of informal caregivers for adult patients in Saudi Arabia. **Methods**: Adult patients who have informal caregivers were invited to participate in a cross-sectional study. The inclusion criteria were patients who were 18 years old or older and permanent Saudi residents. A self-administered online questionnaire was used to identify patients' demographics, roles, responsibilities, and care challenges. Data collection lasted four months. Percentages, means, and standard deviations were reported in the analysis. **Results:** The study included 276 participants, mostly female (68.8%), with a mean age of 55.21 years (SD = 20.3). Over half were married (56.2%) and not employed (81.9%). Common chronic diseases were diabetes and hypertension, with 55.8% using up to five medications. Caregivers were mainly sons or daughters (62%) living with the patient (84.1%). The top caregiver tasks were escorting patients to appointments (63.4%), scheduling doctor appointments (60.1%), and tracking medication refills (59.4%). Common challenges included caregivers lacking time (45.3%), inconsistent care (35.9%), financial constraints (27.5%), and caregivers missing doses (27.9%). The top not encountered challenges were inappropriate medication storage (78.3%), communication barriers (74.3%), improper disposal of injections (72.5%), medication management errors (71.4%), and lack of empathy (70.3%). **Conclusion:** This study highlights the vital role of informal caregivers in managing chronic illnesses in Saudi Arabia. Informal caregivers face challenges such as time constraints and financial limitations. The findings emphasize the need for better support systems, including training programs and improved access to healthcare resources, to enhance care quality for patients.

Keywords: informal caregivers; healthcare recipients; roles; challenges; Saudi Arabia

1. Introduction

Informal caregivers play a crucial role in providing support to individuals with various needs, particularly older adults, encompassing a wide range of tasks that are essential for their care recipients' well-being. Understanding these responsibilities is vital for recognizing the impact of informal caregiving on caregivers and the healthcare system. Key responsibilities include physical assistance, in which caregivers often help with daily activities such as mobility, medication management, and personal hygiene, which are critical for maintaining their care recipient's health [1]. They also serve as navigators in healthcare systems, helping older adults access necessary services and advocating for their needs [2]. Informal caregivers also provide emotional and social support, which are essential for their care recipients' mental well-being [3]. Additionally, they frequently coordinate among various healthcare providers and services to ensure continuity of care and address any gaps in service delivery [2]. The financial impact of caregiving is substantial, with caregivers in the United States delivering approximately 37 billion hours of care each year, amounting to an estimated value of USD 470 billion. This underscores the vital contribution caregivers make to the healthcare system [4].

In Saudi Arabia, patients often rely on family members or domestic workers (e.g. housemaids) to assist them with a wide range of tasks, including those related to their health [5]. A national study revealed that nearly half of all informal caregivers in the country are housemaids, highlighting the significant role they play in the caregiving landscape. Furthermore, the same study found that 66% of patients depend on their caregivers for critical tasks such as medication management. This reliance on informal caregivers underscores the importance of identifying and understanding this group, as it can help pinpoint individuals who are highly dependent on caregivers and ensure they receive the appropriate support they need.

Although substantial international literature has explored the roles and challenges of informal caregivers, much of this research is situated in Western contexts and focuses primarily on family caregivers [6–8]. These studies may not fully reflect the caregiving dynamics in countries like Saudi Arabia, where domestic workers play an unusually prominent role in providing health-related care. In addition, most caregiving literature investigates the views of the caregivers, and limited studies explore the caregiving process from the healthcare recipients' perspective. Understanding the perspectives of care recipients is essential, as they may differ significantly from the caregiver's own perceptions. The voices of care recipients can inform more balanced and patient-centered policy and service development [9].

Despite the critical role of informal caregivers in Saudi Arabia, research on this topic remains limited. Existing studies have primarily focused on the burden experienced by family caregivers [10,11] or have described the demographic characteristics of caregivers and care recipients, along with the scope of care they provide [5,12]. For instance, some studies have explored the emotional, physical, and financial challenges faced by family members who take on caregiving roles, while others have outlined the general responsibilities of caregivers in the Saudi context. However, none of these studies have specifically addressed the tasks and challenges associated with involving informal caregivers—such as housemaids or other domestic workers—in the provision of healthcare to patients.

This gap in the literature highlights the need for a more focused investigation into the roles, responsibilities, and challenges of informal caregivers in Saudi Arabia. By doing so, we can gain a deeper understanding of how these caregivers contribute to the healthcare system, the specific tasks they perform, and the difficulties they encounter. Such insights are crucial for developing targeted interventions and support systems that can improve the quality of care provided to patients and alleviate the burdens faced by informal caregivers.

Therefore, this study aims to determine the roles, responsibilities, and challenges of informal caregivers in Saudi Arabia. By shedding light on these aspects, we hope to contribute to a more comprehensive understanding of the caregiving landscape in the country and inform policies and practices that better support both caregivers and the patients who depend on them. This research is particularly timely and relevant, given the growing reliance on informal caregivers in Saudi Arabia and the need to ensure that their contributions are recognized and supported within the healthcare system.

2. Methodology

2.1. Study Design

A cross-sectional study was conducted in Saudi Arabia to investigate the experiences and perspectives of healthcare recipients toward caregivers. The study utilized an online data collection method through a self-reported questionnaire. The survey was distributed via Twitter, a social media platform, to reach a broad audience efficiently. Data collection spanned four months, ensuring a sufficient sample size and diversity in responses.

2.2. Participants

A convenient sample of healthcare recipients were invited. The use of a convenience sample was justified by the need for rapid data collection and the accessibility of participants through social media platforms like Twitter. The inclusion and exclusion criteria were designed to ensure that the study focused on the experiences of adult healthcare recipients in Saudi Arabia who rely on informal caregivers, thereby providing insights into the dynamics of caregiving within familial or domestic settings. The inclusion criteria for the study required healthcare recipients to be living in Saudi Arabia, aged 18 years or more, and report having a caregiver, either a family member or a domestic worker, at the time of initial screening. Conversely, the exclusion criteria specified that healthcare recipients living outside Saudi Arabia; independent patients; informal caregivers for children; and those with formal caregivers, such as paid nurses, were not eligible to participate in the study.

2.3. Data Collection/Data Source

Recruitment

Twitter was used as the main source to approach the target healthcare recipients. We created an account for this study, highlighting the research problem and potential implications. Then, we posted the survey on a regular basis. We contacted several national accounts related to chronic disease organizations and governmental bodies in health to post the survey to their accounts.

2.4. Instrument

SurveyMonkey [13] was used to create the online survey. The first page gave a brief description of the study's aim. Then, consent to participate in the study was required. To ensure that we targeted the right sample, we asked a few screening questions, which included the country of current residence, the need for caregivers (family or paid domestic worker), and the participant's age. If the participant passed the screening section, the survey questions started appearing afterward. If the participants did not pass some of the screening questions, the survey ended at this point.

The instrument used in this study consisted of three sections. The first section captured the healthcare recipients' demographic data. The second section was a checklist intended to assess the level of caregiver involvement in providing care to the healthcare recipients. The expected caregivers' tasks were derived from published studies [14]. The third section assessed reasons for needing assistance and health-related challenges arising from the caregivers' provision of the patients' healthcare. The total number of roles and responsibilities was 16 and the total number of challenges associated with caregiving was 12. Three Likert scales were used for the second and third sections.

The survey was reviewed by three professionals who determined its validity. It was utilized in a five-participant pilot study to check the clarity and applicability. The study survey is given in Supplementary File S1.

Statistical Analysis: Statistical analyses were conducted using SPSS 22. Descriptive analysis was conducted to describe the data. Numbers and percentages were used to present categorical data and means, and standard deviation was used to represent continuous data. This study was exploratory in nature and did not involve regression or multivariate analyses, as its primary objective was to describe and understand the roles, responsibilities, and challenges of informal caregivers in Saudi Arabia.

2.5. Ethical Considerations

Participation in the study was voluntary. Participants' name were not revealed. The collected data were kept private. The consent page was displayed on the first page of the questionnaire to all participants, clearly indicating the purpose of the study. No incentives or rewards were given to the participants, and their anonymity and confidentiality were guaranteed. Ethical approval was obtained from King Fahad Medical City (IRB number 20-436E).

3. Results

The number of study participants was 276 (68.8% female), with a mean age of 55.21 (SD = 20.3), and the majority had a secondary or low educational level (39.6%) or university educational level or higher (31.9%) (Table 1). More than half of the sample were married (56.2%) and not employed (81.9%). Ninety-seven percent were Saudis from the central region (62.7%), living in an urban region (88%) with a spouse or children (43.8%). Regarding chronic diseases, 62.7% and 46% reported having diabetes and hypertension, respectively (Table S1), and used up to five medications (55.8%) for their chronic illnesses. Most of the patients (68.5%) reported using medications that require caregivers' assistance, such as injections (27.9%) and eye and ear drops (19.2%).

The majority of caregivers were sons or daughters, (62%), lived together with the patient (84.1%), and provided care a maximum of 8 h weekly (55.1%) for more than two years (60.1%).

Table 1. Characteristics of study participants (n = 276).

Variables		N (%)
Age, Years	55.21 SD = 20.3	
Gender	Female	190 (68.8)
	Male	86 (31.2)
Education level	Illiterate	79 (28.6)
	Primary school	33 (12)
	Middle school	27 (9.8)
	Secondary school	49 (17.8)
	University	82 (29.7)
	Postgraduate	6 (2.2)
Marital status	Single	54 (19.6)
	Married	155 (56.2)
	Divorced	11 (4)
	Widowed	56 (20.3)

Table 1. *Cont.*

Variables		N (%)
Employment	Employee	50 (18.1)
	Nonemployee	226 (81.9)
Nationality	Saudi	269 (97.5)
	Non-Saudi	7(2.5)
Region of residence	Central	173 (62.7)
	East	29 (10.5)
	West	50 (18.1)
	North	22 (8)
	South	2 (0.7)
Urban or Rural	Urban	243 (88)
	Rural	33 (12)
Living arrangement	Alone	12 (4.3)
	With spouse	29 (10.5)
	With spouse and children	121 (43.8)
	With older sons/daughter	46 (16.7)
	With family relative	18 (6.5)
	Other	50 (18.1)
Relationship to the caregiver	Spouse	45 (16.3)
	Son or daughter	171 (62)
	Parent	54 (19.6)
	Permeant housekeeper	24 (8.7)
	Temporary housekeeper	11 (4)
	Friend or neighbors	2 (0.7)
	Other relatives	28 (10.1)
Distance between patients and caregiver	Living together	232 (84.1)
	Less than 10 min	14 (5.1)
	11–30 min	17 (6.2)
	More than 30 min	13 (4.7)
Care provided per week on average, hours	≤8	152 (55.1)
	9–19	62 (22.5)
	20–40	62 (22.5)
Length of care	0–3 months	47 (17)
	4–12 months	24 (8.7)
	One to two years	39 (14.1)
	More than two years	166 (60.1)

SD: standard deviation.

Patient-reported reasons for the need for caregiver assistance are illustrated in Figure 1. The most common were having complex health issues and polypharmacy (46.7%), followed by the presence of physical inability to manage health (45.7%), the inability to use technology for booking appointments, and refilling medications (37.3%).

Caregivers' roles and responsibilities were reported by 248 participants. The top three rated roles and responsibilities were escorting the patient to an appointment (63.4%), followed by scheduling doctors appointments (60.1%), and keep tracking of medication refills (59.4%) whereas injecting medication into patients (40.6%), wound ostomy care (42.8%), and helping the patient bathe and maintain personal hygiene (49.6%) were the bottom three rated roles and responsibilities (Table 2).

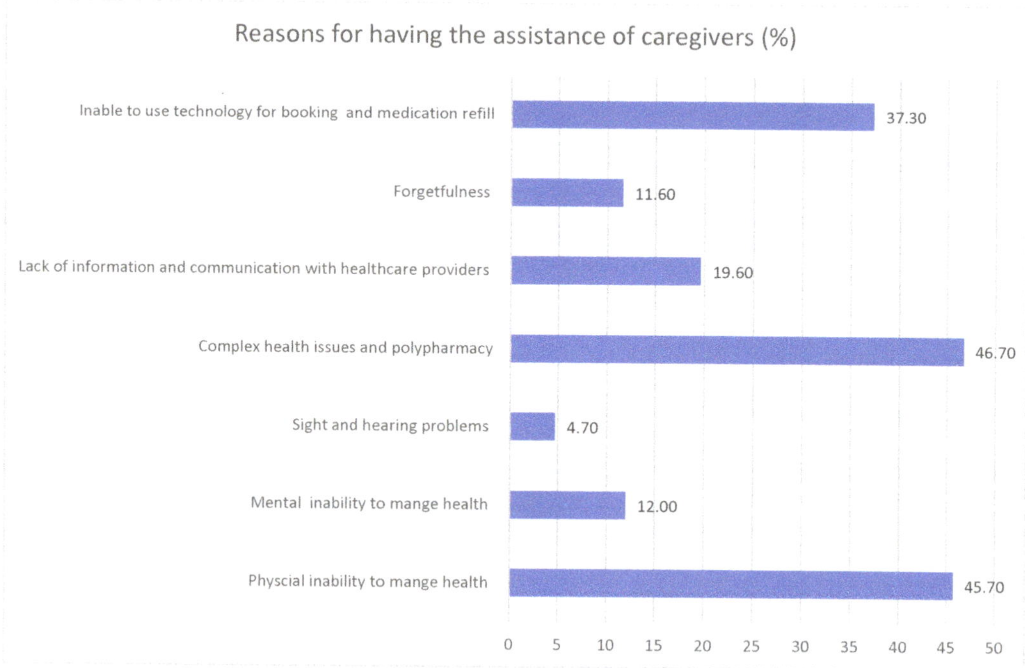

Figure 1. Reasons participants reported for having caregivers' assistance, as percentages.

Table 2. Caregivers' roles and responsibilities ($n = 248$).

Responses	Never Applicable N (%)	Sometimes Applicable N (%)	Always Applicable N (%)
Obtain medication from the pharmacy	25 (9.1)	82 (29.7)	141 (51.1)
Remind you to take medications	28 (10.1)	82 (29.7)	138 (50)
Prepare pill boxes	55 (20.3)	65 (23.6)	127 (46)
Hand you the medications	53 (19.2)	81 (29.3)	114 (41.3)
Write down a report of falling or any medication side effects	40 (14.5)	86 (31.2)	122 (44.2)
Measure patient's blood pressure and sugar	49 (17.8)	78 (28.3)	121 (43.8)
Inject medication into patients	112 (40.6)	47 (17)	89 (32.2)
Keep track of medication refill	22 (8)	62 (22.5)	164 (59.4)
Escort you to an appointment	14 (5.1)	59 (21.4)	175 (63.4)
Schedule doctor appointment	32 (11.6)	50 (18.1)	166 (60.1)
Assist you in performing physiotherapy exercise	92 (33.3)	59 (21.4)	97 (35.1)
Prepare special food for you	47 (17)	73 (26.4)	128 (46.4)
Assist you in eating	55 (20.3)	81 (29.3)	111 (40.2)
Assist you in bathing and personal hygiene	137 (49.6)	40 (14.5)	71 (25.7)
Wound ostomy care	118 (42.8)	51 (18.5)	79 (28.6)
Encourage the patients to adhere to a healthy lifestyle	22 (8)	63 (22.8)	163 (59.1)

The challenges encountered during care (n = 248) are presented in Table 3. Patients reported always or sometimes having challenges with the caregiver because they has no time (45.3%), inconsistent care because the caregiver has other responsibilities (35.9%), the patient being unable to afford a paid domestic worker (27.5%), and the caregiver missing doses (27.9%). Of the most common not encountered challenges, the caregiver stored medication (e.g., insulin) inappropriately (78.3%), had difficulty communicating due to a language barrier (74.3%), inappropriately disposed of injections (72.5%), made an error during medication management (e.g., wrong medication or wrong frequency/dose) (71.4%), or lacked empathy (70.3%).

Table 3. Patient's response regarding challenges encountered during care (n = 248).

Responses	Never Applicable N (%)	Sometimes Applicable N (%)	Always Applicable N (%)
Caregiver made an error during medication management (e.g., wrong medication, wrong frequency/dose)	197 (71.4)	44 (15.9)	7 (2.5)
Caregiver stored medication (e.g., insulin) inappropriately	216 (78.3)	27 (9.8)	5 (1.8)
Inappropriate disposal of injections	200 (72.5)	26 (9.4)	22 (8)
Caregiver missed doses	171 (62)	70 (25.4)	7 (2.5)
Caregiver lacks specialized skills needed (e.g., using injection or nebulizers)	178 (64.5)	49 (17.8)	21 (7.6)
Caregivers are not consistently monitoring my condition	184 (66.7)	53 (19.2)	11 (4)
The caregiver does not understand the assigned task/ limited health literacy	165 (59.8)	66 (23.9)	17 (6.2)
Difficulty in communicating due to language barrier	205 (74.3)	27 (9.8)	16 (5.8)
Inconsistent care because caregiver has other responsibilities	149 (54)	69 (25)	30 (10.9)
Lack of empathy	194 (70.3)	41 (14.9)	13 (4.7)
The caregiver has no time	123 (44.6)	115 (41.7)	10 (3.6)
Inconsistent care because I cannot afford a paid domestic worker	172 (62.3)	44 (15.9)	32 (11.6)

4. Discussion

The study highlights the demographics of healthcare recipients who require informal caregivers in Saudi Arabia and the caregivers' roles, responsibilities, and challenges when they provide care to the recipients. The sample involved a diverse group of participants, primarily middle-aged females with various educational backgrounds, most of whom were married and unemployed. The majority reported chronic health conditions, often managing multiple medications. The caregivers, primarily adult children, lived with the healthcare recipients and contributed several hours of care each week. Healthcare recipients emphasized their need for assistance due to complex health issues and physical limitations. Key caregiver tasks included accompanying patients to appointments and managing scheduling, and common challenges faced included time constraints, inconsistent care, and difficulties in medication management, alongside issues with medication storage and communication barriers.

The use of technology was one of the main reasons for having informal care assistance in the current study. Our results were consistent with a published systematic review that highlighted that age-related physical limitations, such as hearing and poor vision; cognitive disorders, such as poor memory; and limited learning skills were the main barriers to adopting healthcare technologies [15].

Escorting patients to appointments and scheduling were reported in our study as caregiver tasks. This aligned with several studies that reported similar practical caregiver tasks, such as contacting home care services, scheduling appointments, and providing transportation [6–8]. They also kept records of test results and handled multiple medications for older adults with complex needs [6–8].

According to the current study's results on the roles and responsibilities of caregivers, tracking medicine refills, preparing pill boxes, and administering medication to patients were the most reported tasks. This aligns with Reinhard et al., who reported that more than one third of informal caregiver respondents helped with various medication management responsibilities [16].

Caregivers have reported making medication errors, particularly in the storage and administration of medications. These errors include losing pills, administering medications at incorrect times, and missing doses [17]. A study showed that one in eight caregivers involved in medication management acknowledged making mistakes in administering medications [18]. In the current study, a minority of healthcare recipients reported having issues with their caregiver making a mistake during medication management (e.g., incorrect medicine or inappropriate frequency/dosage) or missing a medication dose. In addition, a small number of healthcare recipients reported that their caregiver lacks specialized skills needed (e.g., using injection or nebulizers).

4.1. Limitations

The study has several limitations that should be considered. First, the use of a convenient sample and recruitment through Twitter may introduce sampling bias because the sample might not represent the entire population of healthcare recipients in Saudi Arabia. Additionally, the reliance on self-reported data can lead to response bias, with participants potentially providing inaccurate or socially desirable answers. In addition, technical issues were encountered when the participants filled the online questionnaire and led to incomplete surveys by some respondents.

4.2. Implication

This study's results have several important implications. First, the high prevalence of chronic diseases, such as diabetes and hypertension, among the healthcare recipients highlights the significant burden of these conditions in the population. The reliance on caregivers for medication administration and other health-related tasks underscores the critical role caregivers play in managing chronic illnesses. The findings also indicate that many caregivers are family members, primarily sons or daughters, who provide care despite having other responsibilities, which can lead to inconsistent care and missed doses. The reported challenges, such as caregivers lacking time and the ability to afford paid domestic workers, suggest a need for better support systems for healthcare recipients and caregivers. Additionally, the low incidence of certain problems, such as inappropriate medication storage and communication barriers, suggests that some aspects of caregiving are being managed effectively. However, the overall findings emphasize the need for targeted interventions to support caregivers, improve medication management, and address the specific needs of healthcare recipients with chronic illnesses. This could include training programs for caregivers, better access to healthcare resources, and policies to alleviate the financial burden on families [2,15].

In the Saudi Arabian context, where caregivers often include domestic workers, the caregiving process may be influenced by varying levels of health literacy, education, and language barriers. These factors can hinder effective communication, understanding of medical instructions, and safe medication practices, making culturally and linguistically tailored training programs essential.

This study provides a foundation for future investigations into the quality and safety of informal caregiving, especially when non-family members are involved. Future research should explore the perspectives of caregivers themselves to identify training needs and to develop targeted interventions that address role overload, time constraints, and knowledge gaps. Longitudinal studies are also warranted to evaluate how caregiver-related challenges impact patient outcomes over time. In addition, future studies should examine the influence of demographic factors—such as age, gender, and education level—on caregivers' roles and responsibilities

5. Conclusions

In conclusion, this study highlights the significant roles, responsibilities, and health challenges of informal caregivers in managing the health of patients from the perspective of their recipients in Saudi Arabia. The findings reveal that caregivers, primarily family members, are heavily involved in various health-related tasks, including medication management and attending medical appointments. However, caregivers face numerous challenges, such as time constraints, inconsistent care due to other responsibilities, and financial limitations. These issues underscore the need for enhanced support systems for healthcare recipients and caregivers. Targeted interventions, such as caregiver training programs, improved access to healthcare resources, and policies to reduce the financial burden, are essential to improve the quality of care and support provided to healthcare recipients with chronic illnesses.

Supplementary Materials: The following supporting information can be downloaded at: https://www.mdpi.com/article/10.3390/healthcare13091038/s1, File S1: Study Survey; Table S1: Type of chronic disease and number of medications patients take.

Author Contributions: Conceptualization, S.H.A.; Methodology, N.F.A.; Formal analysis, S.S.A.; Data curation, N.F.A.; Writing—original draft, S.H.A., S.S.A. and N.F.A.; Writing—review and editing, S.H.A. and S.S.A. All authors have read and agreed to the published version of the manuscript.

Funding: This research received no external funding.

Institutional Review Board Statement: This study was approved on 2 July 2020 by the Institutional Review Board (IRB) at King Fahad Medical City (IRB number 20-436E).

Informed Consent Statement: Informed consent was obtained from all subjects involved in the study.

Data Availability Statement: The data will be available for review from the corresponding author upon request.

Acknowledgments: The author is thankful to all the associated personnel who contributed to this study by any means.

Conflicts of Interest: The authors declare that there is no conflict of interest regarding the publication of this paper.

References

1. Weir, R.L.; Hoover, D.L. Providing Physical Assistance for Family or Friends: An Overview for the Home Health Care Professional—Part 1. *Home Health Care Manag. Pract.* **2023**, *35*, 57–63. [CrossRef]
2. Kim, B.; Wister, A.; O'dea, E.; Mitchell, B.A.; Li, L.; Kadowaki, L. Roles and experiences of informal caregivers of older adults in community and healthcare system navigation: A scoping review. *BMJ Open* **2023**, *13*, e077641. [CrossRef] [PubMed]
3. Hejazi, S.S.; Hosseini, M.; Ebadi, A.; Majd, H.A. Family caregiver: The forgotten savior. *Int. J. Community Based Nurs. Midwifery* **2021**, *9*, 346.
4. Raanani, P.; Ledany, R. Make family caregivers visible, valued, and supported: An interview with patients' caregivers' advocate. *Acta Haematol.* **2023**, *146*, 49–53. [CrossRef] [PubMed]
5. Alrashed, A.M. Illustration of informal caregiving within Saudi society: Demography, scope of care and enabling arrangements. *Scand. J. Caring Sci.* **2017**, *31*, 263–272. [CrossRef] [PubMed]
6. Charles, L.; Brémault-Phillips, S.; Parmar, J.; Johnson, M.; Sacrey, L.-A. Understanding how to support family caregivers of seniors with complex needs. *Can. Geriatr. J.* **2017**, *20*, 75. [CrossRef] [PubMed]
7. Ploeg, J.; Matthew-Maich, N.; Fraser, K.; Dufour, S.; McAiney, C.; Kaasalainen, S.; Markle-Reid, M.; Upshur, R.; Cleghorn, L.; Emili, A. Managing multiple chronic conditions in the community: A Canadian qualitative study of the experiences of older adults, family caregivers and healthcare providers. *BMC Geriatr.* **2017**, *17*, 40. [CrossRef] [PubMed]
8. Bunn, F.; Burn, A.-M.; Robinson, L.; Poole, M.; Rait, G.; Brayne, C.; Schoeman, J.; Norton, S.; Goodman, C. Healthcare organisation and delivery for people with dementia and comorbidity: A qualitative study exploring the views of patients, carers and professionals. *BMJ Open* **2017**, *7*, e013067. [CrossRef] [PubMed]
9. McCann, S.; Evans, D.S. Informal care: The views of people receiving care. *Health Soc. Care Community* **2002**, *10*, 221–228. [CrossRef] [PubMed]
10. Alshammari, S.; Alzahrani, A.; Alabduljabbar, K.; Aldaghri, A.; Alhusainy, Y.; Khan, M.; Alshuwaier, R.; Kariz, I. The burden perceived by informal caregivers of the elderly in Saudi Arabia. *J. Fam. Community Med.* **2017**, *24*, 145–150. [CrossRef] [PubMed]
11. Alzahrani, S.H.; Fallata, E.O.; Alabdulwahab, M.A.; Alsafi, W.A.; Bashawri, J. Assessment of the burden on caregivers of patients with mental disorders in Jeddah, Saudi Arabia. *BMC Psychiatry* **2017**, *17*, 202. [CrossRef] [PubMed]
12. Almehmadi, S.; Alrashed, A.M. The experience of informal caregiving within Saudi society: Expressed needs and expectations. *J. Egypt. Public Health Assoc.* **2023**, *98*, 2. [CrossRef] [PubMed]
13. Survey Monkey Inc. Available online: https://www.surveymonkey.com (accessed on 1 June 2020).
14. Lindquist, L.A.; Jain, N.; Tam, K.; Martin, G.J.; Baker, D.W. Inadequate health literacy among paid caregivers of seniors. *J. Gen. Intern. Med.* **2011**, *26*, 474–479. [CrossRef] [PubMed]
15. Bertolazzi, A.; Quaglia, V.; Bongelli, R. Barriers and facilitators to health technology adoption by older adults with chronic diseases: An integrative systematic review. *BMC Public Health* **2024**, *24*, 506. [CrossRef] [PubMed]
16. Reinhard, S.C.; Levine, C.; Samis, S. *Family Caregivers Providing Complex Chronic Care to Their Spouses*; AARP Public Policy Institute: Washington, DC, USA, 2014.
17. Erlen, J.A.; Lingler, J.; Sereika, S.M.; Tamres, L.K.; Happ, M.B.; Tang, F. Characterizing caregiver-mediated medication management in patients with memory loss. *J. Gerontol. Nurs.* **2013**, *39*, 30–39. [CrossRef] [PubMed]
18. Donelan, K.; Hill, C.A.; Hoffman, C.; Scoles, K.; Feldman, P.H.; Levine, C.; Gould, D. Challenged to care: Informal caregivers in a changing health system. *Health Aff.* **2002**, *21*, 222–231. [CrossRef] [PubMed]

healthcare

MDPI

Article

Relationship Between Instagram, Body Satisfaction, and Self-Esteem in Early Adulthood

Cristina Flores Mata [1,*] and Carmina Castellano-Tejedor [1,2,3,4,5,*]

1 Faculty of Psychology, Universidad Internacional de la Rioja, 26006 Logroño, Spain
2 Psynaptic, Psicología y Servicios Científicos y Tecnológicos S.L.P., 08192 Barcelona, Spain
3 Department of Psychology and Education Sciences, Universitat Oberta de Catalunya (UOC), 08018 Barcelona, Spain
4 GIES Research Group, Basic Psychology Department, Autonomous University of Barcelona, 08192 Barcelona, Spain
5 Research Group on Aging, Frailty and Care Transitions in Barcelona (REFiT), Parc Sanitari Pere Virgili & Vall d'Hebron Research Institute (VHIR), 08023 Barcelona, Spain
* Correspondence: floresmatacristina@gmail.com (C.F.M.); carmina.castellano.t@gmail.com (C.C.-T.)

Abstract: Background/Objectives: This study aimed to explore the effects of Instagram use on body satisfaction and self-esteem in young adults 20 to 40 years (N = 95). Given the widespread use of social media and its potential influence on body image, we sought to understand how Instagram use may contribute to body dissatisfaction and self-esteem, particularly through quantitative analysis of self-report measures. **Methods:** A cross-sectional survey design in which the Rosenberg Self-Esteem Scale (RSES), the Body Shape Questionnaire (BSQ), and additional ad hoc questions designed to assess Instagram usage patterns were employed. **Results:** The results indicated that greater Instagram use is associated with increased body dissatisfaction ($p = 0.005$), although it did not significantly affect self-esteem ($p = 0.211$). Gender did not play a significant role in these relationships ($p = 0.173$). Notably, a significant positive correlation was found between body satisfaction and self-esteem, showing that individuals with higher body satisfaction also reported higher self-esteem ($p < 0.001$). Further analyses indicated that users exposed to appearance-centered content were more likely to report body dissatisfaction. **Conclusions:** These findings suggest that Instagram usage, particularly in the context of appearance-focused content, has a considerable impact on body dissatisfaction among young adults but does not appear to influence self-esteem. This highlights the importance of developing interventions focused on promoting healthy social media habits and critical content engagement to mitigate negative impacts on body image. Social media exposure should be a key component in future interventions designed to improve body image and overall psychological well-being.

Keywords: body dissatisfaction; self-esteem; Instagram; body image

1. Introduction

The multidimensional paradigm shift brought about by social networks has altered, among many other aspects, individuals' relationship with themselves concerning body satisfaction and self-esteem. Numerous studies have shown that constant exposure to social networks like Instagram, which bombards its users with images of perfect and idealized bodies on a daily basis, promotes physical comparison behaviors [1], body dissatisfaction [2,3], and low self-esteem [4] due to the pressure generated by unattainable beauty standards that have evolved significantly in recent years and are now greatly influenced by social networks [5]. Instagram's unique emphasis on visual content creates distinct patterns of social comparison and body image concerns that differ from other platforms. Body dissatisfaction, as well as damaged self-esteem, increase the likelihood of suffering from an eating disorder [6,7] or disorders such as muscle dysmorphia or body dysmorphia [3], as well as presenting low emotion regulation [8], depression, or anxiety [9,10]. Additionally, social network addiction increases body dissatisfaction and predisposes one to low self-esteem [3]. For all these reasons, this research is relevant, as it aims to analyze how exposure to Instagram is a risk factor for body satisfaction and self-esteem in early adulthood, as well as to establish gender differences, given that most studies in this area are limited and scarce.

1.1. Self-Esteem: Conceptualization

Self-esteem is a fundamental concept, defined as the subjective appreciation that a person makes of their own worth, influenced by their social environment and personal experiences. Rosenberg [11] defines self-esteem as "the positive evaluation an individual makes of themselves in terms of respect and worth" (p. 30) [11].

Abdel-Khalek [12] defines it simply as general self-satisfaction, while Branden [13] emphasizes its role in preparing individuals for life's challenges based on their confidence and emotional responses to various aspects of their identity and abilities. Self-esteem is multidimensional, affecting various life areas and evolving significantly during key developmental stages, such as adolescence [12]. This period is particularly critical due to significant psychological changes and identity integration, heavily influenced by family, teachers, and peers. Self-esteem is a global evaluation of one's worth, encompassing beliefs, emotions, competencies, and the perceived affection one deserves, ranging from high to low based on the outcome of this evaluative process [12].

1.2. Low Self-Esteem as a Risk Factor

The study of the relationship between self-esteem and gender has been extensive and diverse. The literature states that men tend to have better self-esteem than women, seeing themselves as more valuable and skilled. This trend begins in adolescence and persists until adulthood, balancing out once old age is reached. These differences are due to both sociocultural contexts and genetic and biological processes that go beyond culture [14,15].

People with low self-esteem feel inferior, less important, and less competent, suffer from greater emotional instability, and are more likely to associate with people with low self-esteem, feeling irritated in the presence of people with higher self-esteem [12,13]. Regarding technology use, Casale et al. [16] state that low self-esteem increases smartphone dependency, impulsivity, sensation seeking, and substance use. Liu et al. [17] have evidenced that low self-esteem is a risk factor for the development of mental health problems such as depression, anxiety, or eating disorders, being related to academic stress and suicidal ideation [18], as well as a reduced capacity to cope with problems [12] and a higher likelihood of experiencing burnout syndrome [19].

1.3. Body Satisfaction: Conceptualization

We live in a body-worshiping society. We are surrounded by stimuli that exalt and idealize physical appearance, from media, social networks, the fashion industry, cinema, advertising, and toys to the amount of money and effort invested in improving appearance through diets, physical exercise, and cosmetic enhancements. These factors influence body image, and more specifically, satisfaction with physical appearance [20]. To understand body satisfaction, Taylor [21] emphasizes that it is essential to distinguish between how an individual perceives their body size and the concern they feel about their body shape, as these are not equivalent terms and might not be linked. A person can misjudge how they perceive themselves physically and not feel dissatisfaction with their image and vice versa [21]. Once this distinction is made, body satisfaction can be understood as a person's contentment with various parts of their body or their overall appearance, as well as the comfort they feel with their body in different contexts [22]. Body image satisfaction is a construct closely related to general self-esteem. Authors affirm that women are the most dissatisfied and concerned about their figure, weight, or physical shape [20,23]. However, authors like Baile [24] have shown that gender differences are decreasing, as men also suffer from body image issues, specifically tending to worry more about their muscle mass and being toned and defined. Nevertheless, no significant gender differences were found in how social networks impact body dissatisfaction [25]. Saiphoo and Vahedi [26] state that there is a significant relationship between body dissatisfaction and heavy social media use. Tiggemann et al. [20] highlight that Instagram use increases women's dissatisfaction with their facial features. Lastly, Lowe and Grieve [27] warn about the dangers of following many fashion influencers, as this can negatively affect users' body satisfaction.

1.4. Distorted Perception of Body Image

The construction of body image encompasses perceptual, cognitive, affective, and behavioral aspects [28,29]. The perceptual aspect influences our body satisfaction [30] and refers to how accurately an individual perceives their body size, shape, or weight. Body image is said to be distorted when an individual's evaluation of their image leads to overestimating or underestimating their appearance disproportionately [31]. This occurs when there is a significant difference between a person's actual physical size or shape and their self-evaluation or subjective judgment [32]. Distorted body image can affect physical and psychological health, damaging self-esteem, mood, sense of competence, or social functioning [29], and can even precipitate the development of mental health disorders such as eating disorders or body dysmorphic disorders [33]. In individuals with anorexia, there is perceptual distortion regarding weight or body constitution, as they tend to evaluate themselves as heavier than they actually are. In body dysmorphic disorders, there is significant distress due to perceived physical imperfections that are not noticeable to others. Individuals with muscle dysmorphia show excessive concern about their muscle mass, perceiving themselves as thinner and weaker than they are [33]. The association between social media exposure and distorted body image has been scarcely explored in scientific studies, indicating a need for more research in this specific area. However, Parrillo and Troncoso [34] found significant results regarding Instagram use and its impact on body perception.

1.5. Body Dissatisfaction as a Risk Factor

Those who feel significantly dissatisfied with their physical appearance are more predisposed to engage in strict diets, follow intense exercise routines, undergo surgeries to alter their appearance, and consequently develop mental health issues such as eating disorders, body dysmorphic disorder, or muscle dysmorphia [24,33]. Additionally, stress, low self-esteem, and experiences of bullying have also been shown to trigger body dissatisfaction issues [35]. Exposure to social networks is a risk factor for developing body dissatisfaction, which in turn contributes to a higher risk of developing eating disorders [36]. Romano et al. [37] determined that body dissatisfaction correlates with an increase in binge eating, purging, restriction, excessive exercise, and behaviors aimed at increasing muscle mass. Furthermore, comments about physical appearance from parents during childhood and adolescence are related to greater body dissatisfaction [38]. Dissatisfaction increases the likelihood of experiencing obsessive concern about one or more body parts, as well as paying excessive attention to areas considered defective. This symptomatology is exacerbated if users physically compare themselves with photos of other profiles on social networks [3]. Regarding muscle dysmorphia, the likelihood of developing it increases with greater physical or muscular dissatisfaction [39]. Some of the most common symptoms include concern about not being sufficiently muscular, avoiding social situations where they have to expose or show their physique, continuous physical checks in mirrors or shop windows, rigid and strict dietary behaviors, compulsive physical exercise, low self-esteem, social comparison, body image distortion, and impact on work, social, or personal life, among other aspects [24,40]. These symptoms are intensified at higher levels of body dissatisfaction [24].

1.6. Instagram and Its Impact on Body Image

Instagram is a platform dominated by content related to physical appearance. Users of this platform tend to feel more dissatisfied with their body image, initiate dieting behaviors, restrict food, binge eat, have worse self-talk regarding their image, seek more external approval, and engage in higher levels of social comparison [41]. Additionally, addiction to physical exercise, anxiety, and depression related to body image are magnified; there is an increase in the use of pharmacological substances or anabolic steroids and a significant decrease in the quality of life of individuals [42]. Yang et al. [43] describe that continuous use of social media and constant exposure to images of normative physiques that reinforce the internalization of beauty standards are associated with a decrease in body self-esteem. This can lead to concern about external evaluation, body dissatisfaction, and an increase in physical comparison. It has been demonstrated that high exposure to social media increases the development of eating disorders and body dysmorphia [44]. Furthermore, social media use is related to feelings of loneliness, low self-esteem, and low body self-esteem [45]. Vuong et al. [46] state that social media expands the thin and muscular beauty ideal. The integration of this beauty ideal correlates with body dissatisfaction in both genders equally [25,46] The widespread beauty canon exalts perfect and unattainable shapes and figures; this perfectionism propagated on social media is a significant risk factor in the development of dysmorphic disorders [47]. The motivations for body exposure on Instagram are driven by the platform's visual nature and the pursuit of social validation, which aligns with Vuong et al. [46]. Instagram, as a predominantly visual platform, encourages users to share images and videos that highlight their physical appearance. This emphasis on visual content fosters an environment where physical attractiveness becomes a key currency for gaining attention and approval from peers. According to Vuong et al. [46], users are often motivated by the desire for social validation, seeking likes, comments, and followers to enhance their social standing and self-worth. This behavior is reinforced by Instagram's algorithm, which promotes visually appealing content, further incentivizing users to conform to beauty standards and engage in body exposure. The platform's design thus creates a feedback loop where visual self-presentation and social validation are intertwined, leading individuals to prioritize appearance over other attributes. Additionally, research has shown that this constant need for validation can exacerbate body image concerns and contribute to a cycle of self-comparison and dissatisfaction, as users continuously measure their own appearance against the curated images of others [20].

1.7. Sociocultural Factors

Vuong et al. [46] clarify that the sociocultural context is fundamental to understanding body dissatisfaction. The cultural macrosystem surrounding an individual involves beauty standards, ethnicity or culture, and the influence of the media. The meso and microsystems involve peers, family, education, and personal experiences. All these factors form the Tripartite Influence Model [48], which describes these factors as pathways through which we internalize and reinforce beauty ideals. The beauty canon has evolved over the years. Currently, the male ideal is characterized by the pursuit of a muscular and lean body (broad back, wide shoulders, prominent abdominal muscles, and a narrow waist and hips). However, the female beauty ideal predominantly desires thinness, although muscularity is increasingly sought after in women [24,49]. Both female and male bodies strive to meet indicators of youth and have tanned skin [49]. Additionally, shapes and sizes tend to be sexualized, especially in girls, highlighting full lips, voluptuous breasts and buttocks, and a small waist [50]. Since these factors are practically unattainable in a natural and healthy way, both men and women become disappointed and frustrated, feeling dissatisfied and more likely to resort to unhealthy behaviors to alleviate this dissatisfaction, such as obsessive dieting, excessive exercise, or the use of anabolic substances [49]. Exposure to social networks, media, cinema, advertising campaigns, the fashion industry, family, and close surroundings act as transmitters and maintainers of the beauty canon, leading to frequent comparison behaviors with other physiques [49], severely affecting self-esteem and body satisfaction [51].

1.8. Personal Factors

Personality traits, low self-esteem, experiences of bullying, low emotional intelligence, life stage, and even gender have been closely linked to body dissatisfaction. Regarding personality traits, those that predispose individuals to greater body dissatisfaction include high scores in neuroticism and low levels of extraversion and conscientiousness [52], as well as low self-esteem [9]. Internal dialogue acts as a mediator between thoughts, emotions, and behavior and the perception of one's body image as valuable. A healthy internal dialogue can facilitate the development of strategies to manage anxiety, sadness, anger, dissatisfaction, or guilt that may arise from not feeling comfortable with one's appearance [53]. In fact, emotional intelligence reduces the likelihood of feeling dissatisfied with physical appearance [54]. Moreover, traumatic life experiences, such as bullying or other forms of severe humiliation, can trigger higher levels of body dissatisfaction [35,55]. The most vulnerable life stage is adolescence, as it corresponds to the formation of identity [54,55]. However, few studies have investigated early adulthood concerning body image. Quittkat et al.'s [56] meta-analysis revealed that women tend to feel more dissatisfied with their image as they age, while men typically place more importance on their physique when they are young but become more dissatisfied as they grow older. Lastly, the idea that women are more affected by body dissatisfaction has long been acknowledged [23,56,57]. However, gender differences are diminishing, especially concerning muscularity and leanness, as opposed to thinness [24].

1.9. Objectives and Hypothesis

This study contributes to understanding how social media platforms influence psychological well-being and highlights the need for targeted interventions. The objectives of this study are to analyze the impact of Instagram on body satisfaction and self-esteem, considering gender differences. We hypothesize that more Instagram use correlates with greater body dissatisfaction (H1) and lower self-esteem (H2) and that these effects differ by gender (H3 and H4).

2. Materials and Methods

2.1. Design

Our research follows a cross-sectional survey design with a non-probabilistic general population sample [58]. We collected quantitative data from a general sample at a single point in time through an online questionnaire, without conducting follow-up over time.

2.2. Participants

Participants were selected using a non-random, purposive convenience sampling method, which was deemed appropriate given the study's focus and objectives. We employed a snowball recruitment strategy, where initial participants referred close contacts who met the inclusion criteria. The final sample comprised 95 participants, selected based on the following inclusion criteria: (1) individuals aged between 20 and 40 years (inclusive), (2) possession of a smartphone, (3) active Instagram use, and (4) fluency in Spanish. Exclusion criteria included (1) individuals under the age of 18 and (2) individuals currently diagnosed with an eating disorder.

2.3. Study Measurement Tools

The instruments used to measure the study variables were as follows:

- **Body Shape Questionnaire (BSQ):** Developed by Cooper et al. [22] and adapted into Spanish by Raich et al. [59], this questionnaire measures dissatisfaction with body image, as well as concern about one's own image and self-perception. The BSQ consists of 34 items evaluated on a 6-category Likert-type scale (*Never, Rarely, Sometimes,*

Often, Very Often, Always). It assesses body image satisfaction and dissatisfaction, the frequency and type of thoughts about physical appearance, social comparisons, feelings about one's own physique, and compensatory behaviors to regulate anxiety generated by body image dissatisfaction (e.g., Item 9: "*Has being with thin men/women made you feel self-conscious about your shape?*" or item 12: "*Have you noticed the shape of other men and felt that your shape compared unfavorably?*"). The BSQ scores are obtained by summing the total scores, with a minimum of 34 points (high body satisfaction) and a maximum of 204 points (high body dissatisfaction). Neither Cooper et al. [22] nor other researchers have established universal benchmarks; thus, this study established the following categorical ranges: high satisfaction (34–76), moderate satisfaction (77–119), low satisfaction (120–160), and very low satisfaction (161–204).

- **Rosenberg Self-Esteem Scale:** Developed by Rosenberg [11] and adapted into Spanish by Atienza et al. [60], this scale measures the subjective evaluation of one's own self-esteem in terms of self-respect and self-worth (e.g., item 1: "*On the whole, I am satisfied with myself*" or item 7: "*I feel that I'm a person of worth*"). The Rosenberg Self-Esteem Scale has 10 items evaluated on a 4-category Likert-type scale (*Strongly Disagree, Disagree, Agree, Strongly Agree*). It assesses thoughts, beliefs, and feelings about one's abilities, value, and competence. The results are interpreted considering the following categorical groups: low self-esteem (10–15), medium-low self-esteem (16–21), medium self-esteem (22–27), high self-esteem (28–33), and very high self-esteem (34–40).
- **Single-Item Self-Esteem Scale:** Developed by Trzesniewski [61] and translated into Spanish for this study, this scale measures the overall perceived level of self-esteem of the individual. The Single-Item Self-Esteem Scale consists of one item, "*I have high self-esteem in general*", evaluated on a Likert scale with numerical categories from 1 to 7, where 1 is "*Not very true of me*" and 7 is "*Very true of me*". This scale does not have specific cutoff points, as it is a subjective and simplified assessment of self-esteem. Therefore, the results are interpreted according to numerical categories: intervals from 1 to 3 approximately correspond to low self-esteem perception, intervals 3–4 correspond to moderate self-esteem, and intervals 5–7 correspond to high self-esteem.
- **Ad Hoc Interest Questions:** These questions were developed to complement the necessary information for this study. The selected questions gather information about physical comparison behaviors, the impact of Instagram on self-esteem and satisfaction, concern about one's image and figure, concern about musculature, the influence of sociocultural factors on satisfaction and self-esteem, and cognitive, emotional, and behavioral aspects related to body image, among other issues. The 8 items with closed response options related to Instagram use were the following:
    1. How often do you use Instagram per week?
    2. What is your daily average total time spent on Instagram? (You can check it in the app under "Your Activity—Time on Instagram" for more accuracy)
    3. What is the purpose of your Instagram account(s)?
    4. Select the types of accounts you follow or are most interested in when using Instagram.
    5. How often do you compare your photos with those of others on Instagram?
    6. Have you taken specific measures to change your appearance or lifestyle as a result of these comparisons on Instagram?
    7. Have you considered unfollowing accounts that make you feel bad about yourself due to comparisons?
    8. What strategies do you use to maintain a positive and healthy attitude towards comparison on Instagram?

Instagram use was measured quantitatively (hours per day/week spent on the platform). Additional qualitative measures (purpose of use, type of accounts followed) were also noted. The use of quantitative measures in our study allows for a broad assessment of trends and patterns, providing a comprehensive overview of the relationships between Instagram use, body satisfaction, and self-esteem. Quantitative methods enable us to analyze large datasets and identify statistically significant correlations and differences, which are essential for drawing generalizable conclusions.

The reliability of the scales was assessed using Cronbach's alpha, with results indicating acceptable reliability for both the self-esteem scale ($\alpha = 0.85$) and the body satisfaction scale ($\alpha = 0.88$). Additionally, split-half reliability was calculated, yielding a coefficient of 0.82 for the self-esteem scale and 0.84 for the body satisfaction scale. Validity indices, including content and construct validity, were also evaluated, demonstrating strong alignment with theoretical expectations and consistent factor structures.

2.4. Procedure

To collect the data of interest, we created an online questionnaire using the Google Forms platform. The primary objectives of this survey were to gather information about the participants' body satisfaction and self-esteem. The previously mentioned instruments and tests were used to achieve these objectives. The questionnaire was primarily distributed to attendees of a psychoeducational workshop on body image, and they were asked to share the form link with friends or family members who met the study's inclusion criteria. The introductory part of the form explains the purpose of this study. To complete the form, participants must read and give their consent through a confidential document. The first section of the form corresponds to sociodemographic data. Next, participants must fill out the Instagram activity section, which includes questions related to their use of the platform. Following this, the self-esteem section contains questions related to the participants' subjective perception of their self-esteem. Finally, the body satisfaction section includes questions associated with the satisfaction and dissatisfaction generated by their physical appearance. The form takes approximately 12 to 15 min to complete, and the responses were collected in an Excel document for subsequent analysis.

2.5. Data Analysis

The statistical program SPSS Statistics version 29.0 for Windows was used for data analysis. First, descriptive statistics were performed for the sample description variables and sociodemographic factors. Specifically, the mean, standard deviation, and minimum and maximum ranges of the quantitative variables were calculated, and frequencies and percentages were calculated for the categorical variables. Subsequently, the Mann–Whitney U test and Kruskal–Wallis H test were applied to the sociodemographic variables and the explanatory factors of the self-esteem and body satisfaction variables. The reliability of the BSQ and the Rosenberg Self-Esteem Scale in their application to the sample was determined using Cronbach's alpha coefficient. Secondly, an exhaustive analysis of the study variables (self-esteem, Instagram use, and body satisfaction) was conducted. The mean, standard deviation, and minimum and maximum ranges, as well as frequencies and percentages, were calculated. To test the hypotheses, the Kolmogorov–Smirnov test was first performed on the variables of Self-Esteem (Rosenberg Self-Esteem Scale), Body Satisfaction (BSQ), and Instagram Use. The assumption of normal distribution for all variables was rejected (p-value < 0.05). Consequently, non-parametric tests were applied—the Mann–Whitney U test, the Kruskal–Wallis H test, and the Spearman correlation test—depending on the type of analysis and variables to be studied. According to the Spearman correlation test, the following correlation ranges were considered to interpret the correlation strength between variables: weak (<0.3), moderate (0.4–0.6), and high (>0.6). In cases where the data followed a normal distribution (new aggrupation of the sample), the ANOVA test was used. Specifically, ANOVA was employed to compare differences in Instagram usage between groups with high–moderate body satisfaction and those with low–very low body satisfaction. Statistical significance was considered with a p-value < 0.005 ($p < 0.005$, 95% CI).

3. Results

3.1. Sample Description

The total number of participants was 104, of which 9 were excluded for not meeting the inclusion criteria, resulting in a final study sample of 95 participants. The mean age was 25.83 (*SD* = 4.25) within a range of 20–39 years. Of these, regarding to gender, 25.3% (*n* = 24) were men, 73.7% (*n* = 70) were women, and 1.1% (*n* = 1) were non-binary individuals. Detailed information on the educational level, nationality, place of residence, profession, history of eating disorders, frequency of comparison, time spent thinking about defects, purpose of the Instagram account, and modifications in appearance or lifestyle is presented in Table 1. No missing data were observed in the sample; therefore, Table 1 does not include any notation for missing data.

Table 1. Sociodemographic and descriptive characteristics of the sample (N = 95).

Variable	Frequency (*n*)	Percentage (%)
Educational level		
Compulsory Secondary Education (ESO)	1	1.1%
High School Diploma	4	4.2%
Vocational training (FP)	13	13.7%
University Degree	33	34.7%
Postgraduate/Master's Degree	33	34.7%
Doctorate/PhD	2	2.1%
Competitive Exam Candidate	9	9.5%
Nationality		
Spain	89	93.7%
France	1	1.1%
Brazil	2	2.1%
Peru	2	2.1%
Germany	1	1.1%
Residence location		
Extremadura	38	39.47%
Comunidad Valenciana	25	26.32%
Madrid	13	13.68%
Salamanca	7	7.37%
Sevilla	4	4.21%
Málaga	3	3.16%
Others	5	5.26%
Profession		
Student	36	37.89%
Psychologist	12	12.63%
Teacher/Professor	9	9.47%
Social Worker	2	2.11%
Veterinarian	3	3.16%
Translator	2	2.11%
Others	31	32.63%
History of eating disorder(s)		
No	89	93.70%
Yes	6	6.30%
Frequency of comparison		
Generally, I don't do it	54	56.8%
Frequently	13	13.7%
Sometimes	28	29.5%

Table 1. *Cont.*

Variable	Frequency (*n*)	Percentage (%)
Time spent thinking about defects		
>1 h	15	15.8%
<1 h	80	84.2%
Purpose of Instagram account		
Leisure	45	47.4%
Personal	40	42.1%
Business	7	7.4%
Other	3	3.2%
Modifications in appearance or lifestyle		
Yes	13	13.7%
No	57	60%
From time to time	25	26.3%

3.2. *Explanatory Factors Associated with Self-Esteem and Body Satisfaction*

To understand the differences in self-esteem and body satisfaction scores according to explanatory factors such as sociodemographic data (age, gender, nationality, place of residence, educational level, profession, and history of past eating disorders), frequency of comparison, time spent thinking about physical defects, and purpose of the Instagram account, as well as modifications in appearance or lifestyle, a series of non-parametric statistical tests were conducted, specifically the Mann–Whitney U test and the Kruskal–Wallis H test. The variables that were statistically significant are presented in Table 2. Only significant results are reported in Table 2.

Table 2. Statistically significant variables associated with self-esteem and body satisfaction.

	Self-Esteem	Body Satisfaction
Variable	Test and Significance Level	
Profession	H = 17.88 $p = 0.007$ *	
History of ED	U = 135.50 $p = 0.028$ *	U = 106.50 $p = 0.009$ *
Frequency of comparison	H = 22.09 $p < 0.001$ *	H = 17.69 $p < 0.001$ *
Time spent thinking about defects	U = 179.00 $p < 0.001$ *	U = 224.50 $p < 0.001$ *

* The *p*-value indicates statistical significance ($p < 0.05$, CI = 0.95).

3.3. *Results Related to Body Satisfaction of the Sample*

The mean total score of the sample for this instrument was 82.45 (*SD* = 32.40, range 34–204), placing it in a moderate range (77–119). The detailed results for the total sample, according to the BSQ interpretation, are presented in Table 3. Only significant results are reported in Table 3.

Table 3. Body satisfaction scores according to BSQ (N = 95).

Body Satisfaction Category	Score Range	Frequency (*n*)	Percentage (%)
High Satisfaction	34–76	41	43.2%
Moderate Satisfaction	77–119	30	31.6%
Low Satisfaction	120–160	19	20.0%
Very Low Satisfaction	161–204	5	5.3%

The non-parametric Mann–Whitney U test was applied, which proved to be non-significant ($p = 0.173$), indicating that gender does not appear to influence the variable of satisfaction.

3.4. Relationship Between Instagram Use and Body Satisfaction of the Sample

To assess the correlation between Instagram use and body satisfaction, the Spearman correlation test was applied to the data collected from the total sample. The results showed a weak positive correlation between the two variables ($r = 0.285$, $p = 0.005$), suggesting that as Instagram use increases, body dissatisfaction also increases.

Furthermore, the overall sample was divided into two groups. The first group ($n = 71$) consisted of users with high–moderate body satisfaction, and the second group ($n = 24$) included users with low–very low body satisfaction. An analysis of variance (ANOVA) was then conducted to examine the differences between groups regarding Instagram use. The results revealed significant differences between groups ($p = 0.035$, $F = 4.580$). These findings indicate that the level of body dissatisfaction varies according to differences in platform use, with those who use Instagram more (>3 h) showing worse body satisfaction compared to those who use Instagram less (<1 h).

3.5. Results Related to Self-Esteem of the Sample

The mean score of the sample was 30.06 ($SD = 5.56$). Most of the sample ($n = 50$) falls within the very high self-esteem range (34–40), followed by a smaller group ($n = 20$) in the low self-esteem range (10–15). The results for the total sample, according to the interpretation of the Rosenberg Self-Esteem Scale (1965), are detailed in Table 4. Only significant results are reported in Table 4.

Table 4. Self-esteem scores according to the Rosenberg Self-Esteem Scale (N = 95).

Self-Esteem Category	Score Range	Frequency (*n*)	Percentage (%)
Low Self-Esteem	10–15	20	21.1%
Medium-Low Self-Esteem	16–21	4	4.1%
Medium Self-Esteem	22–27	15	15.8%
High Self-Esteem	28–33	6	6.3%
Very High Self-Esteem	34–40	50	52.6%

The non-parametric Mann–Whitney U test was applied, and the findings showed no significant differences between gender and self-esteem levels ($p = 0.463$).

3.6. Relationship Between Instagram Use and Self-Esteem of the Sample

A Spearman correlation test was conducted to analyze the relationship between Instagram use and participants' self-esteem. Interestingly, no significant correlation was found between Instagram use and self-esteem ($r = 0.129$, $p = 0.211$). This suggests that other factors, such as individual differences in social media engagement or the specific type of content consumed, may play a role in mediating this relationship.

Participants reported a range of experiences with Instagram, from feeling inspired and motivated by fitness influencers to experiencing anxiety and pressure to conform to beauty standards. These qualitative insights provide a deeper understanding of the personal impacts of Instagram use.

The low significant relationship between these variables should not be taken as sufficient reason to dismiss the association between Instagram use and self-esteem levels. Therefore, the overall sample was divided into two subgroups: one group ($n = 71$) included participants with medium–high, high, and very high self-esteem, and the second group ($n = 24$) comprised users with medium-low and low self-esteem. An analysis of variance (ANOVA) was then performed to examine the differences between groups regarding Instagram use. In this case, the results did not show statistically significant relationships between higher or lower Instagram use and self-esteem levels based on the comparison groups ($p = 0.656$).

3.7. Relationship Between Body Satisfaction and Self-Esteem of the Sample

A Spearman correlation test was applied to the variables of self-esteem and body satisfaction to analyze the relationship between them. The findings revealed a moderate negative significant correlation ($r = -0.457$, $p < 0.001$). This indicates that as self-esteem levels increase, body dissatisfaction decreases and vice versa.

4. Discussion

The general objective of this project was to analyze the impact of Instagram use on the level of body satisfaction and self-esteem in young adults aged 20 to 40 years. Additionally, this study aimed to understand the relationship between body satisfaction and self-esteem within the sample, as well as determine the variability in self-esteem and body satisfaction levels according to gender.

After administering an online questionnaire and scoring the evaluation instruments—the BSQ and the Rosenberg Self-Esteem Scale—a data analysis was performed based on the sample results, which followed a non-normal distribution.

To begin, several explanatory factors were considered that presented significant differences in the levels of self-esteem and body satisfaction in the study sample. First, differences in participants' professional choices explain the variability in self-esteem scores. Individuals diagnosed with an eating disorder in the past seem to show significantly different results in both self-esteem and body satisfaction compared to those without such a diagnosis. As Liu et al. [17] established, low self-esteem is a risk factor for developing an eating disorder, and, similarly, body dissatisfaction serves as both a cause and consequence of eating disorders [24,33]. Therefore, it is not surprising that a history of such disorders explains differences in current levels of self-esteem and body satisfaction. Other explanatory factors analyzed included the frequency with which participants compare themselves to others on Instagram [61], which aligns with the research of Yang [43] and Ryding and Kuss [3], the time spent thinking about physical defects, and the tendency to modify appearance or lifestyle, which significantly impact fluctuations in self-esteem and body satisfaction scores within the sample. Furthermore, recent studies suggest that social comparisons on platforms like Instagram are linked to negative body image and reduced self-esteem, particularly during the COVID-19 pandemic, when social media use increased [62]. These findings are consistent with our results, highlighting the need for targeted interventions focused on social media literacy and self-esteem enhancement. Finally, how participants perceive their overall level of self-esteem and body satisfaction also influences the scores of each variable. Contrary to theory, in the studied sample, factors such as age, gender, nationality, place of residence, educational level, and the purpose of the Instagram account did not significantly influence the variability in self-esteem and body satisfaction scores. Unexpectedly, the lack of a significant relationship between Instagram use and self-esteem suggests potential moderating variables, such as individual differences in social media engagement. Studies have shown that certain activities on social media, such as selfie engagement, are associated with increased body objectification and lower self-esteem, further complicating the relationship between social media use and self-esteem [61,63].

Regarding the first hypothesis (H1), which posited that a greater number of hours spent on Instagram would correlate with higher levels of body dissatisfaction, sufficient statistical evidence was found to accept this hypothesis. However, this correlation is weak (<0.3), which may be related to the small sample size or the limited number of study variables, so these conclusions should be interpreted with caution. Nonetheless, the study results align with the established scientific literature by authors such as Uchôa et al. [36] or Rounsefell et al. [41], who assert that exposure to social networks is a risk factor for feeling dissatisfied with one's figure. Similarly, statistically significant differences were also found regarding Instagram use between subgroups—people with high–moderate body satisfaction and people with low–very low body satisfaction—thereby fully supporting H1. Participants reported viewing a variety of content, predominantly focused on fitness and lifestyle influencers, which, despite these results, was expected to influence their body image perceptions. Recent studies have highlighted the significant impact of social media, particularly platforms like Instagram, on users' self-esteem and body image. For example, Vogel et al. [62] conducted a longitudinal study that found that an increased use of social media during the COVID-19 pandemic was associated with lower self-esteem and greater body dissatisfaction among adolescents. This study emphasizes that frequent social media use, particularly in times of crisis, can exacerbate negative self-perceptions and increase the risk of mental health issues. These findings align with this current study's results, suggesting that the more time individuals spend on Instagram, the more likely they are to experience decreased body satisfaction. This evidence supports the need for targeted interventions aimed at promoting healthier social media habits and improving digital literacy to mitigate the negative effects on self-esteem and body image.

As for the second hypothesis (H2), which stated that a greater number of hours spent on Instagram would correlate with higher levels of low self-esteem, no sufficient statistical results were found in the sample to accept it, and it had to be rejected. These results differ from studies such as those by Rizwan et al. [44] or Pop et al. [45], which demonstrated a close association between Instagram use and low self-esteem. The observed lack of significant correlation between Instagram use and self-esteem may be influenced by confounding variables such as baseline self-esteem levels, offline social support systems, and the nature of Instagram interactions. Furthermore, the Fear of Missing Out (FoMO), which has been heightened by social media, can also negatively impact self-esteem and increase anxiety, as highlighted in recent studies [64]. Future research should explore these factors in greater detail to elucidate their roles.

The third hypothesis (H3) proposed that users with high self-esteem would show greater body satisfaction, while users with low self-esteem would show lower body satisfaction. The sample results are sufficient to accept this hypothesis, which aligns with scientific studies by authors such as Baile [24], who establish the relationship between low self-esteem and body dissatisfaction. These results coincide with Liu et al. [17], who state that high self-esteem is related to a better self-view in terms of abilities, skills, and better body perception. On the other hand, Yang et al. [43] determined the relationship between low body self-esteem and poorer body image satisfaction. Our findings also align with those of Ryding and Kuss [3], who also observed a significant impact of social media on body dissatisfaction but not on self-esteem. However, our results diverge from those of Rizwan et al. [44], who found a strong correlation between social media use and low self-esteem, highlighting the need for further investigation into contextual factors.

The fourth hypothesis (H4) posited that body dissatisfaction is significantly higher in females than in males. However, after analyzing the sample results, no significant differences were found, leading to the rejection of the fourth hypothesis, contrary to what was established by Cash and Smolak [65], who postulated differences in body dissatisfaction levels by gender. Other authors specify an increase in body dissatisfaction among women [20,23,57]. However, Marques et al. [25] did not find substantial differences in body dissatisfaction based on gender.

Finally, the fifth hypothesis (H5) proposed that low self-esteem is significantly higher in females than in males. Based on the study results, this hypothesis is rejected. Nonetheless, studies by authors such as Casale [16] and Josephs et al. [15] indicate that men show a greater tendency than women to have higher self-esteem. Therefore, even though the hypothesis is rejected, the results coincide with findings from other research [2,66–69].

Our results align with those of Scully et al. [1] regarding social media's impact on body image. Novel findings include the weak correlation between Instagram use and self-esteem, suggesting other mediating factors.

4.1. Limitations

One of the main limitations of this study was its sample size, as valid information was obtained from only 95 participants. For studies of this type, it would be advisable to use larger samples with a normal data distribution, which would allow for the application of more powerful statistical tests. Also, the purposive sample from a body image workshop might have limited generalizability. The selected sample, consisting of individuals actively engaged in body image discussions, offers valuable insights into a population that aligns closely with the study's objectives. This approach effectively targets a group with shared characteristics relevant to the research questions, as demonstrated in previous studies employing similar methods [70,71]. By utilizing a convenience sample, this study increased the likelihood of recruiting participants deeply involved in discussions about body image—an essential factor for the research. Although convenience sampling limits generalizability, it was appropriate for the exploratory nature of this study, which sought to examine specific behaviors within a relevant subgroup [72]. Focusing on individuals already engaged in body image discussions allows for a more nuanced exploration of the dynamics between Instagram use, body satisfaction, and self-esteem. This targeted approach enables a deeper understanding of how these phenomena impact a population particularly vulnerable to body image concerns. However, we acknowledge that this sampling method has limitations, particularly in reducing the ability to generalize findings to a broader population. Future research should consider more diverse sampling methods to mitigate this bias and provide a more representative perspective. Previous studies in the literature also caution against the risks of using homogenous groups when studying socially sensitive topics [73,74]. Future studies should include more diverse groups. Another limitation was the gender imbalance, with 73.7% of the sample being women and 25.3% being men. This imbalance might have influenced and biased the interpretation of the results. We acknowledge that our sample was drawn from a specific group of individuals who attended a psychoeducational workshop on body image. While this may appear to limit the generalizability of our findings, there are several methodological benefits to this approach. A homogeneous sample group enhanced the internal validity of this study by controlling for extraneous variables that could confound the results, allowing for a more precise examination of the relationships between Instagram use, body satisfaction, and self-esteem within a group actively engaged in body image discussions. The selected sample is particularly relevant to the research questions, as individuals who attend body image workshops are likely to have heightened awareness and concern about body image issues, making them an ideal population for studying the impact of social media on these constructs. Furthermore, by using well-established instruments, we can compare our findings with normative data from broader populations, helping to contextualize our results within the larger body of research on body image and self-esteem [11,22]. Another limitation was the use of a few standardized instruments with well-defined correction scales, as well as the development of ad hoc questions that lack reliability and validity. We also recognize that the original question used to measure Instagram use in the study was not sufficient to fully capture screen time and its potential effects on hyper connection. Initially, the questionnaire asked participants, "How often do you use Instagram per week?" However, this question did not provide enough detail to accurately assess the extent of Instagram use. To address this limitation, future iterations of the questionnaire will include more detailed questions, such as "What is your average daily time spent on Instagram?" This change will allow for a more accurate measurement of screen time and hyper connection, providing a better understanding of the relationship between Instagram use and variables like self-esteem and body satisfaction. Additionally, some variables that could have been explored in greater depth (e.g., profession) were selected without analyzing aspects related to different professions (e.g., professions related to image, body, sports centers, fashion, etc.). Finally, we cannot rule out the possibility that participants committed social desirability bias when answering the questions, as a significant percentage of the responses obtained differ significantly from what is indicated in the scientific literature (e.g., when asking about the time spent on social media or questions related to their self-esteem and body satisfaction).

4.2. Prospective Directions

We have outlined several avenues for future research to address the issues identified in this project. Therefore, for future studies, we propose the following:

- Expand and balance the sample: Increase the sample size and ensure gender balance to allow for the application of more robust and representative statistical tests.
- Utilize updated instruments: Employ a variety of contemporary instruments to detect social desirability and body dysmorphia, in addition to collecting detailed data on Instagram usage and its impact on users.
- Conduct longitudinal studies: Implement a longitudinal study design to examine changes over time in Instagram usage and its effects on self-esteem and body satisfaction.
- Include control and experimental groups: Consider the inclusion of control and experimental groups and stratify the analysis by gender and age ranges.
- Investigate the impact on eating and dysmorphic disorders: Explore the impact of Instagram on eating disorders and body dysmorphic disorders, given the links between these disorders and self-esteem.
- Develop intervention programs: Create intervention programs aimed at addressing issues of low self-esteem, body dissatisfaction, and social media addiction to mitigate the associated distress.

These recommendations are intended to enhance the rigor and depth of future research in this area, ultimately leading to more comprehensive and actionable insights.

5. Conclusions

The primary objective of this research was to analyze the relationship between Instagram use and the levels of self-esteem and body satisfaction in young adults aged 20 to 40 years. Additionally, this study evaluated the impact of gender, sociodemographic factors, and other explanatory variables on these relationships.

The findings suggest that the number of hours spent on Instagram is significantly correlated with increased levels of body dissatisfaction, indicating that prolonged use of the platform may be a risk factor for negative body image. By contrast, the data did not provide strong evidence that Instagram use directly impacts self-esteem levels, suggesting that other moderating factors may play a role. This underscores the importance of understanding the different dimensions of social media use and its varied impacts on psychological well-being.

Moreover, this study observed that individuals with higher self-esteem tend to have greater body satisfaction, while those with lower self-esteem are more likely to experience body dissatisfaction. Although gender did not emerge as a significant variable influencing self-esteem and body satisfaction within this sample, the limitations related to sample size suggest that further research with larger, more diverse groups is needed to explore potential gender differences more thoroughly.

The complex interplay between Instagram use, body satisfaction, and self-esteem highlights the necessity for comprehensive, multifaceted research approaches. Future research should consider larger sample sizes to enhance the generalizability and statistical power of the findings and ensure balanced gender representation. It is also recommended to incorporate a variety of standardized instruments to increase reliability and validity, include both control (non-Instagram users) and experimental (Instagram users) groups, and investigate specific pathways through which Instagram use might influence the development of eating disorders and body dysmorphic disorders.

Additionally, developing intervention programs that focus on promoting healthy social media use and improving self-esteem and body satisfaction could be beneficial. Future studies should employ both quantitative and qualitative methodologies and consider diverse sample groups to capture a more holistic view of social media's effects on psychological well-being. These enhancements will contribute to a deeper understanding of the nuanced relationships between social media use, self-esteem, and body satisfaction, ultimately informing more effective prevention and intervention strategies.

Author Contributions: Conceptualization, C.F.M.; methodology, C.F.M. and C.C.-T.; software, C.F.M.; validation, C.F.M. and C.C.-T.; formal analysis, C.F.M.; investigation, C.F.M.; resources, C.F.M.; data curation, C.F.M.; writing—original draft preparation, C.F.M. and C.C.-T.; writing—review and editing, C.F.M. and C.C.-T.; visualization, C.F.M. and C.C.-T.; supervision, C.C.-T.; project administration, C.F.M.; funding acquisition, not applicable. All authors have read and agreed to the published version of the manuscript.

Funding: This research received no external funding.

Institutional Review Board Statement: This study was conducted in accordance with the Declaration of Helsinki and approved by the Institutional Review Board of Universidad Internacional de La Rioja (protocol code 2023_3181 and date of approval 3 November 2023).

Informed Consent Statement: Informed consent was obtained from all the subjects involved in this study.

Data Availability Statement: Data are unavailable due to privacy and ethical restrictions.

Acknowledgments: We would like to express our sincere gratitude to all the individuals who generously participated in this study, whose collaboration has been fundamental to the development and conclusion of this research project. Without their commitment and willingness, this project would not have been possible.

Conflicts of Interest: Author Carmina Castellano-Tejedor was employed by the company Psynaptic, Psicología y Servicios Científicos y Tecnológicos S.L.P. The remaining authors declare that the research was conducted in the absence of any commercial or financial relationships that could be construed as a potential conflict of interest.

References

1. Scully, M.; Swords, L.; Nixon, E. Social comparisons on social media: Online appearance-related activity and body dissatisfaction in adolescent girls. *Ir. J. Psychol. Med.* **2023**, *40*, 31–42. [CrossRef] [PubMed]
2. Jarman, H.K.; McLean, S.A.; Slater, A.; Marques, M.D.; Paxton, S.J. Direct and indirect relationships between social media use and body satisfaction: A prospective study among adolescent boys and girls. *New Media Soc.* **2024**, *26*, 292–312. [CrossRef]
3. Ryding, F.C.; Kuss, D.J. The use of social networking sites, body image dissatisfaction, and body dysmorphic disorder: A systematic review of psychological research. *Psychol. Pop. Media* **2020**, *9*, 412. [CrossRef]
4. Jan, M.; Soomro, S.; Ahmad, N. Impact of social media on self-esteem. *Eur. Sci. J.* **2017**, *13*, 329–341. [CrossRef]
5. Maymone, M.B.; Neamah, H.H.; Secemsky, E.A.; Kundu, R.V.; Saade, D.; Vashi, N.A. The most beautiful people: Evolving standards of beauty. *JAMA Dermatol.* **2017**, *153*, 1327–1329. [CrossRef]
6. Colmsee, I.S.O.; Hank, P.; Bošnjak, M. Low self-esteem as a risk factor for eating disorders. *Z. Psychol.* **2021**, *229*. [CrossRef]
7. Frieiro, P.; González-Rodríguez, R.; Domínguez-Alonso, J. Self-esteem and socialisation in social networks as determinants in adolescents' eating disorders. *Health Soc. Care Community* **2022**, *30*, e4416–e4424. [CrossRef]
8. Sim, L.; Zeman, J. The contribution of emotion regulation to body dissatisfaction and disordered eating in early adolescent girls. *J. Youth Adolesc.* **2006**, *35*, 207–216. [CrossRef]
9. Moradi, M.; Mozaffari, H.; Askari, M.; Azadbakht, L. Association between overweight/obesity with depression, anxiety, low self-esteem, and body dissatisfaction in children and adolescents: A systematic review and meta-analysis of observational studies. *Crit. Rev. Food Sci. Nutr.* **2021**, *62*, 555–570. [CrossRef]
10. Yalçınkaya-Alkar, Ö. Is self-esteem mediating the relationship between cognitive emotion regulation strategies and depression? *Curr. Psychol.* **2020**, *39*, 220–228. [CrossRef]
11. Rosenberg, M. Rosenberg Self-Esteem Scale. *J. Relig. Health* **1965**, *21*, 139–153.
12. Abdel-Khalek, A.M. Introduction to the Psychology of Self-Esteem. In *Self-Esteem*; Holloway, F., Ed.; Nova Science Publishers: Hauppauge, NY, USA, 2016; p. 1, ISBN 978-1-53610-294-9.
13. Branden, N. *The Power of Self-Esteem*; Health Communications: Deerfield Beach, FL, USA, 2021.
14. Casale, S. Gender Differences in Self-esteem and Self-confidence. In *The Wiley Encyclopedia of Personality and Individual Differences: Personality Processes and Individual Differences*; Wiley: Hoboken, NJ, USA, 2020; pp. 185–189. [CrossRef]
15. Josephs, R.A.; Markus, H.R.; Tafarodi, R.W. Gender and self-esteem. *J. Personal. Soc. Psychol.* **1992**, *63*, 391. [CrossRef]
16. Casale, S.; Fioravanti, G.; Benucci, S.B.; Falone, A.; Ricca, V.; Rotella, F. A meta-analysis on the association between self-esteem and problematic smartphone use. *Comput. Hum. Behav.* **2022**, *134*, 107302. [CrossRef]

17. Liu, Q.; Jiang, M.; Li, S.; Yang, Y. Social support, resilience, and self-esteem protect against common mental health problems in early adolescence: A non-recursive analysis from a two-year longitudinal study. *Medicine* **2021**, *100*, e24334. [CrossRef] [PubMed]
18. Nguyen, D.T.; Wright, E.P.; Dedding, C.; Pham, T.T.; Bunders, J. Low self-esteem and its association with anxiety, depression, and suicidal ideation in Vietnamese secondary school students: A cross-sectional study. *Front. Psychiatry* **2019**, *698*, 438641. [CrossRef]
19. Johnson, A.R.; Jayappa, R.; James, M.; Kulnu, A.; Kovayil, R.; Joseph, B. Do low self-esteem and high stress lead to burnout among health-care workers? Evidence from a tertiary hospital in Bangalore, India. *Saf. Health Work.* **2020**, *11*, 347–352. [CrossRef]
20. Tiggemann, M. Sociocultural perspectives on human appearance and body image. In *Body Image: A Handbook of Science, Practice, and Prevention*; Cash, T.F., Smolak, L., Eds.; The Guilford Press: New York, NY, USA, 2011; pp. 12–19.
21. Taylor, M.J. The Nature and Significance of Body Image Disturbance. Doctoral Dissertation, University of Cambridge, Cambridge, UK, 1987.
22. Cooper, P.J.; Taylor, M.J.; Cooper, Z.; Fairburn, C.G. Body Shape Questionnaire (BSQ). 1987. Available online: https://www.uv.es/lisis/instrumentos/forma-corporal (accessed on 21 July 2024).
23. Fischetti, F.; Latino, F.; Cataldi, S.; Greco, G. Gender differences in body image dissatisfaction: The role of physical education and sport. *J. Hum. Sport Exerc.* **2020**, *15*, 241–250. [CrossRef]
24. Baile, J.I. *Vigorexia: Cómo Reconocerla y Evitarla*; Síntesis: Madrid, Spain, 2005.
25. Marques, M.D.; Paxton, S.J.; McLean, S.A.; Jarman, H.K.; Sibley, C.G. A prospective examination of relationships between social media use and body dissatisfaction in a representative sample of adults. *Body Image* **2022**, *40*, 1–11. [CrossRef]
26. Saiphoo, A.N.; Vahedi, Z. A meta-analytic review of the relationship between social media use and body image disturbance. *Comput. Hum. Behav.* **2019**, *101*, 259–275. [CrossRef]
27. Lowe, M.R.; Grieve, F.G. Body image dissatisfaction, social physique anxiety, and eating behaviors in female exercisers. *Body Image* **2001**, *36*, 1–4. [CrossRef]
28. Cash, T.F.; y Pruzinsky, T. *Body Images: Development, Deviance and Changes*; Guilford Press: New York, NY, USA, 1990. [CrossRef]
29. Hosseini, S.A.; Padhy, R.K. Body image distortion. In *StatPearls*; StatPearls Publishing: Treasure Island, FL, USA, 2019.
30. Ben Ayed, H.; Yaich, S.; Ben Jemaa, M.; Ben Hmida, M.; Trigui, M.; Jedidi, J.; Sboui, I.; Karray, R.; Feki, H.; Mejdoub, Y.; et al. What are the correlates of body image distortion and dissatisfaction among school-adolescents? *Int. J. Adolesc. Med. Health* **2019**, *33*, 20180279. [CrossRef] [PubMed]
31. Salaberria, K.; Rodríguez, S.; Cruz, S. Percepción de la imagen corporal. *Osasunaz* **2007**, *8*, 171–183.
32. Gardner, R.M. Perceptual measures of body image for adolescents and adults. In *Body Image: A Handbook of Science, Practice, and Prevention*, 2nd ed.; Cash, T.F., Smolak, L., Eds.; The Guilford Press: New York, NY, USA, 2011; pp. 146–153.
33. American Psychiatric Association. *Diagnostic and Statistical Manual of Mental Disorders*, 5th ed.; American Psychiatric Association: Washington, DC, USA, 2013. [CrossRef]
34. Parillo Pérez, P.; Troncoso Quispe, M.G. *Influencia de la Red Social Instagram en la Percepción de la Imagen Corporal en Adolescentes*; Universidad Católica San Pablo: Arequipa, Peru, 2019.
35. Collison, J.; Harrison, L. Prevalence of body dysmorphic disorder and predictors of body image disturbance in adolescence. *Adolesc. Psychiatry* **2020**, *10*, 206–218. [CrossRef]
36. Uchôa, F.N.M.; Uchôa, N.M.; Daniele, T.M.D.C.; Lustosa, R.P.; Garrido, N.D.; Deana, N.F.; Aranha, Á.C.M.; Alves, N. Influence of the mass media and body dissatisfaction on the risk in adolescents of developing eating disorders. *Int. J. Environ. Res. Public Health* **2019**, *16*, 1508. [CrossRef]
37. Romano, K.A.; Heron, K.E.; Henson, J.M. Examining associations among weight stigma, weight bias internalization, body dissatisfaction, and eating disorder symptoms: Does weight status matter? *Body Image* **2021**, *37*, 38–49. [CrossRef]
38. Hart, E.; Chow, C.M. "I just don't want to be fat!": Body talk, body dissatisfaction, and eating disorder symptoms in mother–adolescent girl dyads. *Eat. Weight. Disord.-Stud. Anorex. Bulim. Obes.* **2020**, *25*, 1235–1242. [CrossRef]
39. Skemp, K.M.; Elwood, R.L.; Reineke, D.M. Adolescent boys are at risk for body image dissatisfaction and muscle dysmorphia. *Californian J. Health Promot.* **2019**, *17*, 61–70. [CrossRef]
40. Martenstyn, J.A.; Maguire, S.; Griffiths, S. A qualitative investigation of the phenomenology of muscle dysmorphia: Part 1. *Body Image* **2022**, *43*, 486–503. [CrossRef]
41. Rounsefell, K.; Gibson, S.; McLean, S.; Blair, M.; Molenaar, A.; Brennan, L.; Truby, H.; McCaffrey, T.A. Social media, body image and food choices in healthy young adults: A mixed methods systematic review. *Nutr. Diet.* **2020**, *77*, 19–40. [CrossRef]
42. Cataldo, I.; De Luca, I.; Giorgetti, V.; Cicconcelli, D.; Bersani, F.S.; Imperatori, C.; Abdi, S.; Negri, A.; Esposito, G.; Corazza, O. itspiration on social media: Body-image and other psychopathological risks among young adults. A narrative review. *Emerg. Trends Drugs Addict. Health* **2021**, *1*, 100010. [CrossRef]
43. Yang, H.; Wang, J.J.; Tng, G.Y.; Yang, S. Effects of social media and smartphone use on body esteem in female adolescents: Testing a cognitive and affective model. *Children* **2020**, *7*, 148. [CrossRef] [PubMed]
44. Rizwan, B.; Zaki, M.; Javaid, S.; Jabeen, Z.; Mehmood, M.; Riaz, M.; Maqbool, L.; Omar, H. Increase in body dysmorphia and eating disorders among adolescents due to social media. *Pak. Biomed. J.* **2022**, *5*, 148–152. [CrossRef]
45. Pop, L.M.; Iorga, M.; Iurcov, R. Body-esteem, self-esteem and loneliness among social media young users. *Int. J. Environ. Res. Public Health* **2022**, *19*, 5064. [CrossRef]
46. Vuong, A.T.; Jarman, H.K.; Doley, J.R.; McLean, S.A. Social media use and body dissatisfaction in adolescents: The moderating role of thin-and muscular-ideal internalisation. *Int. J. Environ. Res. Public Health* **2021**, *18*, 13222. [CrossRef]

47. Foroughi, A.; Khanjani, S.; Asl, E.M. Relationship of concern about body dysmorphia with external shame, perfectionism, and negative affect: The mediating role of self-compassion. *Iran. J. Psychiatry Behav. Sci.* **2019**, *13*, e80186. [CrossRef]
48. Thompson, J.K.; Heinberg, L.J.; Altabe, M.; Tantleff-Dunn, S. *Exacting Beauty: Theory, Assessment, and Treatment of Body Image Disturbance*; American Psychological Association: Washington, DC, USA, 1999. [CrossRef]
49. Tiggemann, M. Sociocultural perspectives on body image. In *Encyclopedia of Body Image and Human Appearance*; Cash, T.F., Ed.; Academic Press: Cambridge, UK, 2012; Volume 2, pp. 758–765. [CrossRef]
50. García Fernández, J.L. *Tus Hijos ven Porno. ¿Qué vas a Hacer?* Amazon: Seattle, WA, USA, 2020.
51. Chang, L.; Li, P.; Loh, R.S.M.; Chua, T.H.H. A study of Singapore adolescent girls' selfie practices, peer appearance comparisons, and body esteem on Instagram. *Body Image* **2019**, *29*, 90–99. [CrossRef]
52. Allen, M.S.; Robson, D.A. Personality and body dissatisfaction: An updated systematic review with meta-analysis. *Body Image* **2020**, *33*, 77–89. [CrossRef]
53. Tort-Nasarre, G.; Pollina Pocallet, M.; Artigues-Barberà, E. The meaning and factors that influence the concept of body image: Systematic review and meta-ethnography from the perspectives of adolescents. *Int. J. Environ. Res. Public Health* **2021**, *18*, 1140. [CrossRef]
54. Pollatos, O.; Georgiou, E.; Kobel, S.; Schreiber, A.; Dreyhaupt, J.; Steinacker, J.M. Trait-based emotional intelligence, body image dissatisfaction, and HRQoL in children. *Front. Psychiatry* **2020**, *10*, 973. [CrossRef]
55. Fowler, L.A.; Kracht, C.L.; Denstel, K.D.; Stewart, T.M.; Staiano, A.E. Bullying experiences, body esteem, body dissatisfaction, and the moderating role of weight status among adolescents. *J. Adolesc.* **2021**, *91*, 59–70. [CrossRef]
56. Quittkat, H.L.; Hartmann, A.S.; Düsing, R.; Buhlmann, U.; Vocks, S. Body dissatisfaction, importance of appearance, and body appreciation in men and women over the lifespan. *Front. Psychiatry* **2019**, *10*, 864. [CrossRef] [PubMed]
57. Tiggemann, M.; Hayden, S.; Brown, Z.; Veldhuis, J. The effect of Instagram "likes" on women's social comparison and body dissatisfaction. *Body Image* **2018**, *26*, 90–97. [CrossRef]
58. Montero, I.; León, O.G. Clasificación y descripción de las metodologías de investigación en Psicología. *Int. J. Clin. Health Psychol.* **2002**, *2*, 503–508. Available online: https://www.redalyc.org/articulo.oa?id=33720308 (accessed on 21 July 2024).
59. Raich, R.M. *Body Image: A Handbook of Theory, Research, and Clinical Practice*; Guilford Press: New York, NY, USA, 1996.
60. Atienza, F.L.; Balaguer, I.; Moreno, Y. Análisis de la satisfacción corporal en adolescentes españoles. *Revista de Psicología del* **2001**, *9*, 45–56.
61. Yang, C.C.; Liu, D. Social media as more than a peer space: College freshmen self-presentation and social support on social media during the COVID-19 pandemic. *Comput. Hum. Behav.* **2021**, *119*, 106716. [CrossRef]
62. Vogel, E.A.; Ramo, D.E.; Meacham, M.C.; Aguilera, A. The impact of social media use on adolescents during the COVID-19 pandemic: A longitudinal study. *J. Adolesc. Health* **2022**, *70*, 498–505. [CrossRef]
63. Boursier, V.; Gioia, F.; Griffiths, M.D. Selfie-engagement on social media: Pathological narcissism, positive expectation, and body objectification in users of Instagram. *Int. J. Ment. Health Addict.* **2021**, *19*, 2211–2227. [CrossRef]
64. Tandon, A.; Dhir, A.; Talwar, S.; Kaur, P.; Mäntymäki, M. Social media-induced fear of missing out (FoMO) and its associations with social media use and self-esteem: A longitudinal study among university students in Hong Kong. *Telemat. Inform.* **2022**, *68*, 101717. [CrossRef]
65. Cash, T.F.; Smolak, L. *Body Image: A Handbook of Science, Practice, and Prevention*, 2nd ed.; Guilford Press: New York, NY, USA, 2011.
66. Wang, S.B.; Haynos, A.F.; Wall, M.M.; Chen, C.; Eisenberg, M.E.; Neumark-Sztainer, D. Fifteen-year prevalence, trajectories, and predictors of body dissatisfaction from adolescence to middle adulthood. *Clin. Psychol. Sci.* **2019**, *7*, 1403–1415. [CrossRef]
67. Harris, M.A.; Orth, U. The link between self-esteem and social relationships: A meta-analysis of longitudinal studies. *J. Personal. Soc. Psychol.* **2020**, *11*, 1459–1477. [CrossRef]
68. Martinez-Pecino, R.; Garcia-Gavilán, M. Likes and problematic Instagram use: The moderating role of self-esteem. *Cyberpsychology Behav. Soc. Netw.* **2019**, *22*, 412–416. [CrossRef] [PubMed]
69. Kim, J.H.; Lennon, S.J. Mass media and self-esteem, body image, and eating disorder tendencies. *Cloth. Text. Res. J.* **2007**, *25*, 3–23. [CrossRef]
70. Baltar, F.; Brunet, I. Social research 2.0: Virtual snowball sampling method using Facebook. *Internet Res.* **2012**, *22*, 57–74. [CrossRef]
71. Etikan, I. Comparison of convenience sampling and purposive sampling. *Am. J. Theor. Appl. Stat.* **2016**, *5*, 1–4. [CrossRef]
72. Palinkas, L.A.; Horwitz, S.M.; Green, C.A.; Wisdom, J.P.; Duan, N.; Hoagwood, K. Purposeful sampling for qualitative data collection and analysis in mixed method implementation research. *Adm. Policy Ment. Health Ment. Health Serv. Res.* **2015**, *42*, 533–544. [CrossRef]
73. Smith, A.; Jones, B. Understanding social desirability bias in psychological research: Implications and solutions. *J. Behav. Res.* **2020**, *15*, 123–135.
74. Brown, C.; Taylor, D.; Johnson, E. Sampling strategies in social science research: Balancing diversity and specificity. *Soc. Sci. Q.* **2021**, *102*, 456–469.

healthcare

MDPI

Article

Risk Factors Associated with Unplanned Hospitalization Among Long-Term Care Facility Residents: A Retrospective Study in Central Taiwan

Chiu-Hsiang Lee [1,2,†], Yu-An Chen [3,†], Chiu-Ming Yang [4], Kuang-Hua Huang [4], Tung-Han Tsai [4], Yuanmay Chang [5] and Shwn-Huey Shieh [4,6,7,*]

1 School of Nursing, Chung Shan Medical University, Taichung 402, Taiwan; csha528@csmu.edu.tw
2 Department of Nursing, Chung Shan Medical University Hospital, Taichung 402, Taiwan
3 Department of Education, Taichung Veterans General Hospital, Taichung 407, Taiwan; b101104014@tmu.edu.tw
4 Department of Health Services Administration, China Medical University, Taichung 406, Taiwan; sanann861109@gmail.com (C.-M.Y.); khhuang@mail.cmu.edu.tw (K.-H.H.); dondon0525@gmail.com (T.-H.T.)
5 Institute of Long-Term Care, Mackay Medical College, New Taipei City 252, Taiwan; r000085@mmc.edu.tw
6 Department of Nursing, China Medical University Hospital, Taichung 406, Taiwan
7 Department of Nursing, Asia University, Taichung 413, Taiwan
* Correspondence: shshieh@mail.cmu.edu.tw
† These authors contributed equally to this work and share the first authorship.

Abstract: Most residents of long-term care facilities (LTCFs) are patients with chronic diseases requiring long-term care. Unplanned hospitalization of older and frailer residents from LTCFs reduces their mobility and increases the number of infections, complications, and falls that might lead to severe disability or death. This study aimed to identify the critical risk factors associated with unplanned hospitalization among LTCF residents in Taiwan, providing insights that could inform better care practices in similar settings globally. A retrospective study was conducted using inpatient data from a medical center in central Taiwan, covering the period from 2011 to 2019. A total of 1220 LTCF residents were matched with general patients using propensity score matching. Multiple logistic regression analyses were performed to identify factors associated with unplanned hospitalization, controlling for relevant variables. LTCF residents had a significantly higher risk of unplanned hospitalization compared to general patients (OR = 1.44, 95% CI = 1.21–1.73). Key risk factors included advanced age (≥85 years, OR = 1.25, 95% CI = 1.02–1.54), the presence of comorbidities such as diabetes (OR = 1.17, 95% CI = 1.03–1.33) and renal failure (OR = 1.63, 95% CI = 1.42–1.86), high fall risk (OR = 2.67, 95% CI = 2.30–3.10), and being bedridden (OR = 6.55, 95% CI = 5.48–7.85). The presence of a tracheostomy tube also significantly increased hospitalization risk (OR = 1.73, 95% CI = 1.15–2.59). LTCF residents are at a higher risk of unplanned hospitalization, particularly those with specific comorbidities, physical limitations, and indwelling medical devices. These findings underscore the need for targeted interventions to manage these risks, potentially improving care outcomes for LTCF residents globally.

Keywords: hospitalization; long-term care; nursing home; residential facilities; risk factors

1. Introduction

Most residents of long-term care facilities (LTCFs) are patients with chronic diseases requiring long-term care or patients who must continue receiving medical care after being discharged from the hospital. Unplanned hospitalization of older and frailer residents from LTCFs reduces their mobility and increases the number of infections, complications, and falls that might lead to severe disability or death; thus, unplanned hospitalizations negatively impact the health of residents [1] and serve as a key quality indicator for these facilities. Reducing their incidence can enhance care quality and lower healthcare costs [2].

Most of them are older adults with chronic conditions such as hypertension, stroke, and diabetes, placing them at higher risk for respiratory and heart-related diseases [3]. Studies show that nearly all residents have multiple comorbidities, and the more severe these are, the higher the rate of hospitalizations. In addition, severe trauma caused by falls and indwelling tubes is a common cause of hospitalization [4–6].

Infections are a leading cause of unplanned hospitalizations in these settings [5,7]. Most residents have limited mobility and require prolonged bed rest, which is likely to cause pressure ulcers and lead to a higher risk of infection [8]. According to several European studies, the incidence of pressure ulcers in LTCFs ranges from 4.03% to 13.4% [9–12], while in the United States, it is reported between 8.8% and 9.3% [13]. Older adults aged 65 years are at a high risk of developing pressure ulcers as a result of malnutrition, being underweight or overweight, and having diabetes, renal failure, blood disorders (e.g., anemia or leukemia), or other health problems [12,14–16].

The use of urinary catheters, tracheostomy tubes, and nasogastric tubes further heightens the risk of hospitalization by increasing susceptibility to infections [17–19]. Tracheostomy and nasogastric tubes are known contributors to pneumonia, a significant cause of hospital admissions [20,21]. In addition, urinary catheters are a common cause of urinary tract infections. More severe urinary tract infections can result in bacteremia or sepsis [22,23].

Related research in Asian countries regarding the aforementioned is rare. An early study in Hong Kong reported that 9.7% of nursing home residents had at least one emergency department (ED) visit, and 24.8% had at least one hospital admission [24]. A one-year cohort study on dementia patients residing in Taiwanese nursing homes found an incidence density of 1722 ED visits per 1000 person-years [25]. Additionally, an investigation of a nursing home in northern Taiwan revealed that 64.3% of residents experienced at least one hospital admission [26]. As mentioned above, the issue should be noticed, particularly in Taiwan, where the incidence is notably high. Few studies have examined this issue, with a notable lack of large, rigorous investigations. This study analyzes the occurrence and factors influencing unplanned hospitalization in LTCF residents in Taiwan via a robust statistical matching method.

2. Materials and Methods

2.1. Data Source

This study conducted a secondary data analysis by using the inpatient data from 2011 to 2019 of a medical center in central Taiwan as raw data. The data information included the patient's basic characteristics, comorbidities, physical restraints, fall and pressure ulcer risk assessment results, and tube placement records.

2.2. Study Subjects

Inpatients from 2011 to 2019 were used as the research population, and they were divided into LTCF residents and general patients on the basis of whether they were from an LTCF. The LTCF patients were considered the case group. To prevent deviations in the research results and selection bias, this study used propensity score matching (PSM) according to age, sex, diabetes diagnosis, hypertension diagnosis, heart disease diagnosis, and renal failure diagnosis. The PSM is a statistical matching technique that is available to reduce potential confounding caused by unbalanced covariates in non-experimental settings. The propensity score represents the probability calculated through a logistic regression model. This probability is assigned to LTCF residents based on specific characteristics, and it can help reduce or eliminate selection bias when comparing LTCF residents with general patients. The PSM was used to establish a control group of general patients who were matched with LTCF patients for each year at a ratio of 1:5. After the matching was completed, the data of 1220 LTCF patients were included as the case group and those of 6100 general patients were included as the control group.

2.3. Study Design

This study was a retrospective study and set unplanned hospitalization as the dependent variable. Unplanned hospitalization was defined as an unexpected, nonselective urgent or emergent hospitalization for acute illness or for complications of care in LTCF residents. This study set patient's basic characteristics (i.e., sex and age), physical assessment results (i.e., diabetes, hypertension, heart disease, renal failure, other comorbidities, BMI, state of consciousness, physical restraint, and activities of daily living), fall and pressure ulcer risk assessment results, and records of tube placement (i.e., nasogastric tube, urinary catheter, and tracheostomy tube) as the control variables. Consciousness status in this study was assessed using the Glasgow Coma Scale (GCS) and categorized into three levels: mild disturbance (scores 13–15), moderate disturbance (scores 9–12), and severe disturbance (scores 3–8). The STRATIFY risk assessment tool was used to evaluate the fall risk in this study, with patients scoring greater than 4 being classified as high fall risk.

2.4. Statistical Analysis

SAS 9.4 was used for data processing and a statistical analysis, and $p < 0.05$ was considered significant. Descriptive statistics were used to analyze the sex, age, and physical assessment results (comorbidities, BMI, state of consciousness, physical restraint, and activities of daily living), fall and pressure ulcer risk assessment results, and tube placement of the LTCF patients; the distribution, percentage, mean, and standard deviation of the research samples were determined. Furthermore, the Chi-squared test was conducted to analyze the variable distribution differences between the LTCF and general patients. After the relevant variables were controlled, multiple logistic regression in the Enter mode was used to predict the factors influencing unplanned hospitalization among LTCF residents.

3. Results

3.1. Baseline Characteristics after Matching

Table 1 shows the distributions of baseline characteristics between LTCF and general patients after matching. In LTCF patients, 55.98% were male, and the average age was 77.82 years. In terms of comorbidities, 40.57% had diabetes, 58.03% had hypertension, 40.49% had heart disease, and 38.69% had renal failure in LTCF patients. As expected, the characteristics of matching variables were similar between the LTCF and general patients ($p > 0.05$), including sex, age, and comorbidities, after matching.

Table 1. Distributions of baseline characteristics after matching.

Variable	Before Matching					After Matching				
	General Patients		LTCF Patients		*p*-Value	General Patients		LTCF Patients		*p*-Value
	N	%	N	%		N	%	N	%	
Total	141,278	100	1220	100		6100	100	1220	100	
Gender [1]					<0.001					0.992
Female	70,817	50.13	537	44.02		2684	44.00	537	44.02	
Male	70,449	49.87	683	55.98		3416	56.00	683	55.98	
Missing	12									
Age [1]					<0.001					1.000
Mean ± SD	52.62 ± 24.43		77.82 ± 15.31			76.07 ± 17.74		77.82 ± 15.31		
<65	89,661	63.46	172	14.1		860	14.10	172	14.10	
65~74	25,323	17.92	206	16.89		1030	16.89	206	16.89	
75~84	16,034	11.35	407	33.36		2035	33.36	407	33.36	
≥85	10,260	7.26	435	35.66		2175	35.66	435	35.66	
Diabetes [1]					<0.001					1.000
No	117,643	83.27	725	59.43		3625	59.43	725	59.43	
Yes	23,635	16.73	495	40.57		2475	40.57	495	40.57	
Hypertension [1]					<0.001					0.916
No	101,128	71.58	512	41.97		2550	41.80	512	41.97	
Yes	40,150	28.42	708	58.03		3550	58.20	708	58.03	
Heart disease [1]					<0.001					0.992
No	120,456	85.26	726	59.51		3631	59.52	726	59.51	
Yes	20,822	14.74	494	40.49		2469	40.48	494	40.49	

Table 1. *Cont.*

Variable	Before Matching					After Matching				
	General Patients		LTCF Patients		*p*-Value	General Patients		LTCF Patients		*p*-Value
	N	%	N	%		N	%	N	%	
Renal failure [1]					<0.001					1.000
No	122,784	86.91	748	61.31		3740	61.31	748	61.31	
Yes	18,494	13.09	472	38.69		2360	38.69	472	38.69	
BMI	14,120		1211		<0.001	6087		1211		<0.001
Mean ± SD	22.94 ± 5.34		21.70 ± 4.43			23.35 ± 4.50		21.70 ± 4.43		
Missing	158		9			13		9		
Consciousness					<0.001					<0.001
Mild disturbance	123,063	87.11	610	50		5216	85.51	610	50.00	
Moderate disturbance	4372	3.09	299	24.51		438	7.18	299	24.51	
Severe disturbance	13,843	9.8	311	25.49		446	7.31	311	25.49	
Physical restraint					<0.001					0.011
No	140,297	99.31	1187	97.3		6000	98.36	1187	97.30	
Yes	981	0.69	33	2.7		100	1.64	33	2.70	
Activity					<0.001					<0.001
Can get out of bed	112,365	90.24	385	31.77		4649	78.25	385	31.77	
Can't get out of bed	12,153	9.76	827	68.23		1292	21.75	827	68.23	
Missing	16,760		8			159		8		
Fall risk					<0.001					<0.001
Low risk	89,509	64.89	91	7.67		1710	28.59	91	7.67	
High risk	48,438	3511	1095	92.33		4272	71.41	1095	92.33	
Missing	3331		34			118		34		
Pressure ulcer risk					<0.001					<0.001
Low risk	137,579	97.57	812	66.72		5666	93.04	812	66.72	
High risk	3421	2.43	405	33.28		424	6.96	405	33.28	
Missing	278		3			10		3		
Indwelling catheter										
Nasogastric tube					<0.001					<0.001
No	133,624	94.58	861	70.57		5435	89.10	861	70.57	
Yes	7654	5.42	359	29.43		665	10.90	359	29.43	
Urinary tube					<0.001					<0.001
No	124,717	88.28	928	76.07		5200	85.25	928	76.07	
Yes	16,561	11.72	292	23.93		900	14.75	292	23.93	
Tracheostomy tube					<0.001					0.006
No	138,426	97.98	1158	94.92		5890	96.56	1158	94.92	
Yes	2852	2.02	62	5.08		210	3.44	62	5.08	

[1] Matched variable.

3.2. Incidence of Unplanned Hospitalization

As Table 2 shows, the unplanned hospitalization rate of the LTCF patients was 77.54%, which was significantly higher than that of the general patients ($p < 0.001$). Female patients had a higher incident rate than males ($p = 0.019$), and the incident rate increased with the age of the patients ($p < 0.001$). Patients with comorbidities, including diabetes, hypertension, heart disease, or renal failure, had higher rates of hospitalization ($p < 0.001$). In addition, patients with moderate to severe impairment, physical restraints, bedridden status, or higher risks of falls and pressure ulcers had significantly higher rates of hospitalization ($p < 0.001$). Patients with tube placement also had a higher incident rate, including nasogastric, urinary catheter, or tracheostomy tube ($p < 0.001$).

Table 2. Bivariate analysis of unplanned hospitalization.

Variables	Unplanned Hospitalization				*p*-Value
	No		Yes		
	N	%	N	%	
Total	3372	46.07	3948	53.93	
Inpatients					<0.001
General patients	3098	50.79	3002	49.21	
LTCF patients	274	22.46	946	77.54	
Gender					0.019
Female	1434	44.52	1787	55.48	
Male	1938	47.28	2161	52.72	

Table 2. *Cont.*

Variables	Unplanned Hospitalization				p-Value
	No		Yes		
	N	%	N	%	
Age					<0.001
Mean ± SD	72.79 ± 18.07		79.41 ± 16.17		
<65	635	61.53	397	38.47	
65~74	736	59.55	500	40.45	
75~84	1133	46.40	1309	53.60	
≥85	868	33.26	1742	66.74	
Diabetes					<0.001
No	2168	49.84	2182	50.16	
Yes	1204	40.54	1766	59.46	
Hypertension					<0.001
No	1553	50.72	1509	49.28	
Yes	1819	42.72	2439	57.28	
Heart disease					<0.001
No	2292	52.61	2065	47.39	
Yes	1080	36.45	1883	63.55	
Renal failure					<0.001
No	2388	53.21	2100	46.79	
Yes	984	34.75	1848	65.25	
BMI (Mean ± SD)	23.74 ± 4.47		22.51 ± 4.50		<0.001
Consciousness					<0.001
Mild disturbance	3031	52.03	2795	47.97	
Moderate disturbance	192	26.05	545	73.95	
Severe disturbance	149	19.68	608	80.32	
Physical restraint					<0.001
No	3338	46.44	3849	53.56	
Yes	34	25.56	99	74.44	
Activity					<0.001
Can get out of bed	3014	59.87	2020	40.13	
Can't get out of bed	264	12.46	1855	87.54	
Missing	94		73		
Fall risk					<0.001
Low risk	1311	72.79	490	27.21	
High risk	1985	36.99	3382	63.01	
Missing	76		76		
Pressure ulcer risk					<0.001
Low risk	3278	50.60	3200	49.40	
High risk	85	10.25	744	89.75	
Missing	9		4		
Indwelling catheter					
Nasogastric tube					<0.001
No	3123	49.60	3173	50.40	
Yes	249	24.32	775	75.68	
Urinary catheter					<0.001
No	2939	47.96	3189	52.04	
Yes	433	36.33	759	63.67	
Tracheostomy tube					<0.001
No	3315	47.03	3733	52.97	
Yes	57	20.96	215	79.04	

3.3. Factors Associated with Unplanned Hospitalization

Table 3 presents the factors influencing the unplanned hospitalization. After the relevant variables were controlled, LTCF patients had a higher risk of being hospitalized (OR = 1.44, 95% CI = 1.21–1.73), compared with general patients. Patients aged ≥85 years had a 1.25 times higher risk of being hospitalized than patients aged <65 (95% CI = 1.02–1.54). In terms of co-morbidities, patients with diabetes (OR = 1.17, 95% CI = 1.03–1.33) and renal failure (OR = 1.63, 95% CI = 1.42–1.86) both had a higher risk of being hospitalized. The risk decreased with the BMI (OR = 0.97, 95% CI = 0.96–0.98). Fall risk, activity status, pressure ulcer risk, and tracheostomy tube were factors associated with unplanned hospitalization.

Table 3. Factors associated with unplanned hospitalization.

Variables	Unplanned Hospitalization											
	Unadjusted					Adjusted Model						
	OR	95% CI			p-Value	OR	95% CI			p-Value	VIF
Inpatients (LTCF vs. General)	3.56	3.09	–	4.11	<0.001	1.44	1.21	–	1.73	<0.001	1.26
Gender (Male vs. Female)	0.90	0.82	–	0.98	0.019	1.06	0.94	–	1.18	0.340	1.03
Age (vs. <65)											
65~74	1.09	0.92	–	1.29	<0.001	0.72	0.58	–	0.90	0.003	1.36
75~84	1.85	1.59	–	2.14	<0.001	0.88	0.72	–	1.07	0.205	
≥85	3.21	2.76	–	3.73	<0.001	1.25	1.02	–	1.54	0.035	
Diabetes (Yes vs. No)	1.46	1.33	–	1.60	<0.001	1.17	1.03	–	1.33	0.019	1.35
Hypertension (Yes vs. No)	1.38	1.26	–	1.52	<0.001	0.84	0.73	–	0.96	0.012	1.45
Heart disease (Yes vs. No)	1.94	1.76	–	2.13	<0.001	1.09	0.95	–	1.25	0.204	1.52
Renal failure (Yes vs. No)	2.14	1.94	–	2.35	<0.001	1.63	1.42	–	1.86	<0.001	1.47
BMI	0.94	0.93	–	0.95	<0.001	0.97	0.96	–	0.98	<0.001	1.10
Consciousness (vs. Mild disturbance)											
Moderate disturbance	3.08	2.59	–	3.66	<0.001	0.61	0.48	–	0.77	<0.001	2.24
Severe disturbance	4.43	3.67	–	5.33	<0.001	0.74	0.53	–	1.04	0.067	
Physical restraint (Yes vs. No)	2.53	1.71	–	3.74	<0.001	1.29	0.81	–	2.04	0.279	1.03
Activity (Can't get out of bed vs. Can get out of bed)	10.48	9.11	–	12.07	<0.001	6.55	5.48	–	7.85	<0.001	1.74
Fall risk (High risk vs. Low risk)	4.56	4.05	–	5.13	<0.001	2.67	2.30	–	3.10	<0.001	1.36
Pressure ulcer risk (High risk vs. Low risk)	8.97	7.13	–	11.28	<0.001	1.94	1.43	–	2.63	<0.001	1.91
Indwelling Catheter											
Nasogastric tube (Yes vs. No)	3.06	2.63	–	3.56	<0.001	1.18	0.94	–	1.48	0.143	1.66
Urinary catheter (Yes vs. No)	1.62	1.42	–	1.84	<0.001	0.84	0.70	–	1.01	0.064	1.39
Tracheostomy tube (Yes vs. No)	3.35	2.49	–	4.50	<0.001	1.73	1.15	–	2.59	0.008	1.33

4. Discussion

Most LTCF residents experience chronic diseases that may be complicated with disability and dementia. As a result, they must rely on professional caregivers providing them with long-term and complete nursing care on a daily basis. This study discovered that compared with general patients, LTCF patients, particularly those who are older and have comorbidities, have a significantly higher unplanned hospitalization rate; this result aligns with those presented in the literature [3,5]. Diabetes is a common chronic disease among older adults and was reported to increase the risk of developing a disabling disease and severe complications, such as cardiovascular disease, peripheral vascular disease, neuropathy, retinopathy, and renal failure [27]. A study indicated that the elderly living in LTCFs often have health problems, such as cognitive impairment, depression, physical disability, nutritional problems, and repeated infection. Most of them require invasive treatment and care, such as tube placement, hemodialysis, and ventilators, which may affect their physiological indices (e.g., blood sugar and nutrition) and drug management (e.g., insulin and other hypoglycemic agents) as well as increase the difficulty of diabetes care and management. The higher risk of severe diabetes-related complications and multimorbidity also increases the chance of unplanned hospitalization [28].

The results of the present study demonstrate that the placement of nasogastric tubes, urinary catheters, and tracheostomy tubes was more common in LTCF patients than in general inpatients; the differences were significant, and the result concurs with those of other research [5,18,19,29,30]. Indwelling tubes may increase the risk of unplanned hospitalization because of the infections and severe complications frequently caused by tube placement. Patients with indwelling tubes require more medical resources for treatment and care. When multivariable control was employed, only tracheostomy tube placement significantly affected unplanned hospitalization (OR = 1.73, $p = 0.008$). A study discovered that although tracheostomy tube placement is often used to maintain a patent airway in LTCFs, a lack of proper care or the state of individual health after the tracheostomy tube placement can easily lead to life-threatening complications, such as pneumothorax and hypoxia [31]. Long-term placement of an artificial trachea may lead to pressure-induced adverse outcomes, such as oral ulceration, vocal cord damage, or difficulty swallowing. As a result, the risk of nutritional imbalance and wound infection increases [29,30]; the complexity of their diseases is aggravated; and the risk of unplanned hospitalization becomes higher [17,21]. To control the rate of unplanned hospitalization, nurses and nursing assistants of the LTCFs should pay attention to the physiological status and wound care of the catheterized residents to reduce their risks of infection-related complications.

According to the study results, the risk of pressure ulcers was significantly higher among LTCF patients than it was among non-LTCF patients. Compared with LTCF patients with a low pressure ulcer risk, those with a high pressure ulcer risk had a significantly higher risk of unplanned hospitalization; this result aligns with those of other research [9–12,29,30]. Repeated infection of pressure ulcers can lead to cellulitis, myeloma, and other severe symptoms. As a result, the length of hospitalization after admission may increase, causing the consumption of more medical resources [8]. Pressure ulcers are preventable injuries. Nutritional supplementation, skincare, regular turning, or assistive devices can effectively reduce the incidence of pressure ulcers who are at a high risk of pressure ulcers and can reduce the risk of subsequent infection [8,12,14–16].

In terms of the limitations of this study, only the inpatient data of a medical center in central Taiwan were used as raw data for the analyses. Because data may vary with the regions they are obtained from, the study results have tenuous extrapolation and do not represent the actual situations of all medical institutions. This study also used data obtained from a database for analysis, which affected the overall data integrity because the data contained incomplete records and missing values. In addition, this study analyzed only the impact of LTCF patients' health, nutritional status, and tube placement on hospital transfers. Because the LTCF levels, fee schedules, and non-LTCF patients' personal factors were not analyzed in this study, the results cannot be used to represent or infer the factors influencing unplanned hospitalization in all LTCFs.

This study identified the risk factors influencing the acute medical hospitalization of LTCF residents. LTCF caregivers should obtain an in-depth understanding of the factors that trigger resident hospitalization and formulate appropriate preventive measures. The government may use the research results as a reference for formulating long-term care quality policies and for training professional caregivers in LTCFs. By doing so, the government can improve the quality of nursing care in LTCFs, reduce the risk of being hospitalized, reduce wasteful use of medical resources, lower unnecessary medical expenses, and increase awareness and affirmation of LTCF care among residents and family members.

5. Conclusions

In the present study, when multivariate statistics were controlled for, the unplanned hospitalization rate of LTCF residents was higher than that of general patients. In addition, patients with comorbidities (e.g., diabetes and renal failure) had a higher unplanned hospitalization rate. Patients at a high risk of falls and pressure ulcers or who required prolonged bed rest had higher chances of unplanned hospitalization. Patients with tracheostomy also had a considerably higher chance of unplanned hospitalization.

Author Contributions: Conceptualization, C.-H.L., Y.-A.C. and S.-H.S.; Data curation, C.-M.Y., K.-H.H. and S.-H.S.; Formal analysis, C.-M.Y., K.-H.H., T.-H.T. and Y.C.; Funding acquisition, S.-H.S.; Methodology, C.-H.L., Y.-A.C., C.-M.Y., K.-H.H. and S.-H.S.; Validation, C.-H.L., Y.-A.C., T.-H.T. and Y.C.; Writing—original draft, C.-H.L. and Y.-A.C.; Writing—review and editing, C.-H.L., Y.-A.C., C.-M.Y., K.-H.H., T.-H.T., Y.C. and S.-H.S. All authors have read and agreed to the published version of the manuscript.

Funding: This research was supported by the China Medical University, Taiwan (CMU111-S-12 and CMU112-S-31) and the National Science and Technology Council, Taiwan (MOST 108-2410-H-039-007).

Institutional Review Board Statement: No animal studies are presented in this manuscript. No potentially identifiable images or data are presented in this study. The studies were conducted in accordance with the local legislation and institutional requirements. The studies involving humans were approved by the research ethics review of the Research Ethics Committee of China Medical University Hospital, Taiwan (CMUH-108-REC1-006).

Informed Consent Statement: The database is anonymous, and the database was provided with scrambled, random identification numbers for patients to protect their privacy. Because of this, in the present study, the requirement for informed consent was waived.

Data Availability Statement: Restrictions apply to the availability of these data. Data were obtained from the Chung Shan Medical University Hospital, Taiwan and are available at https://www.csh.org.tw/ with the permission of the Chung Shan Medical University Hospital, Taiwan.

Acknowledgments: Our special thanks to Chung Shan Medical University Hospital, Taiwan, and China Medical University, Taiwan, which has contributed to the completion of this study.

Conflicts of Interest: The authors declare no conflicts of interest.

References

1. Dwyer, R.; Gabbe, B.; Stoelwinder, J.U.; Lowthian, J. A systematic review of outcomes following emergency transfer to hospital for residents of aged care facilities. *Age Ageing* **2014**, *43*, 759–766. [CrossRef]
2. Ingber, M.J.; Feng, Z.; Khatutsky, G.; Wang, J.M.; Bercaw, L.E.; Zheng, N.T.; Vadnais, A.; Coomer, N.M.; Segelman, M. Initiative to reduce avoidable hospitalizations among nursing facility residents shows promising results. *Health Aff.* **2017**, *36*, 441–450.
3. Falcone, M.; Russo, A.; Gentiloni Silverj, F.; Marzorati, D.; Bagarolo, R.; Monti, M.; Velleca, R.; D'Angelo, R.; Frustaglia, A.; Zuccarelli, G.C.; et al. Predictors of mortality in nursing-home residents with pneumonia: A multicentre study. *Clin. Microbiol. Infect.* **2018**, *24*, 72–77. [CrossRef]
4. Gordon, A.L.; Franklin, M.; Bradshaw, L.; Logan, P.; Elliott, R.; Gladman, J.R. Health status of UK care home residents: A cohort study. *Age Ageing* **2014**, *43*, 97–103. [CrossRef]
5. Fuller, R.L.; Goldfield, N.I.; Hughes, J.S.; McCullough, E.C. Nursing Home Compare Star Rankings and the Variation in Potentially Preventable Emergency Department Visits and Hospital Admissions. *Popul. Health Manag.* **2019**, *22*, 144–152. [CrossRef]
6. Heinold, S.; Fassmer, A.M.; Schmiemann, G.; Hoffmann, F. Characteristics of outpatient emergency department visits of nursing home residents: An analysis of discharge letters. *Aging Clin. Exp. Res.* **2021**, *33*, 3343–3351. [CrossRef]
7. Gruneir, A.; Bell, C.M.; Bronskill, S.E.; Schull, M.; Anderson, G.M.; Rochon, P.A. Frequency and pattern of emergency department visits by long-term care residents—A population-based study. *J. Am. Geriatr. Soc.* **2010**, *58*, 510–517. [CrossRef]
8. Hofmann, H.; Hahn, S. Characteristics of nursing home residents and physical restraint: A systematic literature review. *J. Clin. Nurs.* **2014**, *23*, 3012–3024. [CrossRef]
9. Gunningberg, L.; Hommel, A.; Baath, C.; Idvall, E. The first national pressure ulcer prevalence survey in county council and municipality settings in Sweden. *J. Eval. Clin. Pract.* **2013**, *19*, 862–867. [CrossRef]
10. Moore, Z.; Johansen, E.; Etten, M.; Strapp, H.; Solbakken, T.; Smith, B.E.; Faulstich, J. Pressure ulcer prevalence and prevention practices: A cross-sectional comparative survey in Norway and Ireland. *J. Wound Care* **2015**, *24*, 333–339. [CrossRef]
11. Courvoisier, D.S.; Righi, L.; Bene, N.; Rae, A.C.; Chopard, P. Variation in pressure ulcer prevalence and prevention in nursing homes: A multicenter study. *Appl. Nurs. Res.* **2018**, *42*, 45–50. [CrossRef]
12. Lopes, T.S.; Videira, L.; Saraiva, D.; Agostinho, E.S.; Bandarra, A.J.F. Multicentre study of pressure ulcer point prevalence in a Portuguese region. *J. Tissue Viability* **2020**, *29*, 12–18. [CrossRef]
13. VanGilder, C.; Lachenbruch, C.; Algrim-Boyle, C.; Meyer, S. The International Pressure Ulcer Prevalence Survey: 2006–2015: A 10-Year Pressure Injury Prevalence and Demographic Trend Analysis by Care Setting. *J. Wound Ostomy Cont. Nurs.* **2017**, *44*, 20–28. [CrossRef]
14. Aygor, H.E.; Sahin, S.; Sozen, E.; Baydal, B.; Aykar, F.S.; Akcicek, F. Features of pressure ulcers in hospitalized older adults. *Adv. Skin. Wound Care* **2014**, *27*, 122–126. [CrossRef]
15. Rasero, L.; Simonetti, M.; Falciani, F.; Fabbri, C.; Collini, F.; Dal Molin, A. Pressure Ulcers in Older Adults: A Prevalence Study. *Adv. Skin. Wound Care* **2015**, *28*, 461–464. [CrossRef]
16. Lai, S.-W.; Liao, K.-F.; Lin, C.-L.; Lin, C.-C.; Lin, C.-H. Longitudinal data of multimorbidity and polypharmacy in older adults in Taiwan from 2000 to 2013. *BioMedicine* **2020**, *10*, 1. [CrossRef]
17. Dwyer, R.; Stoelwinder, J.; Gabbe, B.; Lowthian, J. Unplanned Transfer to Emergency Departments for Frail Elderly Residents of Aged Care Facilities: A Review of Patient and Organizational Factors. *J. Am. Med. Dir. Assoc.* **2015**, *16*, 551–562. [CrossRef]
18. Tsan, L.; Davis, C.; Langberg, R.; Hojlo, C.; Pierce, J.; Miller, M.; Gaynes, R.; Gibert, C.; Montgomery, O.; Bradley, S.; et al. Prevalence of nursing home-associated infections in the department of Veterans Affairs nursing home care units. *Am. J. Infect. Control* **2008**, *36*, 173–179. [CrossRef]
19. Spector, W.D.; Limcangco, R.; Williams, C.; Rhodes, W.; Hurd, D. Potentially Avoidable Hospitalizations for Elderly Long-stay Residents in Nursing Homes. *Med. Care* **2013**, *51*, 673–681. [CrossRef]
20. Blumenstein, I.; Shastri, Y.M.; Stein, J. Gastroenteric tube feeding: Techniques, problems and solutions. *World J. Gastroenterol.* **2014**, *20*, 8505–8524. [CrossRef]
21. Wojkowska-Mach, J.; Gryglewska, B.; Romaniszyn, D.; Natkaniec, J.; Pobiega, M.; Adamski, P.; Grodzicki, T.; Kubicz, D.; Heczko, P.B. Age and other risk factors of pneumonia among residents of Polish long-term care facilities. *Int. J. Infect. Dis.* **2013**, *17*, E37–E43. [CrossRef]

22. Montoya, A.; Mody, L. Common infections in nursing homes: A review of current issues and challenges. *Aging Health* **2011**, *7*, 889–899. [CrossRef]
23. Meddings, J.; Saint, S.; Krein, S.L.; Gaies, E.; Reichert, H.; Hickner, A.; McNamara, S.; Mann, J.D.; Mody, L. Systematic Review of Interventions to Reduce Urinary Tract Infection in Nursing Home Residents. *J. Hosp. Med.* **2017**, *12*, 356–368. [CrossRef]
24. Tang, M.; Woo, J.; Hui, E.; Chan, F.; Lee, J.; Sham, A.; Chau, P.H. Utilization of emergency room and hospitalization by Chinese nursing home residents: A cross-sectional study. *J. Am. Med. Dir. Assoc.* **2010**, *11*, 325–332. [CrossRef]
25. Wang, J.Y.; Yang, Y.W.; Liu, C.H.; Chang, K.C.; Lin, Y.T.; Liu, C.C. Emergency department visits and associated factors among people with dementia residing in nursing homes in Taiwan: A one-year cohort study. *BMC Geriatr.* **2023**, *23*, 503. [CrossRef]
26. Chen, P.W.; Hsiung, H.F.; Cheng, S.H.; Wu, F.L. Factors Associated with Unplanned Hospitalizations of Nursing Home Residents. *Int. J. Gerontol.* **2023**, *17*, 220–225. [CrossRef]
27. de Rekeneire, N.; Volpato, S. Physical function and disability in older adults with diabetes. *Clin. Geriatr. Med.* **2015**, *31*, 51–65, viii. [CrossRef]
28. Munshi, M.N.; Florez, H.; Huang, E.S.; Kalyani, R.R.; Mupanomunda, M.; Pandya, N.; Swift, C.S.; Taveira, T.H.; Haas, L.B. Management of Diabetes in Long-term Care and Skilled Nursing Facilities: A Position Statement of the American Diabetes Association. *Diabetes Care* **2016**, *39*, 308–318. [CrossRef]
29. Marincowitz, C.; Preston, L.; Cantrell, A.; Tonkins, M.; Sabir, L.; Mason, S. Factors associated with increased Emergency Department transfer in older long-term care residents: A systematic review. *Lancet Healthy Longev.* **2022**, 3, e437–e447. [CrossRef]
30. Searle, B.; Barker, R.O.; Stow, D.; Spiers, G.F.; Pearson, F.; Hanratty, B. Which interventions are effective at decreasing or increasing emergency department attendances or hospital admissions from long-term care facilities? A systematic review. *BMJ Open* **2023**, *13*, e064914. [CrossRef]
31. Fiorini, F.R.; Santoro, R.; Deganello, A.; Mannelli, G.; Meccariello, G.; Gallo, O. Is open tracheotomy performed by residents in otorhinolaryngology a safe procedure? A retrospective cohort study. *Eur. Arch. Oto-Rhino-Laryngol.* **2015**, *272*, 1483–1489. [CrossRef]

healthcare

MDPI

Article

Understanding Ethical Concerns Involving Vulnerable Human Participant Populations in Medical Research: Mixed-Method Analysis of Liberian Ebola Survivors' Experiences in PREVAIL I–VII

Jessi Hanson-DeFusco [1,*], Decontee Davis [2], Meghana Bommareddy [3] and Zainab Olayemi Olaniyan [3]

[1] Humanities, Social Sciences, and Communication Department, College of Arts and Sciences, Lawrence Technological University, Southfield, MI 48075, USA
[2] Winifred J. Harley College of Health Sciences, United Methodist University of Liberia, Monrovia 1000, Liberia; ddecontee54@gmail.com
[3] Public Policy and Political Economics Program, School of Economic, Political, and Policy Sciences, University of Texas at Dallas, Richardson, TX 75080, USA; meghana.bommareddy@utdallas.edu (M.B.); zainab.olaniyan@utdallas.edu (Z.O.O.)
* Correspondence: jhansonde@ltu.edu; Tel.: +1-720-548-7241

Abstract: Background: As the number of large-scale outbreaks continues to rise worldwide, clinical trials are increasingly engaging disease-affected peoples within the Minority World (nations with over 80% poverty rates). Yet global health research inadequately addresses potential ethical issues of including impoverished, disease-affected populations and their contextual vulnerabilities in medical research. **Objective:** This paper presents a mixed-method analysis from our 2022 semi-structured survey capturing the experiences of Liberian Ebola Virus Disease (EVD) survivors serving as study participants in the Partnership for Research on Ebola Virus in Liberia (PREVAIL) clinical trials. **Methods:** Firstly, we conducted an extensive literature review of the scholarship related to biomedical research and ethical standards protecting study participants to inform our survey method and design. Applying a theoretical framework on vulnerability, we then qualitatively explored the survey responses of 19 EVD survivors' perceptions and experiences taking part in PREVAIL, including their expectations, treatment, delivered benefits, and quality of care. We further quantitatively codified their statements for underlying themes of reported negative experiences against standard ethical regulations in biomedical research, conducting a statistical analysis to inform generalizability. Most of the 19 survivors reported facing extreme ongoing vulnerabilities related to their disease status, including physical impairments, psychosocial stress, and socio-economic inequity. **Results:** Initially, the survivors tended to experience a sense of hope and pride in volunteering for PREVAIL. One in five participants reported benefiting from PREVAIL's regular medical diagnoses. However, most of their survey responses indicated prevalent negative shared experiences, including continually being confused or misinformed of their study participant rights, roles, and benefits; being burdened by heavy participation transaction costs; and repeated incidents of poor treatment and discrimination by PREVAIL staff after initial recruitment. PREVAIL participant satisfaction ranking is negatively correlated with receiving insufficient financial compensation ($r = -0.51$), extensive time requirements for each medical visit (-0.40), and being poorly treated by clinical staff (-0.67).

Keywords: clinical trials; Ebola survivors; global health; ethical treatment; medical research

1. Introduction

Human participant research plays an ever more vital role in medical breakthroughs to combat contagious diseases [1], especially as the number of global epidemiological threats continues to grow exponentially in recent decades [2]. Large-scale outbreaks can offer researchers access to rare disease-affected populations, including survivors as human participants in clinical trials to aid in medical advancements [1,3,4]. One of the worst pre-COVID-19 health crises was the 2014–2016 West Africa outbreak, the largest recorded Ebola epidemic since 1976 [5,6]. Liberia, one of eleven nations affected, experienced 10,678 Ebola cases with a 55% survival rate [7–9]. At the end of the West African crisis, there was an estimated 17,000 West African Ebola Virus Disease (EVD) survivors, with approximately 5000 survivors residing in Liberia [10–12].

The global shock of the 2014–2016 West African outbreak quickly led to an exponential increase in international support and funding for Ebola biomedical research, from USD 3 million/year before 2015 to USD 116 million between 2015 and 2016 [13–17]. In October 2014, the Partnership for Research on Vaccines and Infectious Diseases in Liberia (PREVAIL) was launched as a large-scale biomedical research initiative, implemented by multiple stakeholders like the Government of Liberia with sponsorship by the US National Institute of Allergy and Infectious Diseases (NIAID). Starting in February 2014, PREVAIL recruited approximately 1500 Liberian survivors and 6000 of their close contacts as human participants in randomized vaccination trials, physical and bodily fluid exams, psychosocial assessments, and natural studies over the next five years [10,18–20]. This study examines the shared experiences of Liberian EVD survivors as human participants in PREVAIL.

1.1. EVD Survivor Participation in PREVAIL

As demonstrated by various HIV/AIDS studies, human participant involvement can offer unique opportunities to people negatively impacted by their disease status and related health impairments to altruistically give of themselves to a greater cause, so that their suffering and loss may not be in vain [4]. Starting in 2014, in meetings with the Liberian Ministry of Health (MOH) and the Ebola Survivors' Network, hundreds of EVD survivors sought opportunities to contribute to any response or research efforts. They were often motivated by the hope of finding a sense of purpose to cope with the effects of survivor's guilt and a need to feel useful. Others wanted to become part of a team comprised of empathetic survivors like themselves with similar shared experiences [5,21–27]. Additionally, most volunteer opportunities came with supplemental benefits like financial stipends and potential for future employment [11,23,27].

In turn, the 2014–2016 outbreak offered medical researchers with the unique prospect of accessing EVD survivors on a large scale to robustly study the effects of Ebola [15,17,28]. PREVAIL initiated its first clinical trial in 2015, and as financial support continued to increase, seven staged studies were executed in total, using different methods, target populations, and sample sizes [10,18–20]. Throughout its various clinical trials, the PREVAIL design included screening all recruited participants for a history of family illness, conducting a physical exam, and performing blood tests. Some were also provided eye examinations. Ebola survivors and those who entered an ETU but may not have had Ebola then were asked to visit a PREVAIL clinic at 3, 6, and 12 months, followed by 6-month visits over 5 years [10,13,14]. A formal research report on PREVAIL notes its various contributions to survivors' longer-term recovery. For instance, the PREVAIL VII clinical trial (evaluating the persistence of Ebola viral RNA in the eye and response to cataract surgery among EVD survivors) concluded that "EVD survivors and controls demonstrated significant visual improvement from cataract surgery" [17] (paragraph 3). Likewise, PREVAIL I, II, IV, and V are reported to have led to crucial epidemiological advancements, including the provision of vaccines against the disease [13,14,29] (list of all staged studies and contributions/key findings summarized in Appendix B). However, there are initial reports of poor implementation and procedural oversight quality and criticism by EVD survivors pertaining to PREVAIL [9,15,29–31].

1.2. Ethical Concerns of Biomedical Research and Vulnerable African Populations

In the past 50 years, "the level of oversight on human participants research has exploded from almost none to what is now an exhaustive system of protections. Still, these oversights and protections are not uniform throughout the world, and many nations, especially poor-resource nations, remain at risk for ethical improprieties" [1] (paragraph 3). Ethical issues in medical research in the Majority World (countries with at least 80% poverty rates) continue to gain attention. Cases include McGown's testing of new drugs and anesthetics without proper authorization in Zimbabwe in the 1990s to the 1996 Pfizer American testing of trovafloxacin against ceftriaxone to treat bacterial meningitis killing eleven Nigerian children [32–36]. Yet despite "documented reports of research abuses in Africa and poor-resource nations in other parts of the world, the majority of incidences related to breaches in ethical conduct most likely go unreported" [33] (p. 961). Additional factors diminishing a person's quality of life (QoL) (e.g., extreme poverty, gender inequity, low education) can make them more susceptible to being less informed of their rights and roles; taken advantage of; and/or inadequately protected from harm, especially when the ethical standards and procedures of a study do not account for their contextual needs [36–39].

Survivors entering PREVAIL tended to face a variety of vulnerabilities. Nearly all Liberian survivors, many of whom came from low-income and low-educational backgrounds, were made more vulnerable by their disease status. Most adult survivors continually struggled with long-term EVD-related physical impairments (e.g., blindness, nerve damage, body pains), poor mental health (e.g., depression, PTSD), and increased socio-economic hardships (e.g., being fired, abandoned, or evicted due to disease status) [23,26,40,41]. PREVAIL further confirmed these vulnerabilities in its third trial, which "determine[d] the long-term consequences of EVD by comparing health outcomes in survivors (966 people) and a control group of uninfected household and community contacts (2350 people)" [42] (p. 1). Yet while there were reports about negative experiences of EVD survivors in medical research, there are few formal investigations linked to their vulnerabilities. We aim to address this research gap by examining Liberian EVD survivors' reported experiences and perspectives as recruited human participants in PREVAIL.

1.3. Rationale and Study Purpose

With this background, our research project applied a mixed method design conducting our 2022 semi-structured survey of 19 Liberians EVD survivor respondents. Applying a theoretical framework of vulnerability, we examined two key questions:

- What are potential underlying themes of EVD survivor experiences as human participants in PREVAIL I–VII?
- To what extent is EVD survivors' quality of life affected by their experiences with PREVAIL?

Our research team first conducted a robust literature review related to biomedical research, human participant involvement, ethics, and Ebola to inform our study design, method, and research framework. Based on the literature and initial PREVAIL and partner reports (such as by USAID/CDC), we hypothesized the following:

H1: Ebola survivors' participation in PREVAIL is linked to improved self-efficacy and psychosocial health.

H2: Survivor participants gained targeted medical support for their specific disease status at PREVAIL clinics.

H3: Any negative experiences involving biomedical research ethical standards during PREVAIL negatively impacts human participants' quality of life.

This article is presented as follows. We first detail our theoretical framework, materials, and methods. We then summarize the qualitative results of common shared experiences reported by 19 EVD survivor respondents of our digital semi-structured survey. Secondly, we supplement the analysis by codifying open-ended statements related to key threads of their experiences against ethical standards for protecting human participants in medical research and then perform a statistical analysis (correlation; bootstrap) to address the generalizability of their experiences against the larger PREVAIL human participant population. We elaborate on the survey results in reference to key findings from our literature review in Section 4 and, lastly, present research implications and recommendations in Section 5.

1.4. Theoretical Framework

This research applied the theoretical framework on vulnerability, which offers both theoretical and practical foundations for ethical human subject research as presented by Gordon (2020). Vulnerable participants require extended protections to safeguard their rights and wellbeing. Vulnerability can be theoretically studied by two approaches; the categorical approach examines which groups and populations are vulnerable, and the contextual approach characterizes various vulnerabilities that may affect the individual person. Study participants in medical research can be made vulnerable in a series of different ways, which, when aggregated, can negatively impact their involvement in biomedical interventions [38]. There are six types of vulnerabilities:

- Medical—involving physical impairments, poor mental health, and poor medical services/access
- Economic—inequitable distribution of social goods and services like financial income or secure housing
- Social—when an individual falls into an undervalued social group because of their health status
- Cognitive—diminished capacity or inability to effectively communicate
- Institutional—vulnerability to hierarchical power dynamics
- Deferential—informal hierarchical power dynamics such as those created by gender or social economic status; imbalances in power dynamics like doctor and patient, or knowledge like researcher and low-educated participants [38].

Ethical codes of medical research specifically concern the need for proper safeguards and operational protocols to be put into place to address all study participant and/or medical patient needs related to their vulnerabilities [37,38,43].

2. Materials and Methods

2.1. Study Design

During January–April 2022, our research team conducted a robust literature review of 331 top-cited scholarship on Google Scholar and PubMed, using key search terms including Ebola, biomedical research, PREVAIL, Liberia, ethical standards, participants in clinical trials, development, and epidemiology to inform the study purpose and design. We additionally mapped standard ethical regulations in biomedical research and medical treatment, applying a theoretical framework on vulnerability in healthcare.

In April, the survey was designed by the research team, including being formally reviewed by a team of Liberian global health experts from the Ministry of Health and University of Liberia to ensure the instrument was contextually relevant and culturally sensitive. The primary investigator (PI) worked as an EVD responder with the MOH, MOG, and ESNL throughout the Liberian crisis. This study builds on some of her previous research on EVD-affected peoples [5,41]. Additionally, one of the co-investigators is an EVD survivor with medical training and field survey experience of EVD survivors.

The survey includes open-ended questions, as well as Likert-scaled ranking questions, capturing both quantitative data and testimonies of their post-EVD-recovery experiences including participating in PREVAIL, governmental support, and sentiments/motivational statements related to their disease status (see Appendix A). The survey used both standard English and Liberian English. A key scale incorporated was the Perceived Psychosocial Stress Scale, which was widely used during the 2014–2016 EVD outbreak [5,27,41]. It captures self-reported stressors like anxiety, withdrawal, anger, and flashbacks [44–46]. The survey was pilot tested with alpha testing on Likert scaling ($\alpha > 0.65$) to verify high inter-rater reliability. All pilot test data were excluded.

The survey was launched on Qualtrics (2023, SAP, USA) through May–July 2022 using a snowball approach on the Liberian Ebola Survivor group and Ebola Information Facebook pages. Snowball sampling (or chain-referral sampling) is a nonprobability sampling method in which initial study participants share the study with acquaintances to expand recruitment. Use of social media in snowballing can be an effective means of facilitating the distribution of the digital survey to hard-to-reach populations [47–49]. An estimated three-in-four survivors use Facebook to communicate with other survivors and survivor information pages [29], thus serving as a strong means of recruiting survey participants.

The digital survey included informed consent that was presented first after clicking on the survey, which participants read and then clicked on "agree to participate" to continue with the survey. The nature of the study required participants to have some level of technology to complete the survey. Eligibility criteria included speaking English; basic literacy; being a Liberian citizen; having documentation of being a survivor of EVD; and being aged 18–65. Participation was anonymous.

2.2. Data Collection and Analysis

During data collection, 33 people clicked on the survey link, with 25 completing the survey on Qualtrics. Six participants' data were excluded due to the participants not having consented or being non-survivors. In total, 19 adult survivor testimonials were included (13 women/6 men, ages 25–49, residing in Montserrado and Margibi (urban/semi-urban counties)).

The first phase of the data analysis was a literature review of 331 top-cited sources, which informed the study design, as well as later analysis of the survey data (see Figure 1). In the second phase, the self-reported responses of the survivors who participated in our survey were qualitatively explored by the entire research team, facilitated by the PI. We employed a generic qualitative inquiry approach, commonly used in mixed method psychological studies using a survey design. Unlike a phenomenological approach, generic qualitative inquiry collects data using semi-structured questions capturing qualitative statements in which participants share their ideas and experiences of real events [50–52]. Compared to the better-known qualitative approaches like phenomenology, grounded theory, or ethnography, the generic qualitative inquiry approach "is clearest when it is defined in the negative: it is research that "is not guided by an explicit or established set of philosophic assumptions in the form of one of the known [or more established] qualitative methodologies" [53] (paragraph 9). Generic studies epistemologically apply a social constructivist lens that explores how participants interpret their personal lived experiences, conceptualize their world/environment, and give meaning to these experiences [51,54]. Studies using this approach can offer rich descriptions of the phenomenon being studied and are commonly quite inductive and include open codes, categories, and thematic analysis [51,55].

We adopt the process recommended by Percy, Kostere, and Kostere (2015) (pp. 76–84) [50]. Qualitative data (open-ended responses) can then be re-structured quantitatively, often converting them into a second binary or categorical variables, based on noted trends (shared experiences or similar opinions/perspectives) among various participant statements. Like how ethnographers and field researchers code their field notes, this approach can allow for a statistical analysis to support qualitative analysis [50–52,56–59]. The purpose of this additional step is to measure the frequency of trends and to assess findings against the general population, especially in studies with limited sampling (small N) [50–52,60].

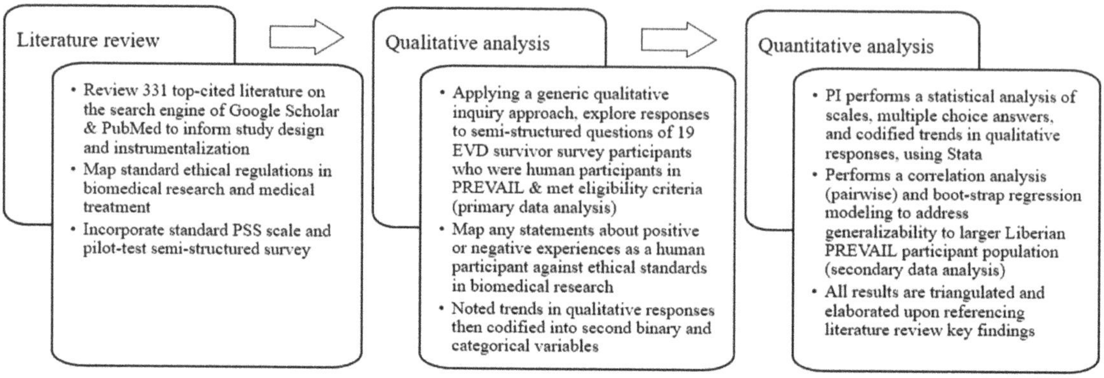

Figure 1. Data analysis phases.

All participant open-ended responses were assessed for naturally occurring trends that were later quantitatively codified. From this, we created binary variables indicating if a person's statements about their experiences mentioned the following (1 yes; 0 no): having no medical provision, receiving no financial compensation, feeling/experiencing poor treatment by PREVAIL staff, experiencing long visits lasting around eight hours each trip, or feeling they experienced unequal/discriminant opportunities to participate in specific PREVAIL medical treatments or studies like eye exams. We used statistical findings, namely Point Biserial correlation analysis and boot-strap modeling, to triangulate survivor statements. Finally, we explored the relevance of this research, its limitations, and possible ethical implications for global health policy and research. The PI performed the statistical analysis in Stata (StataCorp LLC/SE 17/College Station, TX, USA) with data interpretation support from the research team. Underlying themes are summarized using both quantitative and qualitative data in the Results section.

2.3. Ethical Approval

This 2022 research involved a snowball survey approach of Liberians who are Ebola survivors. This project received ethical approval from the University of Texas at Dallas (IRB#22-528).

3. Results

3.1. Qualitative Analysis

Our literature review indicates that EVD survivors and EVD-affected peoples face challenges that transcend all categories of vulnerability, including increased financial hardships, social stigmatization, EVD-related disabilities like blindness, and decreased mental health (see Table 1). PREVAIL documentation notes many of these vulnerabilities among their study participants [13–17]. This analysis assesses to what extent steps were taken to accommodate and safeguard against these vulnerabilities during the seven staged studies [29,30].

Along with a robust review of the literature, our research team also qualitatively explored the open-ended responses of the 19 survey participants to better understand their experiences as human participants in the PREVAIL trials. Overall, there were five main trends among their statements identified by our research team (summarized in Table 2). We then codified their qualitative statements to assess the frequencies with which the survivor participants reported experiencing or commenting on these threads.

Table 1. Types of vulnerability compared to EVD survivors' quality-of-life factors.

Type of Vulnerability	Relation to EVD Survivors' Quality of Life
Medical	EVD survivors continue to struggle with long-term poor psychosocial health, which increases over time [12]. Long-haul physical EVD complications include chronic headaches, cognitive impairment, body aches, impotency, and infertility. In total, 1 in 100 Liberians had regular access to mental health services [5,23]
Economic	Most survivors lost their jobs or a household breadwinner due to the disease [5,41,61,62].
Social	Many female and male survivors were physically attacked, beaten, emotionally abused, shunned, illegally convicted, and labeled by others as tainted, dangerous, or victims of ill fortune [23,29,63,64]
Cognitive	75–90% of EVD survivors experienced complications for several years after primary symptoms were resolved [64,65]. EVD-related cognitive, psychiatric, and physical abnormalities led to additional PREVAIL studies [22,66]
Institutional	Liberia tends to be a society valuing both formal and informal hierarchical structures, including community elders and traditional leaders with heavy influence over the lives of people in their ethnic groups [67,68]. Nearly half of adult Liberians would prioritize supporting the decision of traditional leaders in decision making [69]. Many traditional elders often stigmatized and evicted EVD survivors from their communities for fear of contagion spread or bad juju affecting others [23,70]
Deferential	Informal and formal hierarchies that create institutional and deferential vulnerabilities can limit a participant's true autonomous decision making and place them at risk of exploitation. In low-income settings with limited healthcare systems, patients have less choice or voice in medical care due to high demand and low supply. The Liberia Medical and Dental Council (2016) has stated that Liberia's medical and health services are low-resourced, and after EVD, there were 298 medical doctors responsible for the national population (doctor-per-patient ratio of 1:15,000)

Table 2. Summary results of key areas of interest.

Area of Interest	Summary Results
Long-haul EVD effects	Less child stigmatization; positive feelings of being heroes; high psychosocial stress; long-term EVD physical impairments; unemployment and work and discrimination due to disease status; difficulty receiving medical treatment in public facilities; undervalued social group
Participant experience with PREVAIL	High satisfaction with medical diagnoses provided; medical and compensation benefits for human subjects not clearly established, causing confusion and frustration; common misunderstanding of the trial selection process; diagnosed with medical conditions but many left under the impression that they would receive medical treatment to improve their help; issues with what was promised in the recruitment process
Burden on human participant	Heavy transaction costs falling on impoverished human subjects; issues of inadequate or inconsistent financial support and provisions; time costs to participants appearing greatly miscalculated (estimated 8 h long visits plus transportation time)
Unethical treatment of human subjects	Instances of discriminant or improper treatment by PREVAIL team members; 52% of survey testimonies include at least one negative experience; rumors of unethical practices including coercion and sexual assault
Statistical implications	Significant negative association between PREVAIL participant satisfaction ranking and receiving insufficient financial compensation ($r = -0.51$), extensive time requirements for each medical visit (-0.40), and being poorly treated by clinical staff (-0.67)

3.1.1. Meeting Survivor's Long-Term EVD-Related Needs

One of the major topics that the 19 study participants brought up in their responses was their experiences of receiving specialized treatment (or the hope of it) for their long-term physical impairments resulting from suffering EVD. On the one hand, there is recognition of the medical benefits of being a study participant in PREVAIL. All 19 survey respondents mention how PREVAIL offered free diagnostic benefits to all EVD human participants. The diagnostics were linked to baseline and ongoing monitoring of their physical health but were tailored to their special symptoms and needs. They received detailed diagnosis by PREVAIL medical staff, familiar with EVD and its effects on the human body. In total, 10 out of the 19 survey participants (52%) provided statements indicating satisfaction with the free medical diagnoses they received at PREVAIL clinics. This supports the first hypothesis that survivor participants gained targeted medical support for their specific disease status at PREVAIL clinics.

> "When I was in prevail it was fine for me because after Ebola I never knew of any sickness prevail was able diagnose me of being ill and also give us food to eat each time we visit and transported us"—49-year-old female EVD survivor

> "I [completed] ended the prevail study, even when I was pregnant I was referred for treatment, the study was good for me"—28-year-old female EVD survivor

PREVAIL often offered diagnoses of physical and mental ailments caused by EVD that may have been difficult to receive in normal public health facilities. Additionally, PREVAIL offered supplemental support to pregnant women to safely deliver healthy babies, after many experienced recurrent miscarriages just after recovering from Ebola. A WHO 2015 report implies that "[m]ost pregnant woman infected with EVD will lose the unborn child sometime during the course of the disease. Women who recover from EVD with an intact pregnancy (no rupture of membranes or labour) require comprehensive IPC precautions to prevent exposure to intrauterine contents (i.e., amniotic fluid, placenta and fetus) during childbirth or complication management" [71] (p. 15). Thus, having access to specialized prenatal care because of PREVAIL appeared to offer great relief and was deeply appreciated by pregnant survivors.

Additionally, nearly all 19 survivors indicated that they felt like heroes by participating in EVD response work and PREVAIL. They felt a sense of giving back to a greater good. The statistical analysis indicates that, on average, the 19 survivors reported suffering from 5.25 of a total 7 psychosocial stressors (95%CI 4.65–5.85), or 75% aggregated PSS, as a direct result of their EVD status in 2022. The stressors include anger, withdrawal, sadness, poor sleep and eating habits, flashbacks, and anxiety. The most frequent stressors that they reported facing included anger (94.4%, 95%CI 82.7–99.9%), flashbacks (94.1%, 81.6–99.8%), and anxiety (88.2%, 71.2–98.9%). Yet those who felt like Ebola heroes tended to exhibit less PSS ($r = -0.54$, $p < 0.001$), thus offering support for the positive effects that human participant volunteering can provide. This long-haul stress is elaborated on in a sister publication focused on general experiences of survivors [72]. This finding supports our second hypothesis that Ebola survivors' participation (when positive) in PREVAIL is linked to improved self-efficacy and psychosocial health. Yet these positive effects appeared to wash out when human participants faced negative PREVAIL incidences.

> "Prevail had a good start welcome us with smile and great respect, snacks as breakfast and later lunch as times goes back no snacks was out and we started to overstay... the rumors was about after the five years study we could have benefit (medicine, operations, stipends)...My concern is prevail ended with no benefit for survivors after five years of study"—40-year-old man

> "Prevail has been good... help us to know our health status; my issue is prevail ended the study without any [medical or financial] benefit for survivors" —28-year-old woman

> "[T]he [PREVAIL] study didn't favor us survivors even when [we went] to protest...since than no action... my eyes are having problems and I told the study but no solution had been taking towards that [when promised]"—40-year-old male

Comparatively, our analysis of the survey statements indicates a disconnection between what PREVAIL truly provided to participants compared to what the 19 participants were led to believe that they would receive. Most provided statements implying that they were not made adequately aware of their role, mainly as a human participant in biomedical research versus being included as a medical patient, and the benefits that they were guaranteed. Nearly half of the survey participants made statements of not receiving medical treatment beyond an initial diagnosis, and continually going to clinical appointments in anticipation of receiving medical procedures that would cure their ailments, therapy for mental health issues, or provision of free medication.

Major health research institutions acknowledge the importance of how adults being able to voluntarily consent may be compromised by certain circumstances including "economic or educational disadvantage, and physical handicap" [73] (paragraph 11). Because the source of the problem seemingly lies in their role as participants, we felt it important to specifically map the differences between biomedical research and clinical medicine. We visually present the confusion that the survey participants presented as experiences against this mapping (see Figure 2).

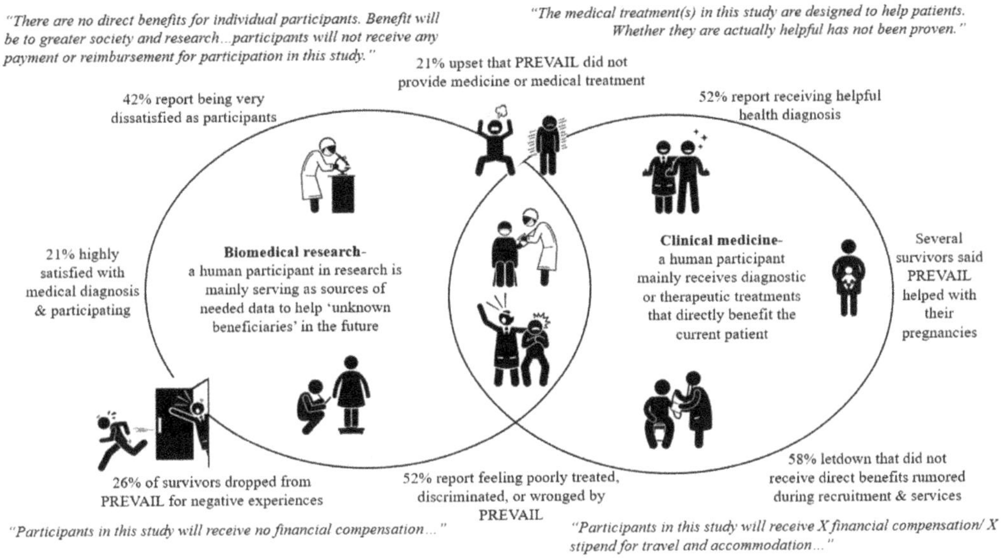

Figure 2. Surveyed Ebola survivors' aggregate PREVAIL experiences compared to standard IRB participant roles and beneficial and statements in biomedical research verses clinical medicine.

While clinical trials can offer medical treatment directly to human participants, there is a standard divide between the specific roles and benefits of the human participant that ethical standards repeatedly assert must be stated clearly in ethical approval documents, including IRB consent forms. Typically, clinical medicine holds the patient as the direct beneficiary of the treatment, with the assumption that, while the effects of treatment may still not be known, the intent is that any benefits will impact the wellbeing of the patient. Comparatively, biomedical research implies that the participant is a needed source of medical information, which will not necessarily benefit the participant but offer knowledge benefiting greater society and future vulnerable populations. These distinctions can be noted in commonly standardized IRB consent forms, in which benefits and compensation are specified. For instance, if a participant will or may be randomly selected for treatment, the potential benefits are specified while highlighting the fact that their effect is yet to be scientifically proven [38,73–75]. Yet in clinical trials or human subject research with no direct benefits, statements like those presented in the Figure need to be stated [73,75]. Our study, however, finds that one in four of the nineteen participants report dropping out of PREVAIL mainly due to negative experiences.

3.1.2. Lack of Clarity of the Participant Role and Selection for Medical Benefits

A review of PREVAIL documents indicates that they clearly define the role of EVD survivors as study participants, with no mention of them as medical patients [14–16,18,28,29,76]. Yet to what extent the 19 survivors understood this role versus what they came to understand it to be (expected or led to believe) appears questionable. Firstly, many of the 19 survivors appeared to have not been made adequately aware of the selection process for some of the randomized trials. Nearly all PREVAIL participants received an initial eye screening, but only specific survivors received more extensive treatment for eye problems [17,77]. Yet in reading the 19 survivors' comments on eyecare treatment, most expected to have the chance at receiving direct medical treatment like uveitis treatment, as a patient would. Statements like those below indicate a high level of confusion and frustration in the eye examination and treatment selection process.

> "[M]y eyes are having problems and I told the study but no solution had been taking towards that"—36-year-old female

> "My concern is prevail took people to the America for eye, since the first group came we have not heard when the other will go America for their eye"—30-year-old female survivor

It also seems that they did not realize that they were study participants with the sole medical benefit of receiving a diagnosis. There was also confusion among survivors about the selection process for randomized control trials, which appeared to have never been fully cleared up by PREVAIL. Many participants anticipated receiving more robust treatment, including being brought to the United States for uveitis studies, of which only a small number ultimately were, causing disappointment and anger among those not selected. With 30% of survivors with uveitis issues going blind [17,77], we posit that many more PREVAIL participants were just as desperate for medical remedies beyond diagnosis.

Secondly, there are also indications that randomized selection processes were compromised by corrupt practices. There were no prompts for issues of corruption, so this finding was surprising. Survivor statements refer to rumors of being able to bribe a staffer for placement in a treatment group instead of the control. There were also rumors of unethical practices including coercion and sexual exploitation.

> "[S]paces [for eye treatment in the US] were sold if you don't have the money, then you end up having sexual abuse with anyone that is in charge"—31-year-old female survivor

> "[S]urvivors could go America for eye and lost [loss] of membrane, but those spaces were sold..."—31-year-old female survivor

There must be a clear distinction between gossip and actual reported facts. The reliability and accuracy of data are often based on the quality of the source [59,60]. However, these statements appear to be more than general gossip but instead secondary-sourced evidence. Several survivors reported directly hearing and knowing an individual person who was victimized by these practices but did not formally come forth to report their experience for fear of retribution.

Thirdly, while diagnoses and prescriptions for ailments were provided, typically the program did not cover costs for medical treatment outside of diagnosis, including any needed hospitalization or medication purchases. Instead, prescriptions were provided by PREVAIL medical staff to individual survivors, unless the person was participating in an experimental trial [14,17]. A total of 21% of the 19 individuals reported feeling let down that PREVAIL did not provide medical care, pay for additional medical treatment, or cover medicines for ailments. These statements indicate an additional ethical concern that these provisions were not concretely communicated and assessed by PREVAIL to all the study participants despite their ongoing financial difficulties and obvious desperation for any support with their ongoing physical and mental health complications.

> "I started 2016, and the was no benefit for survivors, to the extend that PREVAIL will diagnose a[n] illness and give you the update without a treatment, if you the survivors don't have means of getting treatment at a hospital, and that could cause death than you made die from that illness that also was the cause of low enrollment at the study"—31-year-old female survivor

3.1.3. Burden on Study Participants

Initially we hypothesized that participants would receive some financial benefit, such as the provision of stipends and food for attending each clinical appointment, based on reports by PREVAIL. Yet there appears to be heavy transaction costs that fell on some study participants, which appear to be insufficiently addressed by PREVAIL. Most Liberian households are vulnerable to conditions of poverty, and 80% of Liberians have inconsistent work and live on less than USD 1.25/day [78]. All 19 Liberian participants in our study previously had a job before Ebola, yet 7 of the 19 participants (36%) report ongoing issues with unemployment as a direct result of their Ebola status.

> "No money. I'm a single mother that hustling to get food for the kids (4) even finding meals at times is difficult for me so means of sending them to school" —40-year-old female survivor

> "No support being a single mother I can only afford meal for the kids not even regularly a week my kids eat, things actually gone bad for my family"—42-year-old female survivor

PREVAIL reportedly offered varied compensation to participants throughout its different phases. Transportation stipends were provided (around USD 10–20/trip), and, eventually, meals including breakfasts and lunches were also given (at an estimated cost of USD 2/participant per day) [18,29]. But these provisions seemingly changed over time.

Statements like these below imply issues of inadequate or inconsistent financial support and provisions:

> "Prevail had a good start welcome us with smile and great respect, snacks as breakfast and later lunch as times goes back no snacks was out"—40-year-old male survivor

> "[W]hen you go to the study no water to even drink and you have to over stay before getting meal"—36-year-old female survivor

The transaction costs reported by the 19 survivors to be able to participate in the PREVAIL study appear extensive, especially for impoverished, single-parent households (see Figure 3). PREVAIL offered travel stipends based on the distance from clinic sites, with guidelines that each visit would require approximately one to two hours per appointment [20,79,80]. For instance, a recruitment ad for PREVAIL III specifies the following:

> "Participants will have 1 clinic visit. They will have a physical exam. Their vital signs will be measured. They will also have a neurological checkup. The exam will assess their mental status. Their senses, reflexes, and coordination will be tested. They will be observed while walking to assess their gait. This exam will take about 1 h. Participants will have an interview. They will answer questions about any symptoms they have that may be affecting the brain or nervous system. This will take about 1 h" [81] (p. 2).

By contrast, nearly all the survivors in our survey stated that the travel stipend was insufficient, as it only paid for participants, and most visits required up to eight hours a day. Based on the estimates that they provided, we gauge that a single clinical visit could have equated up to USD 20 in transportation per person (often needing to travel with child(ren)); one day's wages for extended examinations over the promised hour time-length; and up to 3 days of wages if transporting from another county, plus accommodations, meals, and potentially family care. PREVAIL's protocols of time and financial costs to participants appear miscalculated, at least for these survivors.

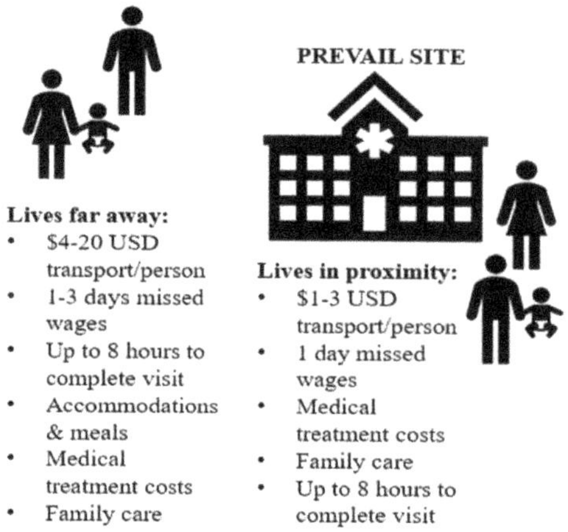

Figure 3. Average transaction costs of Liberian EVD survivors in the PREVAIL study.

> "I was able to end the study, the study started with snacks morning hours and little lunch follow noon hours, but all changes we arrive by 8:00 am and stay till 4:00 for only lunch than change of attitude of prevail staff towards survivors became too harsh"—45-year-old female survivor

PREVAIL offered basic financial compensation, which may have contributed to higher stress among participants. Furthermore, nearly all of the 19 survivors made statements reflecting a misunderstanding or poorly communicated information about their contribution being in-kind and not monetarily compensated beyond the general participant stipend. In total, 58% gave statements reflecting sentiments of frustration at perceived broken promises about direct benefits if they completed the full trial(s).

> "I heard that after the studies survivors was going to benefit and nothing was giving to us from prevail"—43-year-old male survivor

> "[T]he rumors was the end of prevail study survivors was going to have benefit and that was false"—42-year-old female survivor

The literature review could find no documentation by PREVAIL identifying these financial issues in its reports.

3.1.4. Unethical Treatment of Study Participants

Another unanticipated implication of this 2022 study was the magnitude of study participants who reported instances of experiencing discriminant or improper treatment by PREVAIL team members. In total, 52% of written testimonies include at least one negative interaction.

> "I participate in the study and the beginning was fine but later the staffs started using harsh words on us their interest for survivors decrease and cause dissatisfaction for me"—35-year-old male survivor

> "Prevail never treat me well"—27-year-old female survivor

> "[There was a] change of attitude of prevail staff towards survivors became too harsh"—45-year-old female survivor

> "[P]revail [staff] said we survivors are trouble makers"—43-year-old male survivor

> "I want prevail to come back to tell us about out benefits, because the study didn't favor us and survivors even when to protest [to the ESNL and MOH]"—36-year-old female survivor

Statements like these reflect that at first the interactions with PREVAIL staff were pleasant, but as the study continued, the quality of care and treatment of many of the human participants diminished. The next section examines how poor treatment and discriminant experiences impacted their psychosocial health and satisfaction in participating in PREVAIL.

3.2. Statistical Analysis

A correlation analysis triangulated many of these key finds. There is a significant negative association between PREVAIL participant satisfaction ranking and receiving insufficient financial compensation (r = −0.51), extensive time requirements for each medical visit (−0.40), and being poorly treated by clinical staff (−0.67) (see Table 3). Medical treatment provision, unequal treatment opportunities, financial insecurity due to disease status, and major demographics appear non-significant. Those who dropped out of PREVAIL tended to have significantly lower PSS levels than those who stayed until the end (r = −0.45, $p < 0.05$).

Table 3. Point-biserial correlation analysis of PREVAIL experiences among Ebola survivors.

	No Medicine Provision	No Financial Compensation	Treated Poorly by Staff	Long Visits (around 8 h)	Unequal Treatment Opportunities
Satisfaction with PREVAIL (1 low, 3 high)	−0.36	−0.51 **	−0.67 ***	−0.40 *	−0.18
Financial insecurity due to Ebola	−0.13	−0.45 **	−0.15	−0.04	−0.21
Sex (female 1, male 2)	−0.31	−0.21	0.09	−0.15	−0.27
County (Montserrado 1, Margibi 2)	−0.17	−0.05	−0.02	−0.23	0.05

Note: * $p < 0.05$, ** $p < 0.01$, *** $p < 0.001$.

There were approximately 1500 Liberian EVD participants and 6000 close contacts including family members who participated in PREVAIL's various trials. Our study's small sample size (n = 19) limits the causal generalizability of findings to larger populations. Thus, we addressed this statistical limitation by applying bootstrap regression modeling. We noted that the modeling appeared significant (replications = 999). We conducted nonparametric bootstrapping that involved randomized sampling with replacement. This method excludes any assumptions concerning underlying population distribution. It serves as an alternative for hypothesis-testing in small-N studies. By conducting bootstrap regression modeling, we could assess the model parameters' variability and, more so, the extent of random variation within each coefficient related to incremental changes in data values [82–84].

Despite the limited and non-randomized sampling, bootstrap modeling indicated that some findings might be statistically significant. In Table 4, if a survivor experienced poor treatment as a study participant by PREVAIL staff, their overall satisfaction would predictably be 31.67% percent lower (0.95 points out of a total of 3 (high)) than peers who did not ($p < 0.001$). Yet the effects of feeling they had unequal access to additional medical services like sight treatment, along with experiencing long clinic visits, were limited ($p > 0.05$).

Moreover, the EVD survivors self-reported their stress symptoms that they continued to experience as a direct result of their disease status five years after recovery. An additional bootstrap model indicated that those who stated experiencing an incident of being poorly treated or feeling discriminated by PREVAIL staff appeared to have an 18 percent (1.27 points) higher rate of psychosocial stress (SE = 0.63, bias = 0.10, normal CI (0.05–2.50); number of observations = 13; replications = 632, Adj. $R^2 = 0.59$, Wald $\chi^2 = 66.48$, $p = 0.00$).

Table 4. Statistics for bootstrapped regression modeling of 2022 Liberian EVD survivors' satisfaction as study participants in PREVAIL.

	Coefficient			
	Constant	Poor Treatment by PREVAIL Staff (1—yes; 0—no)	Unreasonably Long Clinic Visits (1—yes; 0—no)	Unequal Medical Treatment Access (1—yes; 0—no)
Avg. bootstrap estimate	2.43 ***	−0.95 ***	−0.48	0.31
Bootstrap SE	0.22	0.30	0.42	0.36
Bias	0.02	−0.04	0.01	−0.02
Normal CI	(1.99–2.87)	(−1.54–−0.36)	(−1.31–0.34)	(−0.65–0.72)
Percentile CI	(1.98–2.87)	(−1.56–−0.35)	(−1.25–0.36)	(−0.62–0.74)
Bias-corrected CI	(1.85–2.80)	(−1.44–−0.27)	(−1.26–0.32)	(−0.63–0.74)

Notes: Conducting nonparametric bootstrapping involves randomized sampling with replacement, excluding any assumptions concerning underlying population distribution; serves as an alternative for hypothesis testing in small-N studies; and involves assessing the model parameters' variability and extent of random variation within each coefficient related to incremental changes in data values [82–84]. Two bootstrap confidence intervals (CIs) are shown for each coefficient. Standard error = SE. *** $p < 0.01$. Number of observations = 19; replications = 999. Adj. $R^2 = 0.43$, Wald $\chi^2 = 19.11$, $p = 0.00$.

4. Discussion

Both the qualitative analysis of key literature review findings and the open-ended responses to survey questions, along with the statistical analysis, imply that survivors who participated in PREVAIL experienced some benefits, at least initially. The survivors reported benefiting from free medical diagnoses and an initial sense of purpose for the greater good, including feeling like heroes. However, we question if the benefits of participating in medical trials outweigh the burdens and negative experiences that appear to be commonly shared experiences. The anticipated benefits of participating, often informed by their dire impoverished state and physical impairments because of surviving EVD, were not consistently met. The transaction costs often negatively impacted the survivors' experiences. Likewise, there appear to be critical issues concerning the specific benefits survivors could expect, along with the treatment that they would receive, and what was provided. Often, it seemed to be an issue of the "carrot on the stick", in which misinterpretations of the roles of participants as human subjects rather than medical patients went unchecked, and inconsistent messaging led to rumors of corruption. The participants mostly appeared to have had a positive experience in the beginning of their engagement in PREVAIL, but, over time, their experiences in general worsened. The treatment of participants diminished over time, leading some to experience significantly more psychosocial stress and negative feelings like resentment.

The experiences shared by these 19 survivors provide some initial insights into PREVAIL's operations, as well as the meaning of hardship among study participants as a shared experience. The data from our literature review of 331 sources, combined with the mixed method analysis of the survey data from the 19 Ebola survivors, indicate that this disease-affected population was likely highly vulnerable before PREVAIL was launched. Such scenarios can probably inform contextual vulnerability that can impair a person's ability to fully consent or fully understand the details of clinical research participation without being influenced by these negative factors [6,18,34,37]. Any medical research initiative engaging in recruitment of a vulnerable population should consider how to address their vulnerabilities, including monitoring and evaluating potential unanticipated implementation problems [27,28,37,38].

There are some important factors that the literature review reveals about PREVAIL's ethical preparedness for working with survivors. PREVAIL's timeline appears hurried for protocol development and launch. For example, PREVAIL II's protocol development started in late November 2014, with NIH IRB approval granted on 29 January 2015, the approval of the Liberia National Research Ethics Board (NREB) granted on 13 February, and the "first patient" (only document referring to EVD survivors with this term) examined on 22 March [18]. Standard ethical approval for clinical trials by ethics institutions tend to be longer [37,39,47,56]. The NIH's digital instructions for IRB approval of clinical trials with human participants in international countries "often take a long time" [22]. Moreover, a key document reveals that "there was a great deal of disagreement among researchers over how clinical trials should be designed during the Ebola epidemic, particularly over whether trials should use randomization and concurrent control groups" [57]. PREVAIL was launched after eventual consensus was reached that it would be unethical to deprive patients of a treatment that could possibly prevent or treat Ebola.

PREVAIL studies and documents mention very few of the vulnerabilities that survivors faced in relation to ethical considerations. Instead, most documents include diction like "rapidly appraise", "making progress", and "rapid ethics and regulatory review" [18,20,31,32], possibly reflecting a lack of proper attention before implementation. In general, satisfaction with PREVAIL varied among the 19 survivors, statistically linked to implementation issues like being treated poorly by staff. While some volunteered to help inform the understanding of EVD and to benefit from medical diagnoses, in general most were motivated by desperation for medical service provision, mainly in the hope of some relief from their physical, mental, and socio-economic hardships [6,9,28,34,58]. We do not know the extent to which PREVAIL monitored and evaluated the experiences of its study participants. The comments indicate that at some point, EVD survivors formally protested issues of dissatisfaction, compensation, and medical treatment to GOL and ESNL. Ethical protocols in any EVD-related program that assess for potential negative unintended consequences could play a vital role in better safeguarding participants [6,26,28,59]. As our study implies, EVD survivor participant experiences with recruitment, retention, and treatment varied widely. We posit that implementation standards may have been too loose and inconsistent throughout the different PREVAIL trials, leading these 19 EVD survivors, at least, to feel confused about benefits, their roles as participants, and what to expect.

The survivors' feedback highlights additional vulnerabilities because of their experiences with PREVAIL. Employment with PREVAIL was promised, but most of the participants remarked that few survivors were hired. Stipends and the provision of meals were inconsistent, and there was the likelihood that participating in PREVAIL economically burdened many households. Survivors faced added forms of social vulnerability, as well as deferential vulnerability, in that many of them felt discriminated against, poorly treated by, or lied to by PREVAIL staff, likely damaging their emotional health.

Likewise, their medical vulnerability due to ongoing health issues and the institutional vulnerability of a sick population being targeted repeatedly to volunteer for the study further highlight ethical concerns. Many survivor testimonies reflect the participants' impressions that PREVAIL was designed to provide medical support (even treatment) that would help their own physical health ailments. Only a few appeared to have understood that while there might have been a randomized chance to receive specific treatments like eyecare or vaccines, for the most part, their roles were as sources of data on Ebola. Their blood, statements, and physical exams would inform research contributing mainly to generating collective knowledge that would benefit others in the future. It is questionable to suppose that patients mainly enroll in medical trials solely to support advancing collective knowledge and the benefit of future generations, especially when facing life-threatening diseases. Most EVD survivors were motivated by their personal needs and wellbeing, not altruism. The survivor participants appeared to have felt coerced to participate in the hopes of receiving a direct benefit if they completed the trial. Some indicated that there were issues of corruption and abuse in their dealings with PREVAIL staff, including bribes and trading sexual favors to be placed on prioritization lists for care.

As Salhia and Olaiyaand (2020) indicate, "[t]oday, clinical trials are one of the most heavily regulated practices in the world, and yet still not all people are provided the same oversights and protections, with improprieties disproportionately affecting poor-resource nations and vulnerable populations" [1] (paragraph 1). The ethical hardships that the survey participants report facing as PREVAIL participants highlights the need for the global health community to revisit how we conduct biomedical research in low-income countries, where participants are first made vulnerable due to impoverished circumstances and a lack of healthcare access and then see these compounded by the negative life factors and health impairments that they face after surviving a deadly disease. The NIH and other federal agencies are obligated to adhere to standards of conduct and ethical standards prominent in Western research cultures. Yet high ethical standards and practices can be compromised or hard to ensure in crisis environments, as demands tend to be intense, with limited resourcing, and thus "corners are cut" [3] (paragraph 13). The same factors may also linger even in post-outbreak and recovery phases, living clinical trials open to issues of ethically protecting highly vulnerable research participants in regions like Africa.

Limitations

This study applied a mixed methods approach, merging quantitative analysis with the qualitative exploration of survivors' experiences and the intrinsic meaning behind their experiences as human participants. The main objective of collecting open-ended answers was to capture narratives that explore the essence behind their individual EVD-related experiences [59,60,85]. The generalizability of the statistical findings is limited by the small sample size. This research study (like other small-N studies) tended to provide simplified statistical analyses, establishing correlation patterns but not necessarily causal mechanisms beyond associated relationships. [86–88]. However, as we discussed above, bootstrapping may better inform generalizability, but this has its limitations [59,82,84,85,89]. Future larger-scale and/or randomized control trial studies may better inform the generalizability of these results to the general EVD population.

5. Conclusions

This research reminds the health field of the importance of the unique contextual factors and ethical risks that medical research can have on human participants when implemented in low-income settings beset by poverty-based vulnerabilities. Medical professionals and partners must carefully weigh the benefits of the research against the burdens on participants, many of whom live in extreme poverty and are marginalized due to their disease status. Medical research on hemorrhagic diseases like Ebola plays a critical role in providing deeper understanding of less-known contagions, life-saving vaccinations, and opportunities for those affected by the disease to benefit through participation. PREVAIL led to massive gains in medical knowledge not previously afforded, including vaccination against EVD. PREVAIL also offered survivors targeted medical evaluations and individualized care. Yet the burdens for many EVD survivor participants appear to have outweighed the benefits, leading to increased psychosocial stress, financial hardships, and, in some cases, participant mistreatment.

Ebola biomedical research garnered large international support around the outbreak, including significant increases in funding. Yet when engaging a vulnerable disease-affected population, research must be cautious against rushing the ethical approval process and set up proper measures to safeguard study participants. Likewise, clinical research in low-income settings like Liberia must be careful to clearly communicate the roles, benefits, and processes that participants will undergo, to avoid needless confusion and the sense of being misled. Research and medical interventions like PREVAIL may have been designed with good intentions but were ultimately poorly implemented and at times did not prove adequate to fulfill survivors' needs. The sheer volume of vulnerabilities EVD survivors endured after discharge from ETUs should have served as a clear warning to PREVAIL of participants' desperation to seek any potential solutions to their problems—medically or otherwise. In these circumstances, health organizations must take precautions to clearly understand, articulate, and communicate the different roles, benefits, and needs of participants of vulnerable populations in biomedical research verses medical interventions. They must also consider putting in place frameworks that monitor and safeguard against ethical misconduct and undue burdens on survivor participants, many of whom may have less awareness and resources to protect them.

Author Contributions: Conceptualization, J.H.-D., D.D., M.B. and Z.O.O.; methodology, J.H.-D.; software, J.H.-D.; validation, J.H.-D., D.D., M.B. and Z.O.O.; formal analysis, J.H.-D., D.D., M.B. and Z.O.O.; investigation, J.H.-D., D.D., M.B. and Z.O.O.; resources, J.H.-D.; data curation, J.H.-D., M.B. and Z.O.O.; writing—original draft preparation, J.H.-D., M.B. and Z.O.O.; writing—review and editing, J.H.-D., D.D., M.B. and Z.O.O.; visualization, J.H.-D.; supervision, J.H.-D.; project administration, M.B., D.D. and Z.O.O.; funding acquisition, n/a. All authors have read and agreed to the published version of the manuscript.

Funding: This research received no external funding.

Institutional Review Board Statement: This study was conducted in accordance with the Declaration of Helsinki and approved by the Institutional Review Board at the University of Texas at Dallas (IRB-22-528), approval date: 27 April 2022.

Informed Consent Statement: Informed consent was obtained from all the subjects involved in this study.

Data Availability Statement: The datasets presented in this article are not readily available because of ethical requirements of the IRB to safeguard participant anonymity. Requests to access the datasets should be directed to jhansonde@ltu.edu.

Acknowledgments: We would like to thank the representatives of the Government of Liberia, the Ebola Survivors' Network—Liberia, and the Renewed Energy Serving Humanity (RESH) nonprofit for their support of the research design. This research is dedicated to all EVD survivors and their families.

Conflicts of Interest: D.D. is a Liberian EVD survivor and member of the Ebola Survivors' Network. JHD worked as an Ebola responder in Liberia, including in collaboration with the Ebola Survivors' Network. We wish to acknowledge practitioner experience that may carry weight in our analysis.

Appendix A. Semi-Structured Survey

Q1 Do you consent to participate in this study? Yes, I consent (1); No, I do not (0)

Q2 Have you ever had Ebola? Yes (1) No (0)

Q3 How old are you? (participants must be between 18–65)

Q4 Where do you currently live? (county name)

Q5 What is your gender? Male (1) Female (2) Other (3)

Q6 When did you have (first get infected with) Ebola? What month and year?

Q7 Do you continue to suffer today from any of the following symptoms or negative experiences because of surviving (having) Ebola? (Yes-1, No-0 for all below—Anger, withdrawal, sleeping issues, eating problems (eating too much or too little), anxiety, sadness (sad most days of the week), flashbacks, stigma from others, financial issues or not enough work

Q8 Did you receive assistance (stipend, food stuff, etc.) after being discharged from the ETU? Yes (1) No (0)

Q9 What years did you receive this assistance? Select all years that apply: 2014–2016 (1); 2017–2019 (2), 2020–2021 (3), today (4)

Q10 How satisfied were you with this assistance, on a scale of unhappy face (not at all 1) to smily face (extremely satisfied 5)?

Q11 Did you and/or a family member in your household participate in PREVAIL (Partnership for Resaerch on Ebola Vaccines in Liberia) study? If so, what years? 2014–2017

Q12 (a) If so, did you ever stop participating? Yes (1) No (0) (b) Why? (please explain your experiences with the study, the program, and the quality of care, and any issues you had)

Q13 Did you hear any rumors about PREVAIL that concerned you? Yes (1) No (0), if so, what were the rumors?

Q14 Did you have any other concerns of comments about the PREVAIL study? Yes (1) No (0) Explain

Q15 How much has the government policies supporting Ebola survivors helped you, or not? Did not help at all (1) Somewhat helped (2) Helped a lot (3) Explain

Q16 Were there any promised policies programs for Ebola survivors that were not offered or the quality was very poor? Please explain

Q17 What assistance do you need most today because of being an Ebola survivor?

Q18 Click on the statements that you agree with: I feel like the world has forgotten about Ebola survivors (1); Ebola has changed my life forever (2); Being an Ebola survivor makes me a hero (3)

Q19 Do you have any biological/born or adopted children you care for? Yes (1) No (0)

Q20 If you have children you are responsible for, do they currently go to school? Yes (1) No (0)

Q21 If yes, Is the student welcomed and treated fairly, or do they face issues with stigmatization because they come from an Ebola-affected home?

Q22 If you have kids who are not going to schook, what are the reasons they are not in school?

Q23 Were you working before you got sick with Ebola? Yes (1) No (0)

Q24 Have you had any trouble finding work since, because you are an Ebola survivor? Yes (1) No (0)

Q25 Please explain your work experiences since Ebola ended.

Appendix B

Table A1. PREVAIL Staged Studies and Contributions.

PREVAIL Study	Key Examples of Reported Results
PREVAIL I Double-blind, placebo-controlled RCT of an Ebola vaccine	Among 650 close contacts and contacts of close contacts of EVD cases, 210 (32%) consented and were vaccinated with rVSVAG-ZEBOV-GP. Of those vaccinated, 189 (90%) attended the 1-month follow-up visit; 166 (79%) attended the 6-month visit. No serious adverse events were reported. Among 88 participants without an elevated antibody level at baseline, 77.3% (95% confidence interval, 68.5–86.1) had an antibody response at 1 month [88]
PREVAIL II RCT of the experimental treatment ZMapp	Of the 71 patients who could be evaluated, 21 died, representing an overall case fatality rate of 30%. Death occurred in 13 of 35 patients (37%) who received the current standard of care alone and in 8 of 36 patients (22%) who received the current standard of care plus ZMapp; although the estimated effect of ZMapp appeared to be beneficial, the result did not meet the prespecified statistical threshold for efficacy [85]
PREVAIL III Observational natural history study of Ebola survivors and their close contacts	The stigma questions were administered to 859 EVD survivors at initial visit and 741 (86%) survivors at follow-up. While 63% of survivors reported any stigma at the initial visit, only 5% reported any stigma at follow-up. Over the 18-month period, there was a significant decrease in stigma among EVD survivors (Adjusted Odds Ratio [AOR], 0.02; 95% Confidence Interval [CI], 0.01–0.04) [89]
PREVAIL III Sub-studies: Birth cohort Evaluation of children born to EVD-survivor participants CYTOF Detailed immunological analysis in select survivors and close contacts; Neurology Longitudinal follow-up study of neuropsychological sequelae of EVD; Ophthalmology Longitudinal ophthalmologic (eyecare) follow-up study of a subset of survivors and close contacts; Viral persistence in semen; Assessment of the persistence of Ebola virus in the semen of adult male participants after acute illness Viral persistence in the CNS Assessment of the persistence of Ebola virus in the central nervous system (CNS) of adult participants after resolution of the acute illness	"Most pregnant woman infected with EVD will lose the unborn child sometime during the course of the disease. Women who recover from EVD with an intact pregnancy (no rupture of membranes or labour) require comprehensive IPC precautions to prevent exposure to intrauterine contents (i.e., amniotic fluid, placenta and fetus) during childbirth or complication management" [71] (p. 15). "Neurologic abnormalities following Ebola virus disease involved subcortical structures, cerebellar pathways, and sensory peripheral nerves and were present in most survivors" [90] (p. 2). Recruitment Ad—PREVAIL III: "Participants will have 1 clinic visit. They will have a physical exam. Their vital signs will be measured. They will also have a neurological checkup. The exam will assess their mental status. Their senses, reflexes, and coordination will be tested. They will be observed while walking to assess their gait. This exam will take about 1 h. Participants will have an interview. They will answer questions about any symptoms they have that may be affecting the brain or nervous system. This will take about 1 h" [78] (para. 5). "Signs of uveitis were present in at least 24% of Ebola survivors. . .Optic nerve changes, such as nerve swelling, were present in 10% of survivors and 5% of controls ($p = 0.03$), with color vision deficits occurring in 39% of survivors vs. 13% of controls ($p < 0.001$)" [91] (para. 3).

Table A1. *Cont.*

PREVAIL Study	Key Examples of Reported Results
PREVAIL IV Double-blind, two-phase, two-arm trial RCT of GS-5734 among male Ebola survivors with persistent Ebola virus RNA in their semen	"38 men from July 2016 through June 2018. The mean treatment phase ANRs were 85% (standard deviation [SD] = 24%) and 76% (SD = 30%) in the remdesivir and placebo arms, respectively ($p = 0.270$). The mean follow-up phase ANRs were 96% (SD = 10%) and 81% (SD = 29%) in the remdesivir and placebo arms, respectively ($p = 0.041$). The 5-day remdesivir regimen was well tolerated with no safety concerns… this small trial, remdesivir 100 mg/day for 5 days safely reduced the presence of Ebola virus RNA in the semen of Ebola survivors 2 to 6 months after administration" [16] (para. 3-4).
PREVAIL V (PREVAC) Quadruple blind, placebo-controlled RCT of two Ebola vaccines	"Of the 4789 participants, 2560 (53%) were adults and 2229 (47%) were children. Those < 18 years of age included 549 (12%) aged 1 to 4 years, 750 (16%) 5 to 11 years, and 930 (19%) aged 12–17 years. At baseline, the median (25th, 75th percentile) antibody titer to Ebola virus glycoprotein for 1090 participants was 72 (50, 116) EU/mL" [22] (p. 2). (Involves VSVdeltaG-ZEBOV vaccine and ChAd3-EBO Z vaccine and placebo (later given option to have treatment))
PREVAIL VI Observational study of the genetic factors underlying Ebola risk and response	Some participants will have their blood tested for the infection syphilis and HIV, the virus that causes AIDS. Participants will be told the results and will receive help finding care, if necessary. "The death rate among those with HIV was 12.3% compared to 1.9% in HIV-negative individuals (adjusted odds ratio of 6.87)" [92] (para. 3).
PREVAIL VII Clinical trial to evaluate the persistence of Ebola viral RNA in the eyes and assess the response to cataract surgery of Ebola survivors	"Twenty-two eyes of 22 survivors and 12 eyes of eight controls underwent cataract surgery. All of the aqueous samples tested negative for Ebola viral RNA. Median visual acuity improved from 20/200 at baseline to 20/25 at 1 year in survivors and from count fingers to 20/50 in controls (overall, $p < 0.001$; between groups, $p = 0.07$). After a 1-month course of topical corticosteroids, 55% of survivors and 67% of controls demonstrated at least 1+ anterior chamber cell. Twelve months after surgery, optical coherence tomography revealed a median increase in macular central subfield thickness of 42 µm compared with baseline (overall, $p = 0.029$; between groups, $p = 0.995$) EVD survivors and controls demonstrated significant visual improvement from cataract surgery" [17] (para. 3).

References

1. Salhia, B.; Olaiya, V. Historical Perspectives on Ethical and Regulatory Aspects of Human Participants Research: Implications for Oncology Clinical Trials in Africa. *JCO Glob. Oncol.* **2020**, *6*, 959–965. [CrossRef] [PubMed]
2. Hanson-DeFusco, J.; Shi, M.; Du, Z.; DeFusco, A. Conditioned Learning of Nations-Influence of EVD-Related System Adaptations and COVID-19 Response. Harvard Dataverse: 2022. Available online: https://doi.org/10.7910/DVN/APJNDT (accessed on 24 September 2024).
3. Darrow, W.W. Correction to: Confronting AIDS in the Early 1980s: Biomedicine, Public Health, and the Fourth Estate. *AIDS Behav.* **2023**, *27*, 3535. [CrossRef] [PubMed]
4. Perry, K.E.; Dubé, K.; Concha-Garcia, S.; Patel, H.; Kaytes, A.; Taylor, J.; Javadi, S.S.; Mathur, K.; Lo, M.; Brown, B.; et al. "My Death Will Not [Be] in Vain": Testimonials from Last Gift Rapid Research Autopsy Study Participants Living with HIV at the End of Life. *AIDS Res. Hum. Retroviruses* **2020**, *36*, 1071–1082. [CrossRef] [PubMed]
5. Decosimo, C.A.; Hanson, J.; Quinn, M.; Badu, P.; Smith, E.G. Playing to live: Outcome evaluation of a community-based psychosocial expressive arts program for children during the Liberian Ebola epidemic. *Glob. Ment. Health* **2019**, *6*, e3. [CrossRef] [PubMed]
6. Swanson, K.C.; Altare, C.; Wesseh, C.S.; Nyenswah, T.; Ahmed, T.; Eyal, N.; Hamblion, E.L.; Lessler, J.; Peters, D.H.; Altmann, M. Contact tracing performance during the Ebola epidemic in Liberia, 2014-2015. *PLoS Negl. Trop Dis.* **2018**, *12*, e0006762. [CrossRef]
7. Matanock, A.; Arwady, M.A.; Ayscue, P.; Forrester, J.D.; Gaddis, B.; Hunter, J.C.; Monroe, B.; Pillai, S.K.; Reed, C.; Schafer, I.J.; et al. Ebola virus disease cases among health care workers not working in Ebola treatment units—Liberia, June–August, 2014. *MMWR Morb. Mortal. Wkly. Rep.* **2014**, *63*, 1077–1081.
8. Pillai, S.K.; Nyenswah, T.; Rouse, E.; Arwady, M.A.; Forrester, J.D.; Hunter, J.C.; Matanock, A.; Ayscue, P.; Monroe, B.; Schafer, I.J.; et al. Developing an incident management system to support Ebola response—Liberia, July–August 2014. *MMWR Morb. Mortal. Wkly. Rep.* **2014**, *63*, 930–933.
9. Department of Global Communications. Learning from the Past: UN Draws Lessons from Ebola, Other Crises to Fight COVID-19. 2020. Available online: https://www.un.org/en/coronavirus/learning-past-un-draws-lessons-ebola-other-crises-fight-covid-19 (accessed on 5 October 2022).
10. Routh, J. Study of Ebola Survivors Opens in Liberia-Trial to Examine Long-Term Health Effects of Ebola Virus Disease. 2015. Available online: https://www.nih.gov/news-events/news-releases/study-ebola-survivors-opens-liberia (accessed on 4 September 2024).
11. James, P.B.; Wardle, J.; Steel, A.; Adams, J. Post-Ebola psychosocial experiences and coping mechanisms among Ebola survivors: A systematic review. *Trop. Med. Int. Health* **2019**, *24*, 671–691. [CrossRef]
12. Secor, A.; Macauley, R.; Stan, L.; Kagone, M.; Sidikiba, S.; Sow, S.; Aronovich, D.; Litvin, K.; Davis, N.; Alva, S.; et al. Mental health among Ebola survivors in Liberia, Sierra Leone and Guinea: Results from a cross-sectional study. *BMJ Open* **2020**, *10*, e035217. [CrossRef]

13. NIAID. Partnership for Research on Ebola Virus (PREVAIL) Prevail III: Ebola Natural History Study. 2022. Available online: https://clinicaltrials.gov/ct2/show/NCT02431923 (accessed on 14 December 2023).
14. Dodd, L.E.; Proschan, M.A.; Neuhaus, J.; Koopmeiners, J.S.; Neaton, J.; Beigel, J.D.; Barrett, K.; Lane, H.C.; Davey, R.T. Design of a Randomized Controlled Trial for Ebola Virus Disease Medical Countermeasures: PREVAIL II, the Ebola MCM Study. *J. Infect. Dis.* **2016**, *213*, 1906–1913. [CrossRef]
15. Browne, S.; Carter, T.; Eckes, R.; Grandits, G.; Johnson, M.; Moore, I.; McNay, L. A review of strategies used to retain participants in clinical research during an infectious disease outbreak: The PREVAIL I Ebola vaccine trial experience. *Contemp. Clin. Trials Commun.* **2018**, *11*, 50–54. [CrossRef] [PubMed]
16. Higgs, E.S.; Gayedyu-Dennis, D.; Fischer, W.A., II; Nason, M.; Reilly, C.; Beavogui, A.H.; Aboulhab, J.; Nordwall, J.; Lobbo, P.; Wachekwa, I.; et al. PREVAIL IV: A Randomized, Double-Blind, 2-Phase, Phase 2 Trial of Remdesivir vs Placebo for Reduction of Ebola Virus RNA in the Semen of Male Survivors. *Clin. Infect. Dis.* **2021**, *73*, 1849–1856. [CrossRef] [PubMed]
17. Eghrari, A.O.; Shantha, J.G.; Ross, R.D.; Van Ryn, C.; Crozier, I.; Hayek, B.; Gradin, D.; Roberts, B.; Prakalapakorn, S.G.; Amegashie, F.; et al. Efficacy and Safety Outcomes of Cataract Surgery in Survivors of Ebola Virus Disease: 12-Month Results From the PREVAIL VII Study. *Transl. Vis. Sci. Technol.* **2021**, *10*, 32. [CrossRef] [PubMed]
18. FHI Clinical. Partnership for Research on Vaccines and Infectious Diseases in Liberia (PREVAIL)-Brochure. 2022, pp. 1–4. Available online: https://www.fhiclinical.com/wp-content/uploads/2020/08/Brochure_PREVAIL_20200812_SHARE-2.pdf (accessed on 14 December 2023).
19. NIAID. Research with Human Subjects. 2022. Available online: https://www.niaid.nih.gov/grants-contracts/human-subjects (accessed on 14 December 2023).
20. NIAID. NCT02818582 GS-5734 to Assess the Antiviral Activity, Longer-Term Clearance of Ebola Virus, and Safety in Male Ebola Survivors with Evidence of Ebola Virus Persistence in Semen. 2022. Available online: https://clinicaltrials.gov/study/NCT02818582 (accessed on 14 December 2023).
21. Nyenswah, T.; Fallah, M.; Sieh, S.; Kollie, K.; Badio, M.; Gray, A.; Dilah, P.; Shannon, M.; Duwor, S. Controlling the last known cluster of Ebola virus disease—Liberia, January–February 2015. *MMWR Morb. Mortal Wkly. Rep.* **2015**, *64*, 500–504. [PubMed]
22. Badio, M.; Lhomme, E.; Kieh, M.; Beavogui, A.H.; Kennedy, S.B.; Doumbia, S.; Leigh, B.; Sow, S.O.; Diallo, A.; Fusco, D.; et al. Partnership for Research on Ebola VACcination (PREVAC): Protocol of a randomized, double-blind, placebo-controlled phase 2 clinical trial evaluating three vaccine strategies against Ebola in healthy volunteers in four West African countries. *Trials* **2021**, *22*, 86. [CrossRef]
23. Glayweon, M.; Hanson, J. Ebola Survivors and Their Needs-Survey Assessment. Ministry of Gender: Monrovia, Liberia, 2015.
24. CDC. CDC Releases Detailed History of the 2014–2016 Ebola Response in MMWR. 2016. Available online: https://www.cdc.gov/media/releases/2016/p0707-history-ebola-response.html (accessed on 3 February 2023).
25. Partner Coordination Workshop for the Support of Survivors. *National Package for Resettlement of All EVD Survivors*; Government of Liberia: Monrovia, Liberia, 2015.
26. Bah, A.J.; James, P.B.; Bah, N.; Sesay, A.B.; Sevalie, S.; Kanu, J.S. Prevalence of anxiety, depression and post-traumatic stress disorder among Ebola survivors in northern Sierra Leone: A cross-sectional study. *BMC Public Health* **2020**, *20*, 1391. [CrossRef]
27. MOH/IMS. MOH/IMS Meeting Summary Notes 9/24/2014-5/5/2015. In *Ebola IMS Pillar*; Government of Liberia: Monrovia, Liberia, 2014.
28. Faley, P. Fixing the PREVAIL Ebola project. In Proceedings of the UnwokeID: Unethical Issues in 21st Century International Development, Richardson, TX, USA, 22–24 February 2022; University of Texas at Dallas: Richardson, TX, USA, 2022.
29. Davis, D. Unequal treatment of Ebola survivors in Liberia. In Proceedings of the UnwokeID: Unethical Issues in 21st Century International Development, Richardson, TX, USA, 22–24 February 2022; University of Texas at Dallas: Richardson, TX, USA, 2022.
30. Schwartz, D.A. All the mothers are dead: Ebola's chilling effects on the young women of one Liberian town named Joe Blow. In *Pregnant in the Time of Ebola*; Springer: Cham, Switzerland, 2019; pp. 259–263.
31. Krug, E.G.; Mercy, J.A.; Dahlberg, L.L.; Zwi, A.B. The world report on violence and health. *Lancet* **2002**, *360*, 1083–1088. [CrossRef]
32. Mapitsa, C.B.; Ngwato, T.P. Rooting Evaluation Guidelines in Relational Ethics: Lessons From Africa. *Am. J. Eval.* **2020**, *41*, 404–419. [CrossRef]
33. Astroulakis, N. The development ethics approach to international development. *Int. J. Dev. Issues* **2011**, *10*, 214–232. [CrossRef]
34. Calain, P. The Ebola clinical trials: A precedent for research ethics in disasters. *J. Med. Ethics* **2018**, *44*, 3–8. [CrossRef]
35. Sutton, L.B.; Erlen, J.A.; Glad, J.M.; Siminoff, L.A. Recruiting vulnerable populations for research: Revisiting the ethical issues. *J. Prof. Nurs.* **2003**, *19*, 106–112. [CrossRef] [PubMed]
36. Gordon, B.G. Vulnerability in Research: Basic Ethical Concepts and General Approach to Review. *Ochsner. J.* **2020**, *20*, 34–38. [CrossRef] [PubMed]
37. Public Responsibility in Medicine and Research. Scientific, Regulatory, and Ethical Issues with Experimental Treatments and Ebola Vaccines. 2014. Available online: https://www.youtube.com/watch?v=3cf31hS7tKM (accessed on 7 December 2014).
38. Ministry of Health (MOH). *Mapping of Agencies Supporting Survivors in Response to Ebola*; The Ministry of Health: Monrovia, Liberia, 2015.
39. Hanson, J.; Decosimo, A.; Quinn, M. Diminished Quality of Life among Women affected by Ebola. *J. Soc. Behav. Health Sci.* **2016**, *10*, 11. [CrossRef]

40. Routh, J. Study Finds Ebola Survivors in Liberia Face Ongoing Health Issues. 2019. Available online: https://www.nih.gov/news-events/news-releases/study-finds-ebola-survivors-liberia-face-ongoing-health-issues (accessed on 4 September 2024).
41. US National Bioethics Advisory Commission. *Ethical and Policy Issues in International Research: Clinical Trials in Developing Countries*; National Bioethics Advisory Commission: Bethesda, MD, USA, 2001; Volume 1.
42. Foa, E.B.; Street, G.P. Women and traumatic events. *J. Clin. Psychiatry* **2001**, *62* (Suppl. S17), 29–34.
43. Hembree, E.A.; Foa, E.B. Posttraumatic stress disorder: Psychological factors and psychosocial interventions. *J. Clin. Psychiatry* **2000**, *61* (Suppl. S7), 33–39. Available online: https://www.psychiatrist.com/wp-content/uploads/2021/02/25378_posttraumatic-stress-disorder-psychological-factors.pdf (accessed on 24 September 2024).
44. Foa, E.B.; Riggs, D.S.; Dancu, C.V.; Rothbaum, B.O. PTSD Symptom Scale-Interview (PSS-I). 1993. Available online: https://link.springer.com/article/10.1007/BF00974317 (accessed on 24 September 2024).
45. Chambers, M.; Bliss, K.; Rambur, B. Recruiting Research Participants via Traditional Snowball vs Facebook Advertisements and a Website. *West. J. Nurs. Res.* **2020**, *42*, 846–851. [CrossRef]
46. Leighton, K.; Kardong-Edgren, S.; Schneidereith, T.; Foisy-Doll, C. Using Social Media and Snowball Sampling as an Alternative Recruitment Strategy for Research. *Clin. Simul. Nurs.* **2021**, *55*, 37–42. [CrossRef]
47. Dusek, G.; Yurova, Y.; Ruppel, C.P. Using social media and targeted snowball sampling to survey a hard-to-reach population: A case study. *Int. J. Dr. Stud.* **2015**, *10*, 279–290. Available online: http://ijds.org/Volume10/IJDSv10p279-299Dusek0717.pdf (accessed on 30 November 2023). [CrossRef]
48. Ellis, J.; Hart, D. Strengthening the Choice for a Generic Qualitative Research Design. *The Qualitative Report*, 19 June 2023. [CrossRef]
49. Kahlke, R.M. Generic Qualitative Approaches: Pitfalls and Benefits of Methodological Mixology. *Int. J. Qual. Methods* **2014**, *13*, 37–52. [CrossRef]
50. Percy, W.; Kostere, K.; Kostere, S. Generic qualitative research in psychology. *Qual. Rev.* **2015**, *20*, 76–85. Available online: http://www.nova.edu/ssss/QR/QR20/2/percy5.pdf (accessed on 6 September 2024). [CrossRef]
51. Caelli, K.; Ray, L.; Mill, J. 'Clear as Mud': Toward Greater Clarity in Generic Qualitative Research. *Int. J. Qual. Methods* **2003**, *2*, 1–13. [CrossRef]
52. Merriam, S.B.; Tisdell, E.J. *Qualitative Research: A Guide to Design and Implementation*, 1st ed.; John Wiley and Sons: Hoboken, NJ, USA, 2009.
53. Lim, J. Qualitative methods in adult development and learning: Theoretical traditions, current practices, and emerging horizons. In *The Oxford Handbook of Reciprocal Adult Development and Learning*, 2nd ed.; Oxford University Press: Oxford, UK, 2011; pp. 39–56.
54. Gough, B.; Lyons, A. The Future of Qualitative Research in Psychology: Accentuating the Positive. *Integr. Psychol. Behav. Sci.* **2016**, *50*, 234–243. [CrossRef] [PubMed]
55. Ivankova, N.V.; Creswell, J.W.; Stick, S.L. Using Mixed-Methods Sequential Explanatory Design: From Theory to Practice. *Field Methods* **2006**, *18*, 3–20. [CrossRef]
56. Creswell, J.W. Designing A Mixed Methods Study In Primary Care. *Ann. Fam. Med.* **2004**, *2*, 7–12. [CrossRef]
57. Shadish, W.R.; Cook, T.D.; Campbell, D.T. *Experimental and Quasi-Experimental Designs for Generalized Causal Inference*; Houghton, Mifflin and Company: Boston, MA, USA, 2002.
58. Dunn, W.N. *Public Policy Analysis*; Routledge: New York, NY, USA, 2017. [CrossRef]
59. Calnan, M.; Gadsby, E.W.; Kondé, M.K.; Diallo, A.; Rossman, J.S. The Response to and Impact of the Ebola Epidemic: Towards an Agenda for Interdisciplinary Research. *Int. J. Health Policy Manag.* **2018**, *7*, 402–411. [CrossRef] [PubMed]
60. Van Bortel, T.; Basnayake, A.; Wurie, F.; Jambai, M.; Koroma, A.S.; Muana, A.T.; Hann, K.; Eaton, J.; Martin, S.; Nellums, L.B. Psychosocial effects of an Ebola outbreak at individual, community and international levels. *Bull. World Health Organ.* **2016**, *94*, 210–214. [CrossRef] [PubMed]
61. Davtyan, M.; Brown, B.; Folayan, M.O. Addressing Ebola-related Stigma: Lessons Learned from HIV/AIDS. *Glob. Health Action* **2014**, *7*, 26058. [CrossRef]
62. Tozay, S.; Fischer, W.A.; Wohl, D.A.; Kilpatrick, K.; Zou, F.; Reeves, E.; Pewu, K.; DeMarco, J.; Loftis, A.J.; King, K.; et al. Long-term Complications of Ebola Virus Disease: Prevalence and Predictors of Major Symptoms and the Role of Inflammation. *Clin. Infect. Dis.* **2020**, *71*, 1749–1755. [CrossRef]
63. Chertow, D.S. Understanding long-term effects of Ebola virus disease. *Nat. Med.* **2019**, *25*, 714–715. [CrossRef]
64. Oleribe, O.O.; Salako, B.L.; Ka, M.M.; Akpalu, A.; McConnochie, M.; Foster, M.; Taylor-Robinson, S.D. Ebola virus disease epidemic in West Africa: Lessons learned and issues arising from West African countries. *Clin. Med.* **2015**, *15*, 54–57. [CrossRef]
65. Poni, M. Gov't Engages Traditional Leaders to End Child Marriage. *Number One Citizen Daily Newspaper*, 3 November 2022; pp. 1–4.
66. Hanson-DeFusco, J.; Smith, E.G.; McMaster, A. Efficacy of civil society organizations to mitigate gender-based sexual violence in schools, in Liberia. *J. Civ. Soc.* **2023**, *19*, 310–329. [CrossRef]
67. Hanson, J.; Faley, P.; Quinn, M. Analysis of the Liberian Ebola Survivors Support System (ESSS). *Integr. J. Glob. Health* **2017**, *1*, 2.
68. WHO. WHO Meeting on Survivors of Ebola Virus Disease: Clinical Care of Survivors. 2015. Available online: https://iris.who.int/bitstream/handle/10665/204126/9789241509794_eng.pdf;jsessionid=9C85E2732F8FE0D9740D7E8D1CCB4FD7?sequence=1 (accessed on 7 September 2024).

69. Hanson-DeFusco, J.; Davis, D.; Bommareddy, M.; Olaniyan, Z. Broken Promises: Prolonged Diminished Quality-of-Life among Liberian Ebola Survivors Half a Decade after the 2014-16 West African Outbreak. *J. Soc. Behav. Health Sci.* **2024**, *18*, 130–156. [CrossRef]
70. Institutional Review Board. Informed Consent Guidance. 2022. Available online: https://www.hopkinsmedicine.org/institutional-review-board/guidelines-policies/guidelines/informed-consent-i (accessed on 14 December 2023).
71. Morreim, E.H. Litigation in Clinical Research: Malpractice Doctrines versus Research Realities. *J. Law Med. Ethics* **2004**, *32*, 474–484. [CrossRef] [PubMed]
72. World Medical Association (WMA). Declaration of Helsinki as a Statement of Ethical Principles for Medical Research Involving Human Subjects. 2013. Available online: https://www.wma.net/policies-post/wma-declaration-of-helsinki-ethical-principles-for-medical-research-involving-human-subjects/ (accessed on 14 December 2023).
73. Fallah, M. Clinical Experiences and Data from EVD Survivor Cohorts. 2015. Available online: https://www.jstor.org/stable/pdf/resrep48066.13.pdf (accessed on 29 November 2023).
74. Eghrari, A.O.; Bishop, R.J.; Ross, R.D.; Davis, B.; Larbelee, J.; Amegashie, F.; Dolo, R.F.; Prakalapakorn, S.G.; Gaisie, C.; Gargu, C.; et al. Characterization of Ebola Virus–Associated Eye Disease. *JAMA Netw. Open* **2021**, *4*, e2032216. [CrossRef] [PubMed]
75. OECD Development Centre. Liberia-Social Institutions and Gender Index. 2023. Available online: https://www.genderindex.org/ (accessed on 17 May 2023).
76. NIAID. Partnership for Research on Ebola Vaccines in Liberia (PREVAIL) ClinicalTrials.Gov ID NCT02344407. 2022. Available online: https://clinicaltrials.gov/study/NCT02344407 (accessed on 14 December 2023).
77. NIAID. The Partnership for Research on Ebola Virus in Liberia (PREVAIL). 2022. Available online: https://www.niaid.nih.gov/diseases-conditions/researching-ebola-africa (accessed on 6 April 2023).
78. Billioux. Natural History, Disease Progression, and Long-Term Neurologic Sequelae of Ebola Virus Disease Survivors in PREVAIL III. 2021. Available online: https://www.medifind.com/conditions/seizures/4784/clinical-trial/345631928 (accessed on 7 September 2024).
79. Dwivedi, A.K.; Mallawaarachchi, I.; Alvarado, L.A. Analysis of small sample size studies using nonparametric bootstrap test with pooled resampling method. *Stat. Med.* **2017**, *36*, 2187–2205. [CrossRef]
80. Munoz, R.T.; Pearson, L.C.; Hellman, C.M.; McIntosh, H.C.; Khojasteh, J.; Fox, M.D. Adverse childhood experiences and posttraumatic stress as an antecedent of anxiety and lower hope. *Traumatology* **2018**, *24*, 209–218. [CrossRef]
81. Cheng, Z.; Cai, M.; Tao, H.; He, Z.; Lin, X.; Lin, H.; Zuo, Y. Efficiency and productivity measurement of rural township hospitals in China: A bootstrapping data envelopment analysis. *BMJ Open* **2016**, *6*, e011911. [CrossRef]
82. Hall, D.E.; Hanusa, B.H.; Stone, R.A.; Ling, B.S.; Arnold, R.M. Time Required for Institutional Review Board Review at One Veterans Affairs Medical Center. *JAMA Surg.* **2015**, *150*, 103. [CrossRef]
83. Keusch, M.; Mancher, B. *Integrating Clinical Research into Epidemic Response;* Keusch, G., McAdam, K., Cuff, P., Mancher, M., Busta, E.R., Eds.; National Academies Press: Washington, DC, USA, 2017. [CrossRef]
84. Matangwa, D. Who knows the South best but us? In *Listening to the Voiceless and Hard to Reach: Creating Space and Opportunities for People-Centered Policy Engagement in East Africa." UnwokeID: Unethical Issues in 21st Century International Development;* University of Texas at Dallas: Richardson, TX, USA, 2022.
85. Prevail II Writing Group. A Randomized, Controlled Trial of ZMapp for Ebola Virus Infection. *N. Engl. J. Med.* **2016**, *375*, 1448–1456. [CrossRef]
86. Cook, T.D.; Shadish, W.R.; Wong, V.C. Three conditions under which experiments and observational studies produce comparable causal estimates: New findings from within-study comparisons. *J. Policy Anal. Manag.* **2008**, *27*, 724–750. [CrossRef]
87. Shadish, W.R. Campbell and Rubin: A primer and comparison of their approaches to causal inference in field settings. *Psychol. Methods* **2010**, *15*, 3–17. [CrossRef] [PubMed]
88. Bolay, F.K.; Grandits, G.; Lane, H.C.; Kennedy, S.B.; Johnson, M.P.; Fallah, M.P.; Wilson, B.; Njoh, W.S.; McNay, L.A.; Hensley, L.E.; et al. PREVAIL I Cluster Vaccination Study with rVSVΔG-ZEBOV-GP as Part of a Public Health Response in Liberia. *J. Infect. Dis.* **2019**, *219*, 1634–1641. [CrossRef] [PubMed]
89. Kelly, J.D.; Weiser, S.D.; Wilson, B.; Cooper, J.B.; Glayweon, M.; Sneller, M.C.; Drew, C.; Steward, W.T.; Reilly, C.; Johnson, K.; et al. Ebola virus disease-related stigma among survivors declined in Liberia over an 18-month, post-outbreak period: An observational cohort study. *PLoS Neglected Trop. Dis.* **2019**, *13*, e0007185. [CrossRef] [PubMed]
90. Bowen, L.; Smith, B.; Steinbach, S.; Billioux, B.; Summers, A.; Azodi, S.; Ohayon, J.; Schindler, M.; Nath, A. Survivors of Ebola Virus Disease Have Persistent Neurological Deficits (S53.003). *Neurological* **2016**, *86*, 16. [CrossRef]
91. Shantha, J.G.; Crozier, I.; Yeh, S. An update on ocular complications of Ebola virus disease. *Curr. Opin. Ophthalmol.* **2017**, *28*, 600–606. [CrossRef]
92. Moses, S.J.; Wachekwa, I.; Van Ryn, C.; Grandits, G.; Pau, A.; Badio, M.; Kennedy, S.B.; Sneller, M.C.; Higgs, E.S.; Lane, H.C.; et al. The impact of the 2014 Ebola epidemic on HIV disease burden and outcomes in Liberia West Africa. *PLoS ONE* **2021**, *16*, e0257049. [CrossRef]

healthcare

MDPI

Article

Perceived Well-Being among Adults with Diabetes and Hypertension: A National Study

Leona Yuen-Ling Leung [1], Hon-Lon Tam [2,*], Isaac Sze-Him Leung [3], Alex Siu-Wing Chan [4], Yueheng Yin [5], Xiubin Zhang [6], Aimei Mao [7] and Pak-Leng Cheong [7]

1 School of Nursing and Health Studies, Hong Kong Metropolitan University, Hong Kong SAR, China; lleung@hkmu.edu.hk
2 The Nethersole School of Nursing, The Chinese University of Hong Kong, Hong Kong SAR, China
3 Department of Statistics, The Chinese University of Hong Kong, Hong Kong SAR, China; shleung@cuhk.edu.hk
4 Department of Applied Social Sciences, The Hong Kong Polytechnic University of Hong Kong, Hong Kong SAR, China; chansw.alex@gmail.com
5 School of Nursing, Nanjing Medical University, Nanjing 210029, China; yinyueheng@njmu.edu.cn
6 School of Public Health, National Heart and Lung Institute, Imperial College London, London W12 7RQ, UK; xiubin.zhang@imperial.ac.uk
7 Department of Education, Kiang Wu Nursing College of Macau, Macau SAR, China; maoaimei@kwnc.edu.mo (A.M.); joecheong@kwnc.edu.mo (P.-L.C.)
* Correspondence: hltam@cuhk.edu.hk

Abstract: Perceived health and distresses are associated with the practice of lifestyle modifications, which increases the risk of diabetes and hypertension-related complications. This study aimed to define the characteristics and distribution of perceived health and distresses across the states between people with diabetes and hypertension. Data were derived from a national survey of US adults aged ≥18 years who were interviewed via phone call. Perceived health and distresses were assessed through corresponding questions. An amount of 333,316 respondents (43,911 with diabetes and 130,960 with hypertension) were included in the analysis; 61.8% of people with diabetes and 74.5% of people with hypertension reported having good or better health, while residents in the Southwest region perceived poor health statuses and more distresses. Education level (diabetes: odds ratio [OR] = 0.47–0.79, hypertension: OR = 0.42–0.76), employment status level (diabetes: OR = 1.40–2.22, hypertension: OR = 1.56–2.49), and household income (diabetes: OR = 0.22–0.65, hypertension: OR = 0.15–0.78) were significant factors associated with poorly perceived health among people with diabetes and hypertension, and the use of technology and strategies for policymakers are suggested to improve the perceived health status in this regard.

Keywords: diabetes; hypertension; population surveillance; quality of life

1. Introduction

The World Health Organization (WHO) reported that noncommunicable diseases accounted for 74% of deaths worldwide in 2019 [1], while hypertension and diabetes were the first and the third leading risk factors to cause disease burden globally [2]. Hyperten-sion and diabetes are also major risk factors in various health problems, such as heart diseases, stroke, and kidney diseases [1]. In addition, hypertension and diabetes increase the health expenditure worldwide [3,4]. Different types of pharmacological and non-pharmacological interventions have been developed to manage hypertension and diabetes [5–7]; however, numerous side effects were reported on the use of pharmacological interventions [8], and so non-pharmacological interventions are highly recommended. Among the non-pharmacological interventions, adopting healthy lifestyles is recommended by the WHO to reduce risk of noncommunicable diseases, and different international organizations provide guidelines for management of hypertension and diabetes to reduce risk of complications [5–7,9]. However, a national study of 278,064 individuals found that people with hypertension and diabetes were the least likely to practice healthy lifestyles (odds ratio [OR] = 0.48–0.51) [10], also revealing that people with perceived good or better health were more likely to practice healthy lifestyles (OR = 1.59) [10]. A study of 5123 individuals indicated that people perceived a poor health status when they had physical and mental distress [11]. Another study suggested that perceived health status was related to the practice of healthy lifestyles, physical distress, and mental distress [12].

The mental distress among people with diabetes has been widely discussed in recent years. A systematic review of 55 studies (including 36,998 individuals) found that the prevalence of mental distress among people with diabetes was 36% [13]. A high level of mental distress could lead to poor glycemia control, resulting in an increase in complications and mortality [14]. However, the mental distress among people with hypertension has been less discussed, and the low prevalence (3.2%) might be a possible reason [15]. On the other hand, physical distress could limit people's daily activity [16], but physical distress among people with diabetes and hypertension has not been extensively investigated. Hence, the findings of this study provide valuable information to develop interventions targeted at improving perceived health and reducing physical and mental distress among people with diabetes and hypertension.

Aims

This study aimed to (1) define the characteristics of people with diabetes and hyper-tension, (2) illustrate the distribution of perceived health and distresses across the states, and (3) determine the factors associated with perceived health and distresses at a national level.

2. Materials and Methods

This cross-sectional study was reported in accordance with the Strengthening the Reporting of Observational Studies in Epidemiology guideline [17]. The data were de-identified and publicly available from the US Centers for Disease Control. No institutional review board approval or patient informed consent was required.

2.1. Data Sources

The data from the 2021 Behavioral Risk Factor Surveillance System (BRFSS) survey were used [18]. The survey investigated health-related behaviors and health conditions of noninstitutionalized US adults aged 18 years and above. The surveyor used the random-digit-dialing technique to generate random phone numbers for telephone and mobile phone interviews across all states in the United States. Data collection was conducted throughout the entire year of 2021, while some states continued data collection into early 2022 [18]. Florida was excluded in this annual survey because the data collection time did not fulfil the minimum requirements for inclusion. The median response rate was 44% [18].

2.2. Study Population

Cases for which data regarding sociodemographic variables or health conditions were missing and individuals who refused to answer questions were excluded from the study. We included 333,316/438,693 (75.9%) individuals from the 2021 BRFSS survey.

2.3. Outcome Variables

2.3.1. Sociodemographic Variables

Following a previous study [10], serval sociodemographic variables were extracted from the BRFSS survey. Employment status was recategorized, while the rest of the variables followed the categorizations from the survey.

2.3.2. Perceived Health and Distresses

Related items from the BRFSS survey were extracted to assess individual perceived health and distress. Individuals selected appropriate responses, including 'excellent', 'very good', 'good', 'fair', and 'poor', to indicate their perceived health status. The responses were categorized as 'fair or poor' (including the rating of fair and poor) and 'good or better' (including the ratings of good, very good, and excellent) in regression analysis. Further, perceived distress was assessed by asking individuals about the number of unhealthy days caused by physical distress (related to physical illness and injury) or mental distress (related to stress, depression, and problems with emotions) over the previous 30 days. The number of days of daily activity limitation caused by physical or mental distress was also assessed.

2.4. Data Analysis and Visualization

Data were analyzed using the R statistical software, v. 4.3.2 (R Foundation for Statistical Computing). Logistic regression analysis was used to investigate which sociodemographic characteristics (independent variables) were associated with perceived health status and distresses (dependent variables). All statistical tests were two-tailed, and variables were considered significant at a significance level of <0.05.

The distribution of health status and distresses among people with diabetes and hypertension in different states was visualized using the Geographic Heat Map add-in featured in Excel 2019, v. 16. The blue color was for diabetes, while green was for hypertension. The color would be lighter if the condition was better.

3. Results

We analyzed 333,316 respondents, and 43,911 (13.2%) and 130,960 (39.3%) were diagnosed with diabetes and hypertension, respectively (Table 1). Over 50% of people with diabetes and hypertension were older adults (aged 65 years and older) and retired or unable to work. Regarding the health status, 83.6% (n = 278,783) of individuals were perceived to have good or better health; however, only 61.8% (n = 27,142) and 74.5% (n = 97,534) of people with diabetes and hypertension were reported to have good or better health. Additionally, people with diabetes and hypertension were reported to have more distresses, and people with diabetes reported 7.25 ± 11.05 days and 4.79 ± 9.05 days of physical distress and mental distress in a month, respectively. These distresses could limit their daily activity by 7.89 ± 10.96 days in a month. People with hypertension also reported more distresses than the general population, but the level was less severe than people with diabetes (Table 1).

Table 1. Individual characteristics and health status.

	All	**Diabetes**	**Hypertension**
	N = 333,316	**N = 43,911**	**N = 130,960**
Sex			
Male	159,355 (47.8%)	22,400 (51.0%)	66,956 (51.1%)
Female	173,961 (52.2%)	21,511 (49.0%)	64,004 (48.9%)
Age range (years)			
18 to 24	17,124 (5.1%)	198 (0.5%)	1343 (1.0%)
25 to 34	38,404 (11.6%)	820 (1.9%)	4825 (3.7%)
35 to 44	48,309 (14.5%)	2466 (5.6%)	10,172 (7.8%)
45 to 54	51,345 (15.4%)	5704 (13.0%)	17,084 (13.0%)
55 to 64	65,719 (19.7%)	11,186 (25.4%)	30,378 (23.2%)
65 to 74	67,757 (20.3%)	14,141 (32.2%)	38,704 (29.6%)
75 up	44,658 (13.4%)	9396 (21.4%)	28,454 (21.7%)

Table 1. *Cont.*

	All	Diabetes	Hypertension
	N = 333,316	**N = 43,911**	**N = 130,960**
Residential area			
Urban	284,944 (85.5%)	36,604 (83.4%)	109,565 (83.7%)
Rural	48,372 (14.5%)	7307 (16.6%)	21,395 (16.3%)
Education level			
Attended high school or less	17,652 (5.3%)	3551 (8.1%)	7930 (6.1%)
Graduated from high school	81,692 (24.5%)	12,715 (29.0%)	35,861 (27.4%)
Attended college or above	93,203 (28.0%)	13,622 (31.0%)	38,598 (29.5%)
Graduated from college or above	140,769 (42.2%)	14,023 (31.9%)	48,571 (37.0%)
Employment status			
Employed	182,528 (54.7%)	14,453 (32.9%)	52,282 (39.9%)
Unemployed	34,854 (10.5%)	3320 (7.6%)	9778 (7.5%)
Retired or unable to work	115,934 (34.8%)	26,138 (59.5%)	68,900 (52.6%)
Household income (US dollars)			
Less than 15,000	20,616 (6.2%)	4580 (10.4%)	10,088 (7.7%)
15,000 to <25,000	34,237 (10.3%)	6825 (15.5%)	16,730 (12.8%)
25,000 to <35,000	42,321 (12.7%)	7040 (16.0%)	18,492 (14.2%)
35,000 to <50,000	46,834 (14.1%)	6919 (15.8%)	20,089 (15.3%)
50,000 to <100,000	104,756 (31.4%)	12,077 (27.5%)	39,664 (30.3%)
100,000 to <200,000	66,017 (19.8%)	5430 (12.4%)	20,995 (16.0%)
200,000 or more	18,535 (5.5%)	1040 (2.4%)	4902 (3.7%)
Perceived health			
Excellent	58,798 (17.6%)	1656 (3.8%)	10,722 (8.2%)
Very good	116,103 (34.8%)	8400 (19.1%)	38,373 (29.3%)
Good	103,882 (31.2%)	17,086 (38.9%)	48,439 (37.0%)
Fair	40,593 (12.2%)	11,867 (27.0%)	24,242 (18.5%)
Poor	13,940 (4.2%)	4902 (11.2%)	9184 (7.0%)
Perceived unhealthy day, mean (SD)			
Physical distress	3.80 (8.32)	7.25 (11.05)	5.37 (9.79)
Mental distress	4.23 (8.20)	4.79 (9.05)	4.28 (8.52)
Daily activity limitation	5.18 (8.94)	7.89 (10.96)	6.52 (10.12)

3.1. Perceived Health and Distresses in Different States

The distributions of perceived health and distresses among people with diabetes and hypertension were similar (Figures 1 and 2). People with diabetes and hypertension in the Midwest region were perceived to have the best health statuses and least distresses, while those residing in the Southwest region had the worst perceived health statuses. Attention was required in California, Nevada, Kentucky, and West Virginia, since people with diabetes and hypertension perceived poorer health statuses and more distresses than other states.

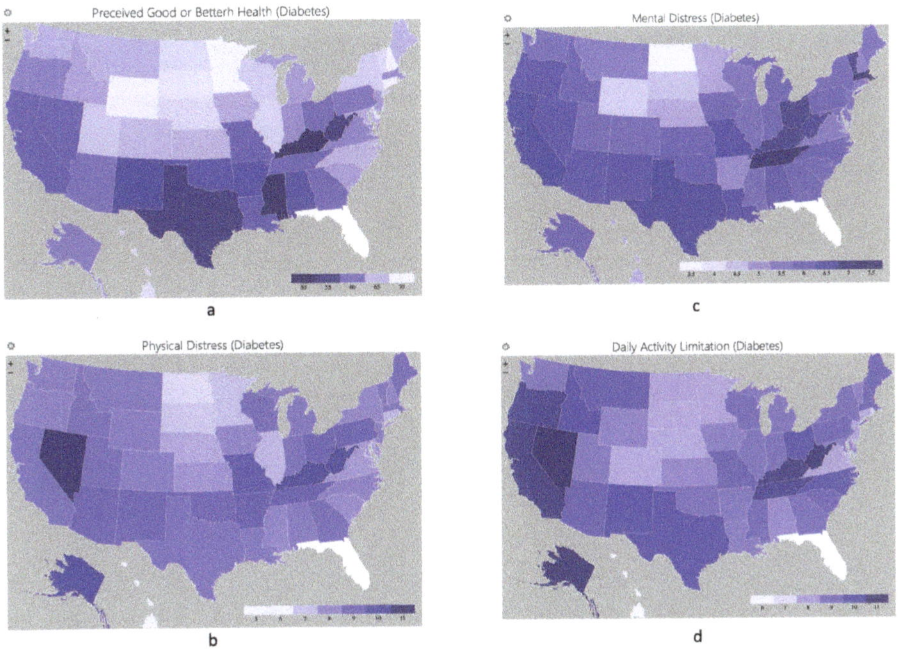

Figure 1. Percentage of perceived good or better health status (**a**), mean days of perceived physical distress (**b**), mental distress (**c**), and daily activity limitation (**d**) among people with diabetes.

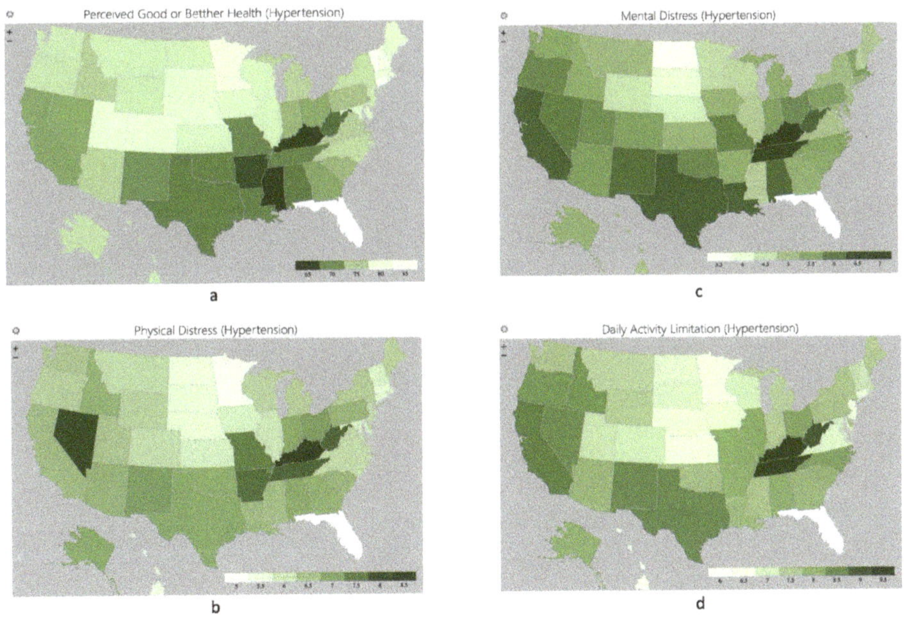

Figure 2. Percentage of perceived good or better health status (**a**), mean days of perceived physical distress (**b**), mental distress (**c**), and daily activity limitation (**d**) among people with hypertension.

3.2. Factors Associated with Perceived Health and Distress

For people with diabetes aged 35–64 years (OR = 0.61–0.72), lower education levels (OR = 0.47–0.79), and household incomes of less than 100,000 (OR = 0.22–0.65) were significant factors in reducing the likelihood of perceived good or better health (Table 2). These factors increased their physical distress significantly. With the exception of lower household income, men (Beta = −1.30) and aging (Beta = −9.09–−1.40) were factors with significantly reduced mental distress among people with diabetes. Compared to those retired or unable to work, people with diabetes and able to work perceived a better health status (OR = 1.40–2.22) with reduced distresses (physical: Beta = −5.04–−2.41, mental: Beta = −2.44–−0.60) and daily activity limitations (Beta = −6.34–−2.06).

Table 2. Factors associated with health status among people with diabetes.

	Perceived Good or Better Health [a]	Physical Distress [b]	Mental Distress [b]	Daily Activity Limitation [b]
	Odds Ratio (95% CI)	Beta (95% CI)	Beta (95% CI)	Beta (95% CI)
Sex: male	0.97 (0.93, 1.01)	0.01 (−0.19, 0.22)	−1.30 (−1.47, −1.14) *	0.69 (0.43, 0.95) *
Age range (years)				
18 to 24	Reference	Reference	Reference	Reference
25 to 34	0.78 (0.55, 1.10)	1.14 (−0.51, 2.80)	−1.40 (−2.75, −0.06) *	0.95 (−0.88, 2.78)
35 to 44	0.61 (0.44, 0.85) *	2.83 (1.28, 4.37) *	−2.27 (−3.52, −1.01) *	1.10 (−0.60, 2.81)
45 to 54	0.63 (0.46, 0.87) *	3.27 (1.76, 4.78) *	−3.47 (−4.70, −2.24) *	1.14 (−0.53, 2.80)
55 to 64	0.72 (0.52, 0.98) *	3.00 (1.50, 4.50) *	−5.09 (−6.31, −3.87) *	0.74 (−0.91, 2.40)
65 to 74	1.13 (0.82, 1.69)	0.07 (−1.44, 1.57)	−7.93 (−9.16, −6.71) *	−2.29 (−3.95, −0.63)
75 up	1.23 (0.89, 1.69)	−0.36 (−1.88, 1.15)	−9.09 (−10.33, −7.86) *	−2.99 (−4.67, −1.32)
Residence in urban areas	1.06 (1.01, 1.12) *	−0.09 (−0.36, 0.18)	0.29 (0.07, 0.50) *	−0.20 (−0.54, 0.14)
Education level				
Attended high school or less	0.47 (0.43, 0.51) *	0.87 (0.44, 1.30) *	−0.22 (−0.57, 0.12)	0.54 (0.02, 1.06) *
Graduated from high school	0.73 (0.69, 0.77) *	0.46 (0.19, 0.74) *	−0.24 (−0.47, −0.02) *	0.23 (−0.12, 0.59)
Attended college or above	0.79 (0.75, 0.84) *	0.76 (0.50, 1.02) *	0.34 (0.13, 0.55) *	0.42 (0.08, 0.75) *
Graduated from college or above	Reference	Reference	Reference	Reference
Employment status				
Employed	2.22 (2.09, 2.35) *	−5.04 (−5.31, −4.76) *	−2.44 (−2.66, −2.21) *	−6.34 (−6.69, −5.99) *
Unemployed	1.40 (1.30, 1.52) *	−2.41 (−2.82, −2.01) *	−0.60 (−0.93, −0.27) *	−2.06 (−2.54, −1.58) *
Retired or unable to work	Reference	Reference	Reference	Reference
Household income (US dollars)				
Less than 15,000	0.22 (0.19, 0.27) *	6.21 (5.46, 6.97) *	4.84 (4.22, 5.46) *	4.78 (3.72, 5.83) *
15,000 to <25,000	0.29 (0.25, 0.35) *	4.47 (3.74, 5.19) *	2.97 (2.37, 3.56) *	3.15 (2.12, 4.18) *
25,000 to <35,000	0.37 (0.31, 0.44) *	3.15 (2.43, 3.86) *	2.01 (1.43, 2.60) *	2.08 (1.06, 3.10) *
35,000 to <50,000	0.46 (0.39, 0.55) *	1.95 (1.25, 2.66) *	1.50 (0.92, 2.08) *	1.36 (0.34, 2.38) *
50,000 to <100,000	0.65 (0.54, 0.77) *	1.07 (0.39, 1.75) *	0.61 (0.06, 1.17) *	0.54 (−0.45, 1.53)
100,000 to <200,000	0.86 (0.71, 1.02)	0.07 (−0.64, 0.77)	0.01 (−0.56, 0.59)	0.21 (−0.82, 1.24)
200,000 or more	Reference	Reference	Reference	Reference

[a] Logistic regression. [b] Linear regression. * Statistical significance, $p < 0.05$.

Table 3 shows the factors associated with health status among people with hypertension. Men (OR = 0.90) aged 25–64 years (OR = 0.48–0.71) with lower education levels (OR = 0.42–0.76) and a household income less than 200,000 (OR = 0.15–0.78) had significantly reduced odds of perceived good or better health. People with hypertension and aged 75 years and above reported less physical distress and daily activity limitations than young adults. Men (Beta = −1.15) and aging (Beta = −8.12––1.70) were alleviating factors, while lower household income increased the mental distress among people with hypertension (Beta = 0.30–5.48). Those aged 65 years and above (Beta = −3.03––2.30) and able to work (Beta = −5.51––2.27) reported less daily activity limitations. No adjustment was made for the regression analyses.

Table 3. Factors associated with health status among people with hypertension.

	Perceived Good or Better Health [a]	Physical Distress [b]	Mental Distress [b]	Daily Activity Limitation [b]
	Odds Ratio (95% CI)	**Beta (95% CI)**	**Beta (95% CI)**	**Beta (95% CI)**
Sex: male	0.97 (0.93, 1.01)	0.01 (−0.19, 0.22)	−1.30 (−1.47, −1.14) *	0.69 (0.43, 0.95) *
Age range (years)				
18 to 24	Reference	Reference	Reference	Reference
25 to 34	0.78 (0.55, 1.10)	1.14 (−0.51, 2.80)	−1.40 (−2.75, −0.06) *	0.95 (−0.88, 2.78)
35 to 44	0.61 (0.44, 0.85) *	2.83 (1.28, 4.37) *	−2.27 (−3.52, −1.01) *	1.10 (−0.60, 2.81)
45 to 54	0.63 (0.46, 0.87) *	3.27 (1.76, 4.78) *	−3.47 (−4.70, −2.24) *	1.14 (−0.53, 2.80)
55 to 64	0.72 (0.52, 0.98) *	3.00 (1.50, 4.50) *	−5.09 (−6.31, −3.87) *	0.74 (−0.91, 2.40)
65 to 74	1.13 (0.82, 1.69)	0.07 (−1.44, 1.57)	−7.93 (−9.16, −6.71) *	−2.29 (−3.95, −0.63) *
75 up	1.23 (0.89, 1.69)	−0.36 (−1.88, 1.15)	−9.09 (−10.33, −7.86) *	−2.99 (−4.67, −1.32) *
Residence in urban areas	1.06 (1.01, 1.12) *	−0.09 (−0.36, 0.18)	0.29 (0.07, 0.50) *	−0.20 (−0.54, 0.14)
Education level				
Attended high school or less	0.47 (0.43, 0.51) *	0.87 (0.44, 1.30) *	−0.22 (−0.57, 0.12)	0.54 (0.02, 1.06) *
Graduated from high school	0.73 (0.69, 0.77) *	0.46 (0.19, 0.74) *	−0.24 (−0.47, −0.02) *	0.23 (−0.12, 0.59)
Attended college or above	0.79 (0.75, 0.84) *	0.76 (0.50, 1.02) *	0.34 (0.13, 0.55) *	0.42 (0.08, 0.75) *
Graduated from college or above	Reference	Reference	Reference	Reference
Employment status				
Employed	2.22 (2.09, 2.35) *	−5.04 (−5.31, −4.76) *	−2.44 (−2.66, −2.21) *	−6.34 (−6.69, −5.99) *
Unemployed	1.40 (1.30, 1.52) *	−2.41 (−2.82, −2.01) *	−0.60 (−0.93, −0.27) *	−2.06 (−2.54, −1.58) *
Retired or unable to work	Reference	Reference	Reference	Reference
Household income (US dollars)				
Less than 15,000	0.22 (0.19, 0.27) *	6.21 (5.46, 6.97) *	4.84 (4.22, 5.46) *	4.78 (3.72, 5.83) *
15,000 to <25,000	0.29 (0.25, 0.35) *	4.47 (3.74, 5.19) *	2.97 (2.37, 3.56) *	3.15 (2.12, 4.18) *
25,000 to <35,000	0.37 (0.31, 0.44) *	3.15 (2.43, 3.86) *	2.01 (1.43, 2.60) *	2.08 (1.06, 3.10) *
35,000 to <50,000	0.46 (0.39, 0.55) *	1.95 (1.25, 2.66) *	1.50 (0.92, 2.08) *	1.36 (0.34, 2.38) *
50,000 to <100,000	0.65 (0.54, 0.77) *	1.07 (0.39, 1.75) *	0.61 (0.06, 1.17) *	0.54 (−0.45, 1.53)
100,000 to <200,000	0.86 (0.71, 1.02)	0.07 (22120.64, 0.77)	0.01 (−0.56, 0.59)	0.21 (−0.82, 1.24)
200,000 or more	Reference	Reference	Reference	Reference

[a] Logistic regression. [b] Linear regression. * Statistical significance, $p < 0.05$.

4. Discussion

This study assessed the factors associated with perceived health, distresses, and limitations at the national level using 2021 BRFSS survey data. People with diabetes and hypertension were reported to perceive less good health and more distresses and limitations than the general population. Geographic variations were noted, with more residents in the Southwest region (and some states) reporting poorer health and more physical and mental distresses than other regions and states. In the regression analysis, education level, employment status, and household income were the factors associated most with perceived poor health, distresses, and limitations.

A previous national study showed that people with diabetes were the least likely to practice a healthy lifestyle [10], with this study identifying the association of sociodemographic variables on perceived health. Future interventions can target these variables to improve their perceived health, aiming to increase the practice of healthy lifestyle and eventually reduce the risk of developing complications [19]. The interventions may be suitable for patients with hypertension, as the associated sociodemographic variables on perceived health were similar to those with diabetes.

A special pattern was noted when people with diabetes and hypertension became older. Compared to those aged 18–24 years, people with diabetes and hypertension reported having the most physical distress and daily activity limitations at age 45–54 years (Tables 2 and 3); however, their physical distress and daily activity limitations were improved when they were aged 65 years and older. The pattern might indicate that the needs of older adults were addressed appropriately at a community level. In 2018, the WHO reported the achievements and outlined the strategies to promote age-friendly cities and communities [20]. A recent review of 27 studies found that the age-friendly community interventions were mainly focused on the improvement of physical and mental health [21]; therefore, our analysis found that older adults with diabetes and hypertension reported less physical and mental distresses than young adults.

Our findings showed that the mean day of having mental distress was similar between the general population and people with hypertension, while those with diabetes were reported to have more mental distress. The linear regression showed that people of an older age reported less mental distress. Some interventions, such as acceptance-based interventions, were reviewed to effectively improve the mental distress among people with diabetes, but most of the participants of the included studies in the reviews were aged 50 years and older [22,23]. The mental distress among young adults with diabetes was concerning, and further studies are suggested to ascertain if the interventions are also effective for them.

Employment status and household income were essential factors in health status among people with diabetes and hypertension. In this study, people who were employed would perceive good or better health and less physical and mental distresses than those unemployed. The findings were in line with a previous study indicating that employment status influenced the perceived health status [24]. Although employed people were perceived to have better health, they were less likely to practice healthy lifestyles, resulting in an increased risk of physical health problems [10], and so workplace-based interventions are suggested. Zhou et al. used a propensity score matching technique to examine the effectiveness of a workplace-based hypertension management program among 12,240 people with hypertension [25]. Participants in the intervention group showed a decreased systolic blood pressure during follow-ups in the 2nd, 4th, 6th, 8th, and 10th years, and the control group showed a decrease only in the 2nd and 4th years. A systematic review of 24 studies showed that workplace-based interventions could significantly reduce body weight [26]. On the other hand, this study found that 67.1% and 60.1% of people with diabetes and hypertension were not working, respectively, indicating that this might be a reason for the low household incomes. In turn, people with low household incomes might spend more time increasing their income by working, paying less attention to their physical health conditions, eventually perceiving a poor health status and more physical and mental distresses.

Since the data collection of this study was conducted during the COVID-19 pandemic, the findings of high physical distress might support that people with diabetes and hypertension were associated with poor outcomes in COVID-19 infection [27]. In turn, the high physical distress might also indicate the outcomes of long COVID among such individuals [28]. With the broad range of symptoms of long COVID, people with diabetes and hypertension might require specific supports that are different from other populations.

4.1. Implications

Our study findings have strong implications for clinical practice, research, and policy making. Geographic variations in perceived health and distresses highlight the need for reviewing current practices at the state level. Although the questions asked in the BRFSS survey to assess physical distress and mental distress are general, the findings of this study provide insights for future studies that may utilize more specific assessments to investigate the physical and psychological needs among people with diabetes and hypertension. On the other hand, uneven distribution of primary care workforces between states could hinder the health promotion for those with chronic health conditions, such as diabetes and hypertension [29,30]. With the rapid increase in smartphone ownership [31], digital interventions, such as webpages and mobile applications, can be integrated into current practice to reduce both physical and mental distresses [32,33]. Also, the use of digital interventions can reduce the influence of uneven distribution of primary care workforces in healthcare services. However, the government should develop strategies to reduce the difference of uneven distribution of primary care workforces between states, and increased training and payment of locum relief may help in this regard [34].

People with diabetes and hypertension aged 45–54 years reported the most physical distress and daily activity limitations; further studies are suggested to investigate their needs and develop specific interventions that reduce physical distress among such individuals. Physical distress caused by long COVID among people with diabetes and hypertension requires further investigation to develop appropriate interventions. On the other hand, we found that young adults with diabetes and hypertension experienced more mental distress. A future study is suggested to explore their source of stressors, such as newly diagnosed health conditions and workplace—family issues, to develop appropriate interventions for them. For example, daily diabetes management may increase mental distress among young adults with diabetes, and so an educational program with psychological components could reduce their mental distress and improve their glycemic control [35].

Although the unemployed rate among people with diabetes and hypertension was lower than that of the general population in this study, an employed status could improve their physical and mental health; therefore, the government needs to take action to reduce the unemployment rates. Tax deduction can be considered to reinforce the companies to provide regular health promotion activities for their employees. On the other hand, people with low household incomes reported poorer health and more distresses, and barriers to health care access might be a possible reason [36]. Notably, 12.6% of adults did not have health insurance in 2021 [37], and the government can engage with non-governmental organizations to increase health insurance coverage [38]. Employment and health insurance coverage might reduce health expenditures caused by complications with hypertension and diabetes [3,4].

4.2. Limitations

The variables in the secondary analysis were limited to the data set used. For example, the majority of people with diabetes and hypertension were older adults, and statistical adjustments to their age in regard to outcome variables were not feasible, as the age is provided in categories in the dataset. All variables were reported by individuals via phone call, which might lead to a reporting bias arising from recollections coming from memory. Data collection was conducted during the COVID-19 pandemic, which may have influenced the respondents of this survey; however, the use of a national data set enhanced the generalizability of our findings.

5. Conclusions

The analysis of the national data set indicated that people with chronic illness were perceived to have poorer health statuses and more physical and mental distresses than the general population, especially those with diabetes. Geographic variations in perceived health and distresses were noted. More attention is suggested to be given to the people with diabetes and hypertension living in the Southwest region. Through regression analysis, some sociodemographic variables, such as age and education level, were identified as significant factors influencing their perceived health and distress. In addition to physical health conditions, several interventions were suggested to strengthen current practice, while policy makers have important roles in addressing several influencing variables.

Author Contributions: Conceptualization, L.Y.-L.L., H.-L.T. and Y.Y.; methodology, L.Y.-L.L., H.-L.T. and I.S.-H.L.; validation, H.-L.T., Y.Y., X.Z. and A.M.; formal analysis, H.-L.T., A.S.-W.C. and I.S.-H.L.; data curation, H.-L.T. and A.S.-W.C.; writing—original draft preparation, L.Y.-L.L., H.-L.T., Y.Y. and X.Z.; writing—review and editing, L.Y.-L.L., H.-L.T., A.M. and P.-L.C.; visualization, H.-L.T., A.S.-W.C. and P.-L.C.; supervision, A.M. All authors have read and agreed to the published version of the manuscript.

Funding: This research received no external funding.

Institutional Review Board Statement: Ethical review and approval were waived for this study due to the data being de-identified and publicly available from the US Centers for Disease Control [18].

Informed Consent Statement: Informed consent was obtained from all subjects involved in the study via the phone call.

Data Availability Statement: The data used in this study (Behavioral Risk Factor Surveillance System 2021) are publicly available [18].

Conflicts of Interest: The authors declare no conflicts of interest.

References

1. WHO. The Top 10 Causes of Death. Available online: https://www.who.int/news-room/fact-sheets/detail/the-top-10-causes-of-death (accessed on 20 February 2024).
2. GBD 2019 Risk Factors Collaborators. Global burden of 87 risk factors in 204 countries and territories, 1990–2019: A systematic analysis for the Global Burden of Disease Study 2019. *Lancet* **2020**, *396*, 1223–1249. [CrossRef]
3. Wierzejska, E.; Giernas, B.; Lipiak, A.; Karasiewicz, M.; Cofta, M.; Staszewski, R. A global perspective on the costs of hypertension: A systematic review. *Arch. Med. Sci.* **2020**, *16*, 1078–1091. [CrossRef]
4. Seuring, T.; Archangelidi, O.; Suhrcke, M. The Economic Costs of Type 2 Diabetes: A Global Systematic Review. *Pharmacoeconomics* **2015**, *33*, 811–831. [CrossRef]
5. Unger, T.; Borghi, C.; Charchar, F.; Khan, N.A.; Poulter, N.R.; Prabhakaran, D.; Ramirez, A.; Schlaich, M.; Stergiou, G.S.; Tomaszewski, M.; et al. 2020 International Society of Hypertension Global Hypertension Practice Guidelines. *Hypertension* **2020**, *75*, 1334–1357. [CrossRef]
6. Williams, B.; Mancia, G.; Spiering, W.; Agabiti Rosei, E.; Azizi, M.; Burnier, M.; Clement, D.L.; Coca, A.; de Simone, G.; Dominiczak, A.; et al. 2018 ESC/ESH Guidelines for the management of arterial hypertension. *Eur. Heart J.* **2018**, *39*, 3021–3104. [CrossRef]
7. American Diabetes Association. Standards of Medical Care in Diabetes—2022 Abridged for Primary Care Providers. *Clin. Diabetes* **2022**, *40*, 10–38. [CrossRef]
8. de Boer, I.H.; Bangalore, S.; Benetos, A.; Davis, A.M.; Michos, E.D.; Muntner, P.; Rossing, P.; Zoungas, S.; Bakris, G. Diabetes and Hypertension: A Position Statement by the American Diabetes Association. *Diabetes Care* **2017**, *40*, 1273–1284. [CrossRef]
9. WHO. Noncommunicable Diseases. Available online: https://www.who.int/news-room/fact-sheets/detail/noncommunicable-diseases (accessed on 20 February 2024).
10. Tam, H.L.; Chair, S.Y.; Leung, I.S.H.; Leung, L.Y.L.; Chan, A.S.W. US Adults Practicing Healthy Lifestyles before and during COVID-19: Comparative Analysis of National Surveys. *JMIR Public Health Surveill.* **2023**, *9*, e45697. [CrossRef]
11. Axon, D.R.; Jang, A.; Son, L.; Pham, T. Determining the association of perceived health status among united states older adults with self-reported pain. *Aging Health Res.* **2022**, *2*, 100051. [CrossRef]

12. Tinajero-Chávez, L.I.; Mora-Romo, J.F.; Bravo-Doddoli, A.; Cruz-Narciso, B.V.; Calleja, N.; Toledano-Toledano, F. Design, Development, and Validation of the Self-Perceived Health Scale (SPHS). *Healthcare* **2023**, *11*, 2007. [CrossRef]
13. Perrin, N.E.; Davies, M.J.; Robertson, N.; Snoek, F.J.; Khunti, K. The prevalence of diabetes-specific emotional distress in people with Type 2 diabetes: A systematic review and meta-analysis. *Diabet. Med.* **2017**, *34*, 1508–1520. [CrossRef]
14. Young-Hyman, D.; de Groot, M.; Hill-Briggs, F.; Gonzalez, J.S.; Hood, K.; Peyrot, M. Psychosocial Care for People with Diabetes: A Position Statement of the American Diabetes Association. *Diabetes Care* **2016**, *39*, 2126–2140. [CrossRef]
15. Ojike, N.; Sowers, J.R.; Seixas, A.; Ravenell, J.; Rodriguez-Figueroa, G.; Awadallah, M.; Zizi, F.; Jean-Louis, G.; Ogedegbe, O.; McFarlane, S.I. Psychological Distress and Hypertension: Results from the National Health Interview Survey for 2004–2013. *Cardiorenal Med.* **2016**, *6*, 198–208. [CrossRef]
16. Duenas, M.; Salazar, A.; de Sola, H.; Failde, I. Limitations in Activities of Daily Living in People with Chronic Pain: Identification of Groups Using Clusters Analysis. *Pain. Pract.* **2020**, *20*, 179–187. [CrossRef]
17. von Elm, E.; Altman, D.G.; Egger, M.; Pocock, S.J.; Gotzsche, P.C.; Vandenbroucke, J.P.; STORBE Initiative. The Strengthening the Reporting of Observational Studies in Epidemiology (STROBE) statement: Guidelines for reporting observational studies. *Prev. Med.* **2007**, *45*, 247–251. [CrossRef]
18. 2021 BRFSS Survey Data and Documentation. Available online: https://www.cdc.gov/brfss/annual_data/annual_2021.html (accessed on 20 February 2024).
19. Li, Y.; Schoufour, J.; Wang, D.D.; Dhana, K.; Pan, A.; Liu, X.; Song, M.; Liu, G.; Shin, H.J.; Sun, Q.; et al. Healthy lifestyle and life expectancy free of cancer, cardiovascular disease, and type 2 diabetes: Prospective cohort study. *BMJ* **2020**, *368*, l6669. [CrossRef]
20. WHO. The Global Network for Age-Friendly Cities and Communities. Available online: https://www.who.int/publications/i/item/WHO-FWC-ALC-18.4 (accessed on 20 February 2024).
21. Hong, A.; Welch-Stockton, J.; Kim, J.Y.; Canham, S.L.; Greer, V.; Sorweid, M. Age-Friendly Community Interventions for Health and Social Outcomes: A Scoping Review. *Int. J. Environ. Res. Public. Health* **2023**, *20*, 2554. [CrossRef]
22. Schmidt, C.B.; van Loon, B.J.P.; Vergouwen, A.C.M.; Snoek, F.J.; Honig, A. Systematic review and meta-analysis of psychological interventions in people with diabetes and elevated diabetes-distress. *Diabet. Med.* **2018**, *35*, 1157–1172. [CrossRef]
23. Ngan, H.Y.; Chong, Y.Y.; Chien, W.T. Effects of mindfulness- and acceptance-based interventions on diabetes distress and glycaemic level in people with type 2 diabetes: Systematic review and meta-analysis. *Diabet. Med.* **2021**, *38*, e14525. [CrossRef]
24. Park, S.; Chan, K.C.; Williams, E.C. Gain of employment and perceived health status among previously unemployed persons: Evidence from a longitudinal study in the United States. *Public. Health* **2016**, *133*, 83–90. [CrossRef]
25. Zhou, Y.F.; Chen, S.; Wang, G.; Chen, S.; Zhang, Y.B.; Chen, J.X.; Tu, Z.Z.; Liu, G.; Wu, S.; Pan, A. Effectiveness of a Workplace-Based, Multicomponent Hypertension Management Program in Real-World Practice: A Propensity-Matched Analysis. *Hypertension* **2022**, *79*, 230–240. [CrossRef]
26. Mulchandani, R.; Chandrasekaran, A.M.; Shivashankar, R.; Kondal, D.; Agrawal, A.; Panniyammakal, J.; Tandon, N.; Prabhakaran, D.; Sharma, M.; Goenka, S. Effect of workplace physical activity interventions on the cardio-metabolic health of working adults: Systematic review and meta-analysis. *Int. J. Behav. Nutr. Phys. Act.* **2019**, *16*, 134. [CrossRef]
27. Hosseinzadeh, R.; Goharrizi, M.; Bahardoust, M.; Alvanegh, A.G.; Ataee, M.R.; Bagheri, M.; Navidiyan, E.S.; Zijoud, S.R.H.; Heiat, M. Should all patients with hypertension be worried about developing severe coronavirus disease 2019 (COVID-19)? *Clin. Hypertens.* **2021**, *27*, 3. [CrossRef]
28. Davis, H.E.; McCorkell, L.; Vogel, J.M.; Topol, E.J. Long COVID: Major findings, mechanisms and recommendations. *Nat. Rev. Microbiol.* **2023**, *21*, 133–146. [CrossRef]
29. Zhang, D.; Son, H.; Shen, Y.; Chen, Z.; Rajbhandari-Thapa, J.; Li, Y.; Eom, H.; Bu, D.; Mu, L.; Li, G.; et al. Assessment of Changes in Rural and Urban Primary Care Workforce in the United States from 2009 to 2017. *JAMA Netw. Open* **2020**, *3*, e2022914. [CrossRef]
30. Tam, H.L.; Chung, S.F.; Wang, Q. Urban-rural disparities in hypertension management among middle-aged and older patients: Results of a 2018 Chinese national study. *Chronic Illn.* **2023**, *19*, 581–590. [CrossRef]
31. Pew Research Center. Smartphone Ownership Is Growing Rapidly around the World, but Not Always Equally. Available online: https://www.pewresearch.org/global/2019/02/05/smartphone-ownership-is-growing-rapidly-around-the-world-but-not-always-equally (accessed on 20 February 2024).
32. Babbage, C.M.; Jackson, G.M.; Davies, E.B.; Nixon, E. Self-help Digital Interventions Targeted at Improving Psychological Well-being in Young People with Perceived or Clinically Diagnosed Reduced Well-being: Systematic Review. *JMIR Ment. Health* **2022**, *9*, e25716. [CrossRef] [PubMed]
33. Nicholl, B.I.; Sandal, L.F.; Stochkendahl, M.J.; McCallum, M.; Suresh, N.; Vasseljen, O.; Hartvigsen, J.; Mork, P.J.; Kjaer, P.; Søgaard, K.; et al. Digital Support Interventions for the Self-Management of Low Back Pain: A Systematic Review. *J. Med. Internet Res.* **2017**, *19*, e179. [CrossRef]
34. Russell, D.; Mathew, S.; Fitts, M.; Liddle, Z.; Murakami-Gold, L.; Campbell, N.; Ramjan, M.; Zhao, Y.; Hines, S.; Humphreys, J.S.; et al. Interventions for health workforce retention in rural and remote areas: A systematic review. *Hum. Resour. Health* **2021**, *19*, 103. [CrossRef]
35. Ngan, H.Y.; Chong, Y.Y.; Loo, K.M.; Chien, W.T. Preliminary efficacy of an acceptance-based diabetes education (ACT-DE) programme for people with type 2 diabetes on diabetes distress and self-care behaviours: A pilot randomised controlled trial. *J. Context. Behav.* **2023**, *30*, 50–60. [CrossRef]

36. Lazar, M.; Davenport, L. Barriers to Health Care Access for Low Income Families: A Review of Literature. *J. Community Health Nurs.* **2018**, *35*, 28–37. [CrossRef] [PubMed]
37. Terlizzi, E.P.; Cohen, R.A. Geographic Variation in Health Insurance Coverage: United States, 2021. *Natl. Health Stat. Rep.* **2022**, *176*, 1–19.
38. Sanadgol, A.; Doshmangir, L.; Majdzadeh, R.; Gordeev, V.S. Engagement of non-governmental organisations in moving towards universal health coverage: A scoping review. *Glob. Health* **2021**, *17*, 129. [CrossRef] [PubMed]

healthcare

MDPI

Article

Enhancing Quality of Life and Sexual Functioning in Female Androgenetic Alopecia: Therapeutic Potential of Hair Follicle-Derived Stem Cells

Katarzyna Krefft-Trzciniecka, Hanna Cisoń, Alicja Pakiet, Danuta Nowicka * and Jacek C. Szepietowski

Department of Dermatology, Venereology and Allergology, Wrocław Medical University, 50-368 Wrocław, Poland; jacek.szepietowski@umw.edu.pl (J.C.S.)
* Correspondence: danuta.nowicka@umw.edu.pl

Abstract: Background: The study aimed to examine the impact of stem cell treatment on quality of life (QoL) and sexual functioning in women with androgenetic alopecia (AGA). Methods: Twenty-three women underwent a single session of autologous cellular micrografts (ACMs). The World Health Organization Quality of Life Brief Version (WHOQOL-BREF) and Female Sexual Function Index (FSFI) were used before and after 6 months. Results: The AGA severity decreased by an average of 1 point on the Ludwig scale ($p = 0.004$) after treatment. FSFI scores indicated sexual dysfunction in over half of the women at baseline, but they improved significantly post-treatment for arousal [median (IQR): 4.8 (1.5) vs. 5.10 (0.9); $p = 0.035$] and satisfaction [4.4 (1.4) vs. 4.8 (1.8); $p = 0.025$]. QoL scores improved after treatment in psychological health (57.96 ± 19.0 vs. 69.35 ± 14.0; $p = 0.031$) and environment (72.96 ± 13.4 vs. 81.09 ± 12.6; $p = 0.007$), but not in physical health and social relationships. No associations were found between the WHOQOL-BREF or FSFI domains versus age and AGA severity. Conclusions: AGA reduces QoL and impacts sexual functioning in women with AGA. The high treatment burden arises from the chronic and progressive nature of AGA, coupled with limited treatment effectiveness. Effective treatments for AGA, like ACM, are urgently needed to enhance patient-reported outcomes along with clinical results.

Keywords: stem cell therapy; regenerative therapy; androgenetic alopecia; quality of life; female sexual function

1. Introduction

Androgenetic alopecia (AGA) is a condition characterized by gradual and ongoing hair loss with an unpredictable pattern of progression [1]. A female pattern of hair loss can cause various psychological problems that reduce quality of life. The loss of self-confidence and decreases in self-esteem are common reactions to hair loss, especially in women [2]. The World Health Organization (WHO) explains that quality of life is a subjective assessment of the perception of reality through the lens of culture and the value system observed by its targets [3,4]. In European culture, physical appearance is highly valued, which is why AGA is such a significant problem [5].

In several studies, alopecia has been shown to have a psychosocial impact on both men and women, but the effects can be more severe and devastating on women [6]. Concerning the male population, the disease affects social functioning and emotional well-being, with pronounced detrimental effects observed among young men [7]. Camacho et al. [8] deduced that depression in the course of AGA was more common in women than in men and was most often described as a "minor". Moreover, Russo et al. [9] concluded that women with AGA are characterized by greater social anxiety and social phobia compared to men with this disease. AGA is usually considered a benign process, mainly cosmetic, but numerous studies confirm that AGA can be a complication and manifestation of underlying systemic diseases, which further increases the patient's anxiety [10]. Gonul et al. [2] examined and compared the quality of life in patients with AGA and alopecia areata using the Hairdex, an instrument developed to assess the quality of life in patients with hair loss. The results are very interesting and surprising, because, among people with AGA, hair loss had a more adverse impact on their emotions, functioning, and symptoms, compared to those with alopecia areata. A similar study was conducted by Jun et al. [11], who used the Hair Specific Skindex-29 to examine quality of life in patients with AGA and alopecia areata, identifying risk factors associated with its deterioration. Patients with AGA were more likely to report a symptomatic decline in quality of life ($p = 0.033$), while patients with alopecia areata showed significantly worse functional quality of life than AGA patients ($p = 0.013$).

Hair has been a significant aspect of identity and image for decades, holding sociological and psychological importance for a person's appearance and personality [12,13]. Sexual health encompasses the physical, emotional, and mental well-being associated with sexuality, while impaired sexual health may have a significant impact on quality of life [14]. Sexual functions are closely linked to other aspects of behavior and cannot be considered independent phenomena. Sexuality has attracted considerable attention throughout human civilization and exerts a significant impact on people's quality of life [13,15]. Quality of life and sexual health are multidimensional and share a bidirectional relationship.

AGA is a hair loss disorder mediated by dihydrotestosterone, which induces the miniaturization of hair follicles and transforms the final hair into vellus hair [16]. The pathogenesis of this condition also involves oxidative stress and microinflammation occurring around the hair follicles [17]. In women with AGA, hair loss can manifest clinically in a variety of ways. The two most common patterns are diffuse hair loss in the central front and posterior regions (Ludwig type—severity is evaluated on the Ludwig scale in three steps) or hair loss in the central part of the front scalp (Olson type), also known as front accentuation or "Christmas tree type" patterns [18–20]. Yu et al. [21] showed that the way people with AGA perceive their disease has a significant impact on health outcomes of other diseases. They also found that all patients considered alopecia to be a major concern with a considerable emotional impact. Patients reported relatively poor control over the disorder and its treatment, as well as a limited understanding of its course.

Minoxidil (topical administration) for female and male pattern hair loss and finasteride (oral administration) only for male pattern hair loss are the two drugs approved by the U.S. Food and Drug Administration (FDA) for the treatment of AGA [22]. Iamsumang et al. [23] reviewed studies involving oral and topical finasteride used in women. Although there are few studies available, their analysis concluded that finasteride was effective and safe for the treatment of female pattern hair loss. However, larger studies are needed to further validate these findings. The literature reports on the efficacy and safety of numerous other therapies, including platelet-rich plasma, dutasteride (systemic administration) (not approved by the FDA for alopecia), hair transplants, oral minoxidil, and low-level laser therapy [22].

Recently, regenerative medicine therapies have been gaining popularity. The goal of regenerative medicine is to restore the normal function of cells and organs by replacing and regenerating damaged cells or organs. Stem cells, cytokines, growth factors from either stem cells or hematopoietic tissues, and gene therapies are used for this purpose. Stem cells possess unique abilities such as self-renewal and the ability to exhibit anti-inflammatory and immunomodulatory effects. These characteristics make them applicable in the treatment of alopecia [24]. For the treatment of AGA, most reports focus on adipose-derived stem cells and hair follicle stem cells, while only a few studies are available on the use of bone marrow stem cells and Wharton's jelly stem cells [25].

In this study, we aimed to investigate whether the stem cell treatment of AGA affects quality of life and sex life. Additionally, we sought to examine the correlation between sexual functioning and the quality of life among women with AGA after treatment.

2. Materials and Methods

2.1. Participants

This study was conducted through face-to-face surveys at the Clinic of Dermatology, Venerology and Allergology of Wroclaw Medical University, during which, participants completed questionnaires. Twenty-three female patients aged between 18 and 65 (mean 40 ± 12) years and diagnosed with AGA were included in the study.

Inclusion criteria were determined through clinical examination by dermatologists and assessed using the Ludwig scale. The distribution of the patients according to Ludwig's female pattern hair loss classification showed that patients were classified as follows: Grade I—60.9%; Grade II—30.4%; and Grade III—8.8%. The primary exclusion criteria for this study included immunosuppression, cancer, severe chronic disease, pregnancy, breastfeeding, age under 18 years, hormonal contraception, hyperprolactinemia, hypothyroidism, active inflammation of the scalp, coagulation disorders, lignocaine allergy, and unstable emotional state. Patients with a positive antinuclear antibody (ANA) 3 test were also excluded. Additionally, patients who had received oral (finasteride, dutasteride, minoxidil, antiandrogens) or topical (minoxidil, prostaglandin analogs, corticosteroids) AGA-targeted treatment in the past 6 months were excluded. The study did not include patients who had used medical devices such as low-level laser therapy or undergone procedures such as platelet-rich plasma injections or micro-needling.

The patients received a single session of autologous cellular micrografting (ACM) obtained with the Regenera Activa® device (Human Brain Wave SRL, Turin, Italy). Before and 6 months after the therapy, all participants completed two questionnaires: the World Health Organization Quality of Life Brief Version (WHOQOL-BREF) and the Female Sexual Function Index (FSFI). We used validated Polish versions of the FSFI and WHOQOL-BREF questionnaires. Both the FSFI and WHOQOL-BREF have a 4-week recall period. All participants provided written, informed consent prior to the enrollment and received instructions on how to complete the study questionnaires. The study was approved by the Bioethics Committee of Wroclaw Medical University (KB-1074/2021, approval date: 3 January 2022).

2.2. ACM Procedure

Under local anesthesia, five 2.5 mm diameter punch biopsies were collected from the scalp skin behind the patient's ear. The collected samples were placed in medical devices (Class I, Rigneracons CE certified; Human Brain Wave SRL, Turin, Italy) and coated with 2 mL of sterile physiological solution. Then, the cell suspension was produced by turning the Rigeneracons at 80 RPM for 2 min. The suspension was then diluted with an additional 2 mL of sterile physiological solution. The resulting solution was injected into the scalp hair area using a 1 mL syringe and 30 mm needles. A volume of 0.1 mL was injected per point, with about 1 cm intervals between the needles.

2.3. Instruments

2.3.1. World Health Organization Quality of Life Brief Version (WHOQOL-BREF)

The WHOQOL-BREF [26,27] is a self-report questionnaire that assesses quality of life in four domains: physical health (7 elements), psychological health (6 elements), social relationships (3 elements), and environment (8 elements). Each item is scored on a 1–5 Likert scale. After collecting filled questionnaires, the domain scores were transformed to a scale of 0 to 100, where higher scores indicate a higher quality of life. The recall period for this questionnaire is 4 weeks.

2.3.2. Female Sexual Function Index (FSFI)

The FSFI is a 19-element measure, composed of six different areas of female sexual function, namely: desire (2 items), arousal (4 items), lubrication (4 items), orgasm (3 items), satisfaction (3 items), and pain (3 items). Total FSFI scores range from 2 (lowest possible score) to 36 (highest score) [28]. This scale is widely used as both a screening and outcome measurement tool for female sexual function, with a 4-week recall period [29]. The FSFI has a clinical cutoff score of 26.55 points total, as proposed by Wiegel et al. [30]. This score currently serves as the clinical standard for differentiating between patients with and without sexual dysfunction. In individual domains, scores below the median were considered indicative of dysfunction for that particular domain, i.e., for desire ≤ 3.6, for arousal ≤ 4.8, for lubrication ≤ 5.1, for orgasm ≤ 4.4, for satisfaction ≤ 4.4, and for pain ≤ 5.6.

2.4. Data Analysis

Variables with normal distributions were presented as mean ± standard deviation (SD), and those without normal distribution were presented as medians with the interquartile range (IQR) in parentheses. Box plots were used to illustrate the distribution of different domains of the WHOQOL-BREF and FSFI among patients. To investigate the differences in patients before and after treatment, paired *t*-tests (for WHOQOL-BREF domains) or Wilcoxon signed rank tests (for FSFI domains) were performed depending on the distribution of the variables, which was checked with the Shapiro–Wilk test. The correlation between WHOQOL-BREF and FSFI was assessed with Spearman's correlation coefficients. The effect size was calculated as described by Cohen [31]. For variables that underwent a paired *t*-test with Cohen's d statistic, $d = (M_1 - M_2)/SD_{pooled}$, where M_1 and M_2 are the means of the compared groups and SD_{pooled} is a pooled standard deviation of the two groups ($SD_{pooled} = \sqrt{[(SD_1{}^2 + SD_2{}^2)/2]}$. For variables that underwent Wilcoxon signed rank tests, effect size was calculated with r, defined as $r = z/\sqrt{n}$, where z is a z-score and n is a sum of the grouped sizes. All calculations were performed using SigmaPlot 14.5 (Systat, Software Inc., San Jose, CA, USA).

3. Results

The results included data from all 23 patients with AGA. Table 1 presents the characteristics of the study patients. Following the ACM treatment, the severity of AGA significantly decreased by an average of 1 point on the Ludwig scale ($p = 0.004$). We did not detect any association between the WHOQOL-BREF or FSFI domains and age or AGA severity.

Table 1. Age and androgenetic alopecia severity in patients.

Age	**N**	**Mean (SD)**
<30 years	9	28 (2)
>30 years	14	47 (10)
Androgenetic alopecia severity	**N Before**	**N After**
Ludwig score 1	7	15
Ludwig score 2	14	7
Ludwig score 3	2	1

Before treatment, 11 patients had scores below 26.55, indicating sexual dysfunction, and this number decreased to 6 patients with sexual dysfunction after 6 months following the ACM session. At baseline, the majority of the patients experienced sexual dysfunction in specific domains, with 65% of patients reporting below the median for desire and arousal, 61% below the median in lubrication and pain, and 57% below the median with regard to orgasm and satisfaction. The FSFI results are summarized in Figure 1. After ACM treatment, patients reported significantly higher arousal with a median of 4.8 (1.5) before and 5.10 (0.9) after treatment ($p = 0.035$, effect size $r = -0.31$, indicating medium effect), as well as satisfaction with a median of 4.4 (1.4) before and 4.8 (1.8) after treatment ($p = 0.025$, effect size $r = -0.324$) as measured by the FSFI. The total FSFI score, as well as the desire, lubrication, orgasm, and pain indexes, did not differ significantly between study points.

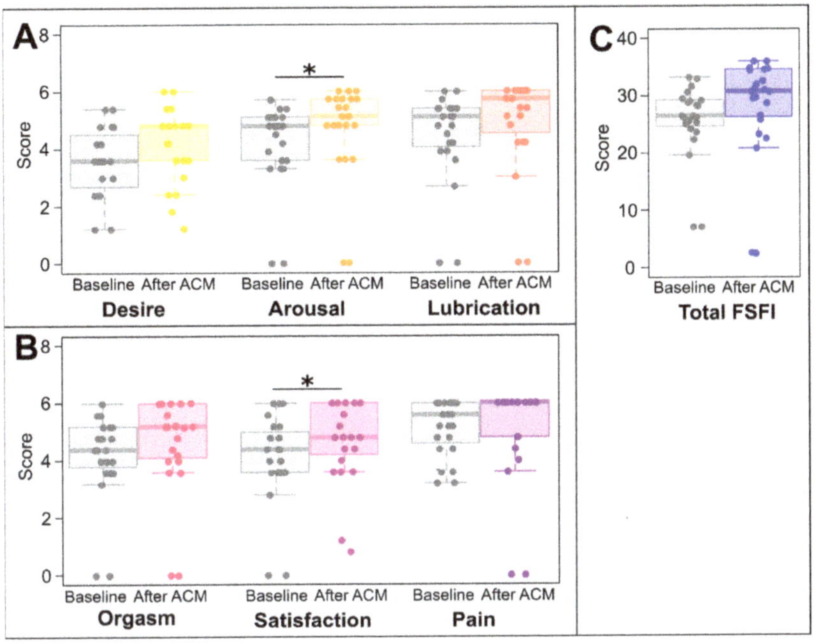

Figure 1. Female Sexual Satisfaction Index scores. Domains (**A**,**B**) and total score (**C**). * $p < 0.05$; values from Wilcoxon Signed Rank test; ACM, autologous cellular micrograft procedure.

Among the WHOQOL-BREF domains (summarized in Figure 2), the AGA patients reported the lowest quality of life in the physical health domain. The assessment with WHOQOL-BREF showed that 6 months after the ACM procedure, the patients experienced higher quality of life in psychological health (mean before 57.96 ± 19.0 vs. mean after 69.35 ± 14.0; $p = 0.031$, the effect size measured by Cohen's d was d = 0.68, indicating a medium effect) and environment (mean before 72.96 ± 13.4 vs. mean after 81.09 ± 12.6; $p = 0.007$, Cohen's d was 0.63). There were no significant changes in reported physical health and social relationships.

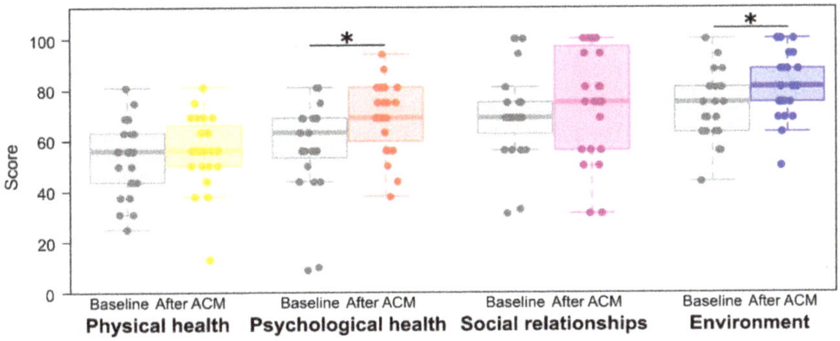

Figure 2. WHOQOL-BREF scores. * $p < 0.05$ from two-tailed t test; ACM, autologous cellular micrograft procedure.

The analysis of correlations between WHOQOL-BREF scores and FSFI results revealed that, across all domains, overall quality of life and sexual health were moderately to strongly positively correlated (Table 2). The strongest associations (above 0.7 Spearman's rho) were found between FSFI arousal and social relationships and FSFI satisfaction and social relationships.

Table 2. Correlations between sexual health and quality and life domains.

	Physical Health	Psychological Health	Social Relationships	Environment
Desire	0.26	0.46 *	0.56 **	0.28
Arousal	0.53 **	0.48 **	0.71 **	0.52 **
Lubrication	0.34 *	0.55 **	0.69 **	0.47 **
Orgasm	0.48 **	0.47 *	0.63 **	0.40 *
Satisfaction	0.54 **	0.46 *	0.76 **	0.35 *
Pain	0.33 *	0.52 **	0.59 **	0.44 *

Shown are Spearman's correlation coefficients. * $p < 0.05$, ** $p < 0.001$.

4. Discussion

Our analyses indicated that female patients with AGA had a reduced quality of life in the physical health domain, which, however, was not dependent on ACM treatment. The applied therapy significantly improved patients' quality of life in the mental health and environmental domains.

Researchers emphasize that women with AGA experience reduced quality of life, a finding consistent with our study. Moorthy et al. [32] also employed the WHO-BREF scale to assess quality of life, using a similar approach employed in our study. Additionally, they used the Hairdex questionnaire, a hair- and scalp-specific measurement tool designed to assess the specific effects of hair loss on the quality of life of patients. This questionnaire consists of 48 items categorized into five domains: symptoms, functions, emotions, self-confidence, and stigma. Their study included 170 patients with AGA of both sexes. The study found that in women under 30, the physical health and mental health domains were most impaired. Among singles, the symptom and emotion domains were affected, while those with less education exhibited impairment in all domains except physical health. Another study conducted by Reid et al. [33] discovered that patients often view their hair loss as more distressing in terms of quality of life than dermatologists perceive it to be. While physician and patient ratings of clinical severity align, the study found that clinical severity alone does not predict the impact of the disease on a patient's quality of life, hence the importance of employing additional validated tools to assess quality of life and using advanced devices to monitor disease progression. In a recent systematic review, Aukerman and Jafferany [5] investigated the psychosocial consequences of AGA and concluded that female patients experience severe dissatisfaction with their hair, leading to a decline in overall body image. Furthermore, dissatisfaction with one's body image significantly contributes to reduced desire and arousal [34]. In the present study, desire was the most affected area of sexual function at baseline, and it did not improve after therapy. However, we observed significant improvements in the domains of arousal and satisfaction, suggesting that ACM treatment has a positive effect on the sexual health of female AGA patients. These two FSFI domains exhibited the strongest association with the social relationships domain of WHOQOL-BREF. The latter did show some improvement after ACM treatment, although it was not statistically significant. Van der Donk et al. [35], based on their study on a group of 58 women, concluded that women with AGA often feel less attractive. Positive perceptions of one's attractiveness are associated with higher sexual satisfaction, higher sexual frequency, and more sexual partners [36]. Improving AGA through treatment and enhancing patients' appearance can boost their self-esteem, thereby influencing their sex lives. Our analysis of the associations between sexual health scores and quality of life indices also suggests that improvements in physical, and psychological health, as well as social relationships and environmental factors, are all linked with better sexual function. Biondo et al. [37], similarly to Reid et al. [33], hypothesized that women with AGA often rate their condition as more severe than their physicians do. However, their study, which examined disparities in perceptions of hair loss severity between patients and clinicians, revealed that women seeking treatment for AGA often underestimate the severity of their disease. Therefore, the findings of Biondo et al. suggest that it can be worthwhile to raise awareness among patients about alopecia and initiate effective treatment, as untreated AGA can progress and negatively affect both quality of life and sexual function. Tas et al. [38] used the ASEX scale, a tool designed to assess the sexual functioning of patients with AGA according to the severity of the disease. This scale assesses five domains: drive, arousal, penile erection/vaginal lubrication, ability to reach orgasm, and orgasmic satisfaction. Their analysis showed that the likelihood of patients developing psychosexual disorders increases with disease progression. Consequently, patients with AGA, especially those in advanced stages, should be referred to psychological or sexology counseling. While mental status becomes improved, the pain domain of the FSFI does not change in response to AGA treatment. Dyspareunia, defined as pain during sexual intercourse, has a complex etiology [39]. Leeners et al. [40] showed that dyspareunia often occurs alongside other psychiatric disorders, with depression being the most common. Depression is an illness frequently associated with AGA, implying a possible overlap of these conditions within our study group.

The availability of studies examining the effect of a specific therapeutic method in relation to the quality of life in women with AGA is limited. While most studies have focused on quality of life in the AGA population, it seems interesting to explore the impact of specific treatments on both quality of life and sexual functioning. Due to limited FDA-approved treatments, experimental and off-label treatments are commonly explored for this condition.

Pharmacotherapy is often used for treating AGA in women; however, many of the agents have not been approved by the FDA for this specific indication. Zhuang et al. [41] conducted a study involving 31 patients diagnosed with AGA to assess the impact on quality of life and clinical improvement after 12 months of using 2% topical minoxidil. They used the Visual Analog Scale (VAS) and the Dermatologic Quality of Life Index (DLQI). The results indicated that hair loss is significantly associated with a reduced quality of life, and the use of topical minoxidil was observed to improve this condition. In another study, Yamazaki et al. [42] investigated how 1 mg of oral finasteride taken for 6 months affected the quality of life of 27 men with AGA aged between 19 and 76 years. They used WHOQOL-BREF, the DLQI, the State–Trait Anxiety Inventory (STAI), and VAS scales. The comparison of WHOQOL-BREF scores before and after the administration of 1 mg of finasteride showed an overall improvement in the quality of life in the study group, although the improvement in individual domains was not statistically significant. It is worth noting that while finasteride treatment is well established in men, only a small number of studies focus on the use of 5 α-reductase inhibitors in female pattern hair loss, which is considered as an off-label treatment. Seale et al. [43] emphasized the potential side effects that 5 α-reductase inhibitors may cause in women when used as an oral treatment for female pattern hair loss and frontal fibrosing alopecia. However, the frequency of sexual function impairment after the administration of dutasteride or finasteride in the identified studies varied. Two studies reported that the daily administration of 5 mg of finasteride contributed to treatment discontinuation due to decreased libido. The occurrence of post-finasteride syndrome in women was not determined in that review. However, post-finasteride syndrome, which includes, among other adverse side effects, sexual dysfunction secondary to 5 α-reductase inhibitors, is well described among male patients and includes the loss of libido and erectile dysfunction [44]. Although finasteride is not yet FDA-approved for female patients, its potential as an alternative treatment is being considered [23]. To date, the limited data available seem to indicate very few side effects of 5 α-reductase inhibitors on sexual function in women [43]. To our knowledge, there are no published studies evaluating the effect of AGA treatment on women's sexual functioning, and the available data on the association of AGA and impaired sexual function are contradictory. Sancak et al. [14] evaluated the correlations between female sexual dysfunction and AGA in premenopausal women, finding that the presence of AGA significantly impaired their sexual function. Conversely, Eyada et al. [45] found no correlation between the incidence of sexual function impairment and AGA.

Topical preparations for AGA are characterized by a lower frequency of side effects, but their high treatment burden limits patient adherence and, consequently, effectiveness. In a study by Zac and da Costa [46], quality of life, treatment satisfaction, and dermatoscopic criteria were evaluated among female patients with AGA undergoing treatment with topical 5% minoxidil. The study concluded that treatment with 5% minoxidil had positive psychological benefits. Interestingly, patient satisfaction and quality of life were not found to be related to age, alopecia severity, or hair shaft reduction per follicle unit. Another study conducted by Moorthy et al. [32] on 170 women with AGA showed that female AGA was associated with significantly reduced quality of life, particularly among young, less educated, and single women. This suggests that the potential benefits of treatment could be age-dependent. In our analysis, we considered the association between age and found no correlation between improvements in quality of life after treatment with hair follicle stem cells and the age of the patients. Vastarella et al. [47] retrospectively studied the effect of oral minoxidil at a dose of 0.5 mg to 2 mg daily in women diagnosed with AGA. The study group consisted of 12 women with AGA (Ludwig scale I-3-III) with a mean age of 36.7 ± 18.8 years. The Women with Androgenetic Alopecia Quality of Life Questionnaire (WAA-QoL) was used to assess quality of life, showing a statistically significant improvement after 24 weeks compared to baseline. The median WAA-QoL score was 70.33 at baseline and decreased to 25.58 at 24 weeks ($p < 0.01$).

There are only a few studies that have investigated quality of life among women with AGA treated with platelet-rich plasma. Meyers et al. [48] conducted a study examining the effect of platelet-rich plasma treatments on the quality of life of 92 female and male patients with pattern hair loss. Using the Hairdex 48 scale, they found that this type of treatment is effective in improving the overall quality of life. The study also revealed a decrease in the domains of symptoms, emotions, and functioning, with improvements demonstrated in the domains of stigma and self-confidence. A study conducted by Bruce et al. [49] was a randomized, controlled pilot trial investigating the efficacy of platelet-rich plasma in comparison to topical minoxidil foam for the treatment of AGA among women. The secondary outcome of this study included the measurement of quality of life using a 16-item questionnaire administered at baseline and after the 12-week treatment period. Notably, no improvements were observed after minoxidil treatment, whereas the platelet-rich plasma group demonstrated significant improvement in aspects such as self-consciousness about people looking at their hair, feelings of jealousy, ability to socialize with people, and satisfaction with overall hair appearance.

Hair transplants involve the surgical transplantation of hair follicles from a donor area, typically the back or sides of the scalp, to areas with hair loss. This procedure is invasive and expensive but effective, providing natural-looking results. Nilforoushzadeh et al. [50] conducted a survey involving 35 men to assess quality of life and self-esteem before and after hair transplant surgery. They used the Rosenberg Self-Esteem Scale (RSES) and the DLQI and demonstrated a statistically significant difference in self-esteem and quality of life before and after the restoration surgery. Additionally, the study revealed a statistically significant relationship between educational achievement and quality of life. This study suggests that as self-esteem improves, patients' quality of life also improves, emphasizing the close connection between self-esteem and a satisfying physical appearance. Xiao et al. [51] investigated health utility measures among patients with AGA after a hair transplant. They compared 31 patients with alopecia with 237 otherwise healthy people. After the hair transplant, the improvement in time trade-off—a technique used to measure the experienced quality of life for economic analyses—was significantly greater for patients with AGA (+0.08 ± 0.12 vs. +0.02 ± 0.09; $p = 0.0070$) and significantly more often exceeded the minimal clinically important difference (45.2% vs. 16.9%; $p = 0.0006$).

A limitation of our study is undoubtedly the small sample size and the lack of a placebo group. A major challenge is to find women with AGA who are willing to abstain from other types of treatment for 6 months. In the future, we aim to investigate how stem cell therapy affects quality of life and sexual functioning in men affected by the disease. It also seems interesting to compare this therapy with others, especially with FDA-approved drugs, in terms of their impact on quality of life. Another important limitation of our study is that the quality of life of our female patients may be affected by factors other than AGA, which were not controlled for. We lacked sufficient information to account for factors that could influence quality of life, such as socialized frequency and marital status. Certainly, collaboration with psychiatrists and psychotherapists, who would be able to professionally assess the mental state of the patients, could have ruled out other potential causes of lowered mood or dissatisfaction with sexual life. Another limitation of our work is the inability to interpret the interesting and surprising result of improved quality of life in the environmental domain. Unfortunately, due to the lack of information about the demographics of the patients, we were not able to interpret its reliably. This area requires further research.

5. Conclusions

Dermatologists need to recognize the tremendous impact that AGA has on the quality of life and sexual functioning of women affected by the condition. The assessment of quality of life and sexual functioning in women with AGA is increasingly important for assessing the effects of the disease on patients and the required treatment. The chronic and progressive nature of AGA, coupled with limited treatment effectiveness, contributes to substantial suffering for those affected. Therefore, there is a pressing need for novel and effective treatments for AGA. Highlighting the potential advantages of a multidisciplinary approach that includes dermatologists, endocrinologists, and psychologists, this study offers optimism regarding the ability of new stem cell treatments to diminish the severity of AGA. This, in turn, holds the promise of enhancing the overall quality of life for individuals affected by the condition.

Author Contributions: Conceptualization, K.K.-T., H.C., A.P., D.N. and J.C.S.; data curation, K.K.-T., H.C. and A.P.; formal analysis, K.K.-T. and H.C.; investigation, K.K.-T., H.C. and A.P.; methodology, K.K.-T., D.N. and J.C.S.; resources, K.K.-T., D.N. and J.C.S.; writing—original draft, K.K.-T., H.C. and A.P.; writing—review and editing, K.K.-T., H.C., D.N. and J.C.S. All authors have read and agreed to the published version of the manuscript.

Funding: This study was funded by the Department of Dermatology, Venereology, and Allergology at Wrocław Medical University through subsidy No SUBZ.C260.24.003.

Institutional Review Board Statement: The study was conducted in accordance with the Declaration of Helsinki and approved by the Bioethics Committee at Wroclaw Medical University (approval no. KB-1074/2021, approval date: 3 January 2022).

Informed Consent Statement: Informed consent was obtained from all subjects involved in the study.

Data Availability Statement: The data that support the findings of this study are available on request from the corresponding author.

Conflicts of Interest: The authors declare no conflicts of interest.

References

1. Alhanshali, L.; Buontempo, M.G.; Lo Sicco, K.I.; Shapiro, J. Alopecia Areata: Burden of Disease, Approach to Treatment, and Current Unmet Needs. *Clin. Cosmet. Investig. Dermatol.* **2023**, *16*, 803–820. [CrossRef]
2. Gonul, M.; Cemil, B.C.; Ayvaz, H.H.; Cankurtaran, E.; Ergin, C.; Gurel, M.S. Comparison of quality of life in patients with androgenetic alopecia and alopecia areata. *An. Bras. Dermatol.* **2018**, *93*, 651–658. [CrossRef] [PubMed]
3. Post, M.W. Definitions of quality of life: What has happened and how to move on. *Top. Spinal Cord Inj. Rehabil.* **2014**, *20*, 167–180. [CrossRef]
4. Fuhrer, M.J. Subjectifying quality of life as a medical rehabilitation outcome. *Disabil. Rehabil.* **2000**, *22*, 481–489. [CrossRef]

5. Aukerman, E.L.; Jafferany, M. The psychological consequences of androgenetic alopecia: A systematic review. *J. Cosmet. Dermatol.* **2023**, *22*, 89–95. [CrossRef]
6. Davis, D.S.; Callender, V.D. Review of quality of life studies in women with alopecia. *Int. J. Women's Dermatol.* **2018**, *4*, 18–22. [CrossRef] [PubMed]
7. Adamowicz, R.; Zalecki, P.; Dukiel, A.; Nowicka, D. Association between Androgenetic Alopecia and Psychosocial Disease Burden: A Cross-Sectional Survey among Polish Men. *Dermatol. Res. Pract.* **2022**, *2022*, 1845044. [CrossRef] [PubMed]
8. Camacho, F.M.; Garcia-Hernandez, M. Psychological features of androgenetic alopecia. *J. Eur. Acad. Dermatol. Venereol.* **2002**, *16*, 476–480. [CrossRef]
9. Russo, P.M.; Fino, E.; Mancini, C.; Mazzetti, M.; Starace, M.; Piraccini, B.M. HrQoL in hair loss-affected patients with alopecia areata, androgenetic alopecia and telogen effluvium: The role of personality traits and psychosocial anxiety. *J. Eur. Acad. Dermatol. Venereol.* **2019**, *33*, 608–611. [CrossRef]
10. Chen, S.; Xie, X.; Zhang, G.; Zhang, Y. Comorbidities in Androgenetic Alopecia: A Comprehensive Review. *Dermatol. Ther.* **2022**, *12*, 2233–2247. [CrossRef]
11. Jun, M.; Keum, D.I.; Lee, S.; Kim, B.J.; Lee, W.S. Quality of Life with Alopecia Areata versus Androgenetic Alopecia Assessed Using Hair Specific Skindex-29. *Ann. Dermatol.* **2018**, *30*, 388–391. [CrossRef] [PubMed]
12. Gupta, S.; Goyal, I.; Mahendra, A. Quality of Life Assessment in Patients with Androgenetic Alopecia. *Int. J. Trichology* **2019**, *11*, 147–152. [CrossRef] [PubMed]
13. Sidi, H.; Puteh, S.E.; Abdullah, N.; Midin, M. The prevalence of sexual dysfunction and potential risk factors that may impair sexual function in Malaysian women. *J. Sex. Med.* **2007**, *4*, 311–321. [CrossRef]
14. Sancak, E.B.; Oguz, S.; Akbulut, T.; Uludag, A.; Akbas, A.; Kurt, O.; Akbulut, M.F. Female sexual dysfunction in androgenetic alopecia: Case-control study. *Can. Urol. Assoc. J.* **2016**, *10*, E251–E256. [CrossRef]
15. Nazarpour, S.; Simbar, M.; Ramezani Tehrani, F.; Alavi Majd, H. Quality of life and sexual function in postmenopausal women. *J. Women Aging* **2018**, *30*, 299–309. [CrossRef] [PubMed]
16. Adil, A.; Godwin, M. The effectiveness of treatments for androgenetic alopecia: A systematic review and meta-analysis. *J. Am. Acad. Dermatol.* **2017**, *77*, 136–141.e5. [CrossRef]
17. Khantham, C.; Linsaenkart, P.; Chaitep, T.; Jantrawut, P.; Chittasupho, C.; Rachtanapun, P.; Jantanasakulwong, K.; Phimolsiripol, Y.; Sommano, S.R.; Prom, U.T.C.; et al. Antioxidation, Anti-Inflammation, and Regulation of SRD5A Gene Expression of Oryza sativa cv. Bue Bang 3 CMU Husk and Bran Extracts as Androgenetic Alopecia Molecular Treatment Substances. *Plants* **2022**, *11*, 330. [CrossRef]
18. Olsen, E.A. The midline part: An important physical clue to the clinical diagnosis of androgenetic alopecia in women. *J. Am. Acad. Dermatol.* **1999**, *40*, 106–109. [CrossRef]
19. Ludwig, E. Classification of the types of androgenetic alopecia (common baldness) occurring in the female sex. *Br. J. Dermatol.* **1977**, *97*, 247–254. [CrossRef]
20. Venning, V.A.; Dawber, R.P. Patterned androgenic alopecia in women. *J. Am. Acad. Dermatol.* **1988**, *18*, 1073–1077. [CrossRef]
21. Yu, N.L.; Tan, H.; Song, Z.Q.; Yang, X.C. Illness perception in patients with androgenetic alopecia and alopecia areata in China. *J. Psychosom. Res.* **2016**, *86*, 1–6. [CrossRef]
22. Devjani, S.; Ezemma, O.; Kelley, K.J.; Stratton, E.; Senna, M. Androgenetic Alopecia: Therapy Update. *Drugs* **2023**, *83*, 701–715. [CrossRef]
23. Iamsumang, W.; Leerunyakul, K.; Suchonwanit, P. Finasteride and Its Potential for the Treatment of Female Pattern Hair Loss: Evidence to Date. *Drug Des. Dev. Ther.* **2020**, *14*, 951–959. [CrossRef]
24. Shimizu, Y.; Ntege, E.H.; Sunami, H.; Inoue, Y. Regenerative medicine strategies for hair growth and regeneration: A narrative review of literature. *Regen. Ther.* **2022**, *21*, 527–539. [CrossRef]
25. Krefft-Trzciniecka, K.; Pietowska, Z.; Nowicka, D.; Szepietowski, J.C. Human Stem Cell Use in Androgenetic Alopecia: A Systematic Review. *Cells* **2023**, *12*, 951. [CrossRef]
26. WHOQOL Group. Development of the World Health Organization WHOQOL-BREF quality of life assessment. The WHOQOL Group. *Psychol. Med.* **1998**, *28*, 551–558. [CrossRef]
27. Bonomi, A.E.; Patrick, D.L.; Bushnell, D.M.; Martin, M. Validation of the United States' version of the World Health Organization Quality of Life (WHOQOL) instrument. *J. Clin. Epidemiol.* **2000**, *53*, 1–12. [CrossRef]
28. Meston, C.M. Validation of the Female Sexual Function Index (FSFI) in women with female orgasmic disorder and in women with hypoactive sexual desire disorder. *J. Sex. Marital. Ther.* **2003**, *29*, 39–46. [CrossRef] [PubMed]
29. Sanchez-Sanchez, B.; Navarro-Brazalez, B.; Arranz-Martin, B.; Sanchez-Mendez, O.; de la Rosa-Diaz, I.; Torres-Lacomba, M. The Female Sexual Function Index: Transculturally Adaptation and Psychometric Validation in Spanish Women. *Int. J. Environ. Res. Public Health* **2020**, *17*, 994. [CrossRef] [PubMed]
30. Wiegel, M.; Meston, C.; Rosen, R. The female sexual function index (FSFI): Cross-validation and development of clinical cutoff scores. *J. Sex Marital. Ther.* **2005**, *31*, 1–20. [CrossRef] [PubMed]
31. Cohen, J. A power primer. *Psychol. Bull.* **1992**, *112*, 155–159. [CrossRef]
32. Moorthy, S.; Yu, L.; Peng, L.; Shen, L.; Han, Y.; Zhang, Z.; Li, Y.; Huang, X. Quality of Life and Its Association with Androgenetic Alopecia Patients in Shanghai: A Cross-Sectional Study. *Clin. Cosmet. Investig. Dermatol.* **2022**, *15*, 2883–2893. [CrossRef]

33. Reid, E.E.; Haley, A.C.; Borovicka, J.H.; Rademaker, A.; West, D.P.; Colavincenzo, M.; Wickless, H. Clinical severity does not reliably predict quality of life in women with alopecia areata, telogen effluvium, or androgenic alopecia. *J. Am. Acad. Dermatol.* **2012**, *66*, e97–e102. [CrossRef]
34. Quinn-Nilas, C.; Benson, L.; Milhausen, R.R.; Buchholz, A.C.; Goncalves, M. The Relationship Between Body Image and Domains of Sexual Functioning Among Heterosexual, Emerging Adult Women. *Sex. Med.* **2016**, *4*, e182–e189. [CrossRef]
35. van der Donk, J.; Passchier, J.; Knegt-Junk, C.; van der Wegen-Keijser, M.H.; Nieboer, C.; Stolz, E.; Verhage, F. Psychological characteristics of women with androgenetic alopecia: A controlled study. *Br. J. Dermatol.* **1991**, *125*, 248–252. [CrossRef]
36. Amos, N.; McCabe, M. The importance of feeling sexually attractive: Can it predict an individual's experience of their sexuality and sexual relationships across gender and sexual orientation? *Int. J. Psychol.* **2017**, *52*, 354–363. [CrossRef] [PubMed]
37. Biondo, S.; Goble, D.; Sinclair, R. Women who present with female pattern hair loss tend to underestimate the severity of their hair loss. *Br. J. Dermatol.* **2004**, *150*, 750–752. [CrossRef]
38. Tas, B.; Kulacaoglu, F.; Belli, H.; Altuntas, M. The tendency towards the development of psychosexual disorders in androgenetic alopecia according to the different stages of hair loss: A cross-sectional study. *An. Bras. Dermatol.* **2018**, *93*, 185–190. [CrossRef] [PubMed]
39. Tayyeb, M.; Gupta, V. Dyspareunia. In *StatPearls*; StatPearls Publishing: Treasure Island, FL, USA, 2023.
40. Leeners, B.; Hengartner, M.P.; Ajdacic-Gross, V.; Rossler, W.; Angst, J. Dyspareunia in the Context of Psychopathology, Personality Traits, and Coping Resources: Results From a Prospective Longitudinal Cohort Study From Age 30 to 50. *Arch. Sex. Behav.* **2015**, *44*, 1551–1560. [CrossRef] [PubMed]
41. Zhuang, X.S.; Zheng, Y.Y.; Xu, J.J.; Fan, W.X. Quality of life in women with female pattern hair loss and the impact of topical minoxidil treatment on quality of life in these patients. *Exp. Ther. Med.* **2013**, *6*, 542–546. [CrossRef] [PubMed]
42. Yamazaki, M.; Miyakura, T.; Uchiyama, M.; Hobo, A.; Irisawa, R.; Tsuboi, R. Oral finasteride improved the quality of life of androgenetic alopecia patients. *J. Dermatol.* **2011**, *38*, 773–777. [CrossRef]
43. Seale, L.R.; Eglini, A.N.; McMichael, A.J. Side Effects Related to 5 alpha-Reductase Inhibitor Treatment of Hair Loss in Women: A Review. *J. Drugs Dermatol.* **2016**, *15*, 414–419. [PubMed]
44. Pereira, A.; Coelho, T.O.A. Post-finasteride syndrome. *An. Bras. Dermatol.* **2020**, *95*, 271–277. [CrossRef] [PubMed]
45. Eyada, M.M.K.; Abd-Elhamid, A.-A.S.; Elboghdady, R.A.F.; Gadallah, A.M.; Azab, M. Assessment of Female Sexual Dysfunction in Patients with Premenopausal Female Pattern Hair Loss. *Adv. Sex. Med.* **2020**, *10*, 86–103. [CrossRef]
46. Zac, R.I.; da Costa, A. Patient Satisfaction and Quality of Life Among Adult Women with Androgenetic Alopecia Using 5% Topical Minoxidil. *J. Clin. Aesthet. Dermatol.* **2021**, *14*, 26–30. [PubMed]
47. Vastarella, M.; Cantelli, M.; Patri, A.; Annunziata, M.C.; Nappa, P.; Fabbrocini, G. Efficacy and safety of oral minoxidil in female androgenetic alopecia. *Dermatol. Ther.* **2020**, *33*, e14234. [CrossRef] [PubMed]
48. Meyers, A.; Jin, A.; Kwiecien, G.J.; Gatherwright, J.; Khetarpal, S.; Zins, J.E. Platelet-Rich Plasma for Treatment of Hair Loss Improves Patient-Reported Quality of Life. *Aesthetic Plast. Surg.* **2023**, *47*, 1528–1534. [CrossRef]
49. Bruce, A.J.; Pincelli, T.P.; Heckman, M.G.; Desmond, C.M.; Arthurs, J.R.; Diehl, N.N.; Douglass, E.J.; Bruce, C.J.; Shapiro, S.A. A Randomized, Controlled Pilot Trial Comparing Platelet-Rich Plasma to Topical Minoxidil Foam for Treatment of Androgenic Alopecia in Women. *Dermatol. Surg.* **2020**, *46*, 826–832. [CrossRef]
50. Nilforoushzadeh, M.A.; Golparvaran, M.; Yekaninejad, M.S. Assessment of quality of life and self-esteem in male patients with androgenetic alopecia before and after hair transplantation. *J. Cosmet. Dermatol.* **2023**, *22*, 2283–2287. [CrossRef]
51. Xiao, R.; Burks, C.A.; Yau, J.; Derakhshan, A.; Liu, R.H.; Senna, M.M.; Yasuda, M.R.; Jowett, N.; Lee, L.N. Health Utility Measures Among Patients with Androgenetic Alopecia after Hair Transplant. *Aesthetic Plast. Surg.* **2023**, *47*, 631–639. [CrossRef]

healthcare MDPI

Article

Exploring the Link between Social Support and Patient-Reported Outcomes in Chronic Obstructive Pulmonary Disease Patients: A Cross-Sectional Study in Primary Care

Izolde Bouloukaki [1,*], Antonios Christodoulakis [1,2], Katerina Margetaki [1], Antonia Aravantinou Karlatou [1] and Ioanna Tsiligianni [1]

[1] Department of Social Medicine, School of Medicine, University of Crete, 71003 Heraklion, Greece; christodoulakisa@icloud.com (A.C.); katmargetaki@hotmail.com (K.M.); toniakoinerg2@gmail.com (A.A.K.); i.tsiligianni@uoc.gr (I.T.)

[2] Department of Nursing, School of Health Sciences, Hellenic Mediterranean University, 71410 Heraklion, Greece

* Correspondence: izolthi@gmail.com; Tel.: +30-2810-394607

Abstract: We aimed to explore the link between social support and various patient-reported outcome measures (PROMs) in primary care patients with COPD. This was a cross-sectional study with 168 patients with COPD from six primary care centers in Crete, Greece. We collected data on sociodemographic characteristics, medical history, disease-specific quality of life, the COPD Assessment Test (CAT), fatigue, the Fatigue Severity Scale (FSS), phycological parameters, Patient Health Questionnaire-9, General Anxiety Disorder-7, sleep complaints, the Pittsburg Sleep Quality Index, the Athens Insomnia scale (AIS), and the Epworth Sleepiness Scale. Social support was measured using the Multidimensional Scale of Perceived Social Support (MSPSS). Out of 168 patients with COPD, 114 (68.9%) exhibited low levels of social support. Low social support (MSPSS total ≤ 5) was positively associated with COPD symptoms (CAT score ≥ 10) (OR = 3.97, 95%CI:1.86–8.44; $p < 0.01$), fatigue (FSS ≥ 36) (OR = 2.74, 95%CI:1.31–5.74; $p = 0.01$), and insomnia symptoms (AIS ≥ 6) (OR = 5.17 95%CI:2.23–12.01; $p < 0.01$), while the association with depressive symptoms (PHQ-9 ≥ 10) was marginally significant (OR = 3.1, 95%CI:0.93–10.36; $p = 0.07$). Our results suggest that lower levels of social support are positively associated with PROMs in patients with COPD. Therefore, our findings show an additional way to improve the overall health of patients with COPD in primary care by putting social support at the epicenter of actions.

Keywords: social support; PROMs; COPD; primary care

1. Introduction

Chronic obstructive pulmonary disease (COPD) is a highly prevalent and progressive respiratory disease, resulting in substantial morbidity and mortality [1–3]. The worldwide prevalence of COPD is approximately 10.3%, but this number may increase as smoking becomes more common in low- and middle-income countries and as the population ages in high-income countries [4]. In Greece, it has been approximated that around 8.4–10.6% of the Greek population is affected by COPD, with a particularly pronounced impact on the elderly and those residing in rural regions [5,6]. This is important, since COPD is characterized by severe symptoms such as coughing, breathlessness, increased sputum production, and reduced physical activity [7,8]. Additionally, symptoms such as persistent fatigue, unintentional weight loss, and disrupted sleep patterns, including insomnia, can further exacerbate their emotional well-being [9–11].

Sleep disturbances are a relatively common symptom of COPD that can have detrimental effects on the quality of life of the patients [12]. For example, chronic insomnia is frequently reported, with up to half of the patients indicating difficulties in initiating sleep, maintaining sleep, or achieving restorative sleep [13]. The significant impact of these sleep disturbances further increases the already heightened risk of anxiety and depression, doubling the likelihood of experiencing them [14]. In addition, the combination of depression and sleep disturbances in patients with COPD leads to a five-fold increase in the likelihood of hospitalization [14]. All these symptoms significantly affect the emotional well-being of patients and elicit feelings of anxiety and depression that ultimately lead to a sense of social isolation [11]. Despite the aforementioned, an assessment of sleep disturbances is not a standard practice in patients with COPD [14].

Healthcare professionals assess the symptoms of patients with COPD by utilizing patient-reported outcome measures (PROMs) during clinical practice [15–19]. These standardized questionnaires provide valuable insights into patients' perceptions of their health and disease [20]. Furthermore, by utilizing PROMs, healthcare professionals can gain a better understanding of a patient's health status and where to intervene when necessary [18]. This understanding allows healthcare professionals to address the multiple aspects of COPD, such as physical, emotional, and social, and thus deliver better quality care to their patients. However, despite the fact that PROMs are highly valuable, they do not fully capture the important aspects of COPD, such as social support [21], which seems to be positively associated with mental health, quality of life, and self-efficacy in these patients [17].

The concept of social support refers to the expectation that one's social network is readily available to offer both emotional and practical assistance when needed [22]. Additionally, it involves providing emotional, informational, and practical assistance to individuals through social networks, including family, friends, peers, healthcare professionals, and community organizations [23]. The available evidence indicates that social support has the potential to enhance stress management and self-esteem, foster medication adherence [22,24], and affect and improve the efficacy of therapeutic interventions [25], quality of life [26], and the well-being of patients with COPD [27]. Furthermore, social support seems to improve the patients' physical health, alleviate symptoms of depression and anxiety, and reduce hospitalization and mortality rates [28,29]. This could mean that social support has the potential to influence PROMs, given its association with all these aspects and symptoms of COPD, including the sleep disturbances [21,30,31]. Considering the potential influence of adequate social support on patients with COPD [32], it is logical to assume that higher levels of perceived social support could positively impact a range of PROMs for these patients [32]. Nevertheless, there is a lack of comprehensive studies in the literature that sufficiently explore the association between perceived social support and self-reported health in patients with COPD using PROMs, particularly in primary care settings [33]. Therefore, our study aimed to explore the link between social support and various PROMs among patients with COPD in primary care settings.

2. Materials and Methods

2.1. Design and Sample

The present cross-sectional study invited patients with COPD from six primary care centers in Crete, Greece. To be eligible for inclusion, patients were required to meet the following criteria: (a) be 40 years of age or older and have a physician-diagnosed COPD confirmed with spirometry, (b) have an educational background beyond elementary school, and (c) provide written informed consent. We excluded patients who had severe neurological or mental disorders, were pregnant, experienced a recent exacerbation of COPD, demonstrated limited comprehension of the Greek language, or did not wish to participate.

2.2. Procedure

During their visit, patients with COPD were provided with information regarding the objectives of the study. Following their agreement to participate, they proceeded to submit written consent and anonymously completed the questionnaires. To mitigate the influence of social desirability bias, the participants were instructed to deposit their study materials in an opaque container that was placed outside the office.

The study adhered to the guidelines specified in the Declaration of Helsinki and received approval from the University of Crete Research Ethics Committee (REC-UOC) (Protocol Number: 183/13.12.2022).

2.3. Data Collection

A comprehensive evaluation of the participants was conducted, which assessed various demographic parameters, such as age, gender, BMI, exercise habits, tobacco and alcohol use, educational status, and comorbidities. COPD-specific quality of life was assessed using the COPD Assessment Test (CAT). The assessment of fatigue involved the use of the Fatigue Severity Scale, while psychological factors were measured using the Patient Health Questionnaire-9 and General Anxiety Disorder-7 questionnaire. Subjective sleep quality and sleep-related complaints were evaluated using the Pittsburgh Sleep Quality Index, the Athens Insomnia Scale, and the Epworth Sleepiness Scale. The multidimensional scale of perceived social support was used to quantify social support. The evaluation for each participant lasted approximately 20–30 min.

2.4. Study Tools and Outcomes

2.4.1. Multidimensional Scale of Perceived Social Support (MSPSS)

The MSPSS is a widely used tool designed to assess an individual's perception of the availability of social support [34]. This scale measures the extent of support received from three specific sources: family, friends, and a significant other. It is comprised of twelve items and three subscales. The total mean scores range from 1 to 7. Higher scores indicate a higher level of perceived social support. The present study employed the total mean score and a cutoff point of 5 or below to determine the presence of low social support [35]. The MSPSS exhibits a high level of internal consistency reliability, as indicated by a Cronbach's alpha of 0.85–0.91 [36]. The questionnaire has been translated and culturally adapted into Greek [37], and our study has achieved excellent internal consistency with a Cronbach's alpha of 0.96.

2.4.2. COPD Assessment Test (CAT) Questionnaire

The CAT is a simple-to-complete questionnaire that assesses the self-reported impact of COPD on health status. The CAT consists of eight items (cough, phlegm, chest tightness, breathlessness, limited activities, confidence in leaving home, sleeplessness, and energy), that the patient rates on a scale of 0 to 5 [16]. The score ranges from 0 to 40, with higher values indicating poorer health status. A cutoff point of 10 or above is used to determine the presence of poor health status. It has been also validated in Greek [38] and exhibited a Cronbach's alpha of 0.78 in our study population.

2.4.3. Patient Health Questionnaire (PHQ-9)

PHQ-9 is a self-report questionnaire that consists of nine items. These items reflect the criteria used in diagnosing depressive disorder according to the Diagnostic and Statistical Manual of Mental Disorders (DSM) 4th edition (DSM-IV) [39] but are theoretically in line with the 5th version of the DSM (DSM-5) [40]. The PHQ-9 has a score range of 0 to 27, with higher scores indicating more severe depressive symptoms. The cutoffs of 5, 10, 15, and 20 correspond to mild, moderate, moderately severe, and severe depressive disorders, respectively. The present study employed a cutoff point of 10 or above to determine the presence of depressive symptoms. The initial validation study of the PHQ-9 showed high reliability in a large sample of primary care patients, with a Cronbach's alpha coefficient of 0.89 [39]. Subsequent studies in various populations have demonstrated an adequate internal consistency (α = 0.70–0.93) [41–46]. It has also been validated in Greek [47] and exhibited a Cronbach's alpha of 0.86 in our study population.

2.4.4. General Anxiety Disorder (GAD-7)

The GAD-7 is a validated instrument that evaluates seven symptoms related to generalized anxiety disorder, as described in the DSM-IV [48]. The total score ranges from 0 to 21, with higher values indicating greater disturbance. Scores of 5, 10, 15, or higher represent mild, moderate, or severe impairment, respectively. In our study, we considered a threshold above 10 to be a marker for the presence of GAD, indicating the existence of anxiety symptoms at moderate and severe levels. The GAD-7 has been found to have good-to-excellent reliability in different populations, with Cronbach's α values ranging from 0.8 to 0.97 [49–55]. The Greek version of the GAD-7 [56] was employed in the current study and yielded a Cronbach's alpha of 0.93.

2.4.5. Pittsburgh Sleep Quality Index (PSQI)

The PSQI is a widely recognized questionnaire for its ability to distinguish between poor and good sleep quality. The PSQI is a nineteen-item self-rated questionnaire used to evaluate subjective sleep quality and quantity, sleep habits associated with quality, and the occurrence of sleep disturbances among adults within a one-month interval [57]. The score range is 0 to 21. The higher the score, the more pronounced the adverse effects on the sleep quality. A global score of $\geq$6 indicates poor sleep quality. Additionally, it has been translated and validated in Greek and used for assessing sleep quality in a Greek sample [58, 59]. Previous studies have demonstrated satisfactory levels of internal consistency, with Cronbach's alphas ranging from 0.70 to 0.83 [59–63]. Our study population achieved an acceptable [64] Cronbach's alpha of 0.67.

2.4.6. Athens Insomnia Scale (AIS)

The AIS is a Greek questionnaire and was designed as a standardized assessment tool to measure the level of sleep difficulty, following the guidelines of the International Classification of Diseases-10 edition (ICD-10). It is a self-assessment psychometric tool comprising eight items. The total score ranges from 0 to 24, and a score equal to or greater than 6 indicates the likelihood of insomnia [65]. In both clinical and community samples, the AIS exhibited exceptional internal consistency, with Cronbach's alphas ranging from 0.81 to 0.86, thereby confirming its efficacy in measuring insomnia symptoms [66]. For our population, Cronbach's alpha was 0.85.

2.4.7. Epworth Sleepiness Scale (ESS)

The ESS is presently the most extensively employed subjective assessment tool for measuring daytime sleepiness in clinical settings [67]. The scale ranges from 0 to 24, and anything below 10 is considered to be within the normal range. The Cronbach's alpha values of previously published studies on ESS were analyzed using reliability generalization meta-analysis, and the cumulative Cronbach's α ranged from 0.80 to 0.83, indicating a high level of reliability. In our study, the Greek version of the ESS was utilized [68], yielding a Cronbach's α of 0.75 for this particular population.

2.4.8. Fatigue Severity Scale (FSS)

The FSS is used by providing individuals with nine statements concerning the severity, frequency, and impact of fatigue on daily life (physical functioning, exercise and work, and family or social life) and asking them to rate their agreement. The FSS score is obtained by finding the average of the scores given to each item, with higher scores reflecting more severe fatigue. Scores < 36 were considered normal. A score that surpasses the specified threshold ($\geq$36) indicates a substantial detrimental impact of fatigue on daily life activities (maximum score of 63) [69]. The FSS has been translated and culturally adapted to Greek [70]. Furthermore, the FSS has been validated in various populations, and the findings suggest that it has satisfactory concurrent validity and internal consistency, with Cronbach's alphas ranging from 0.89 to 0.96. The Cronbach's alpha for our population was 0.99.

2.5. Statistical Analysis

Participants who had completed the MSPSS questionnaire (N = 168) were included in our analysis. For all continuous variables with a normal distribution, the results are reported as the mean ± standard deviation (SD), whereas for variables without a normal distribution, the median (25–75th percentile) is presented. Categorical variables are presented in terms of the absolute numerical value and the corresponding percentage. To conduct comparisons between groups, we utilized a two-tailed *t*-test for independent samples (when data followed a normal distribution) or a Mann–Whitney U-test (when data did not follow a normal distribution) for continuous variables. Furthermore, the Chi-square test was employed for categorical variables. Continuous scales were correlated using the Pearson's correlation coefficient.

In order to assess the associations between the MSPSS and the studied PROMs, we employed linear regression for the continuous MSPSS scales and logistic regression for the dichotomized MSPSS scales. Each PROM was then fitted into a separate model. In each model, we also included factors that were associated ($p < 0.05$) with both the MSPSS and PROMs. Thus, all models were adjusted for age, gender, marital status, and level of education. We further adjusted for obesity and the presence of any other chronic diseases in a sensitivity analysis. Multicollinearity among the predictors was assessed using collinearity statistics to ensure that the collinearity between the predictor variables was within the acceptable range, as indicated by the tolerance value variance inflation factor (VIF < 3 for each model). The results were deemed significant if the *p*-values were less than 0.05. Data were analyzed using the Stata software (version 13).

3. Results

3.1. Patient Characteristics

A total of 191 patients with COPD were initially invited to participate in the study; however, 170 patients (89%) agreed to participate. Moreover, the study questionnaires were completed by 168 patients, yielding an effective response rate of 88%. The average age of the patients included in the study was 68 years (range 41–90 years). Among the participants, 68% were male, 41% were obese (BMI ≥ 30 kg/m2), and 40% were married. A significant portion of the participants exhibited a low level of education (48%), a slightly smaller percentage had a middle education (35%), and only 17% had a high level of education. In terms of smoking habits, 46% of the participants were actively smoking during the survey, whereas 44% had quit smoking. At least one chronic disease was present in 89% of the patients. The sociodemographic characteristics and health status of the 168 participants are provided in Table 1.

Table 1. Demographic characteristics of the participants (n = 168) according to social support status.

Characteristics	Overall	High Support MSPPS > 5	Low Support MSPPS ≤ 5	*p*-Value
	N = 168 (100%)	**N = 54 (32.1%)**	**N = 114 (68.9%)**	
Age (years)	68.4 ± 9.0	66.3 ± 8.1	69.4 ± 9.3	0.040
Age group 40–50 years	8 (4.8)	3 (5.6)	5 (4.4)	
Age group 51–64 years	53 (31.5)	22 (40.7)	31 (27.2)	0.175
Age group ≥ 65 years	107 (63.7)	29 (53.7)	78 (68.4)	
Gender				
Male	114 (67.9)	39 (72.2)	75 (65.8)	
Female	54 (32.1)	15 (27.8)	39 (34.2)	0.404
BMI	29.8 ±6.1	29.6 ±4.9	29.8 ±6.7	0.841
BMI ≥ 30	69 (41.1)	20 (37.0)	49 (43.0)	0.464
Have a spouse				
Yes	40 (23.8)	8 (14.8)	32 (28.1)	
No	128 (76.2)	46 (85.2)	82 (71.9)	0.060

Table 1. *Cont.*

Characteristics	Overall	High Support MSPPS > 5	Low Support MSPPS ≤ 5	*p*-Value
	N = 168 (100%)	N = 54 (32.1%)	N = 114 (68.9%)	
Smoking				
Active	76 (45.5)	21 (38.9)	55 (48.7)	
Former	74 (44.3)	28 (51.9)	46 (40.7)	0.395
Never	17 (10.2)	5 (9.3)	12 (10.6)	
Pack Years	65.1 ±37.2	60.7 ±39.4	67.3 ±36.1	0.309
Alcohol (units/week)	0.0 (0.0, 7.0)	2.0 (0.0, 10.0)	0.0 (0.0, 7.0)	0.137
Physical Exercise (min/week)	0.0 (0.0, 210.0)	0.0 (0.0, 210.0)	0.0 (0.0, 200.0)	0.276
Education level				
Primary level	78 (47.9)	22 (41.5)	56 (50.9)	
Secondary level	57 (35.0)	15 (28.3)	42 (38.2)	0.009
Higher level	28 (17.2)	16 (30.2)	12 (10.9)	
Comorbidities				
Asthma	29 (17.3)	20 (17.5)	9 (16.7)	0.888
Arterial Hypertension	89 (53.0)	25 (46.3)	64 (56.1)	0.233
CVD	54 (32.1)	21 (38.9)	33 (28.9)	0.198
Diabetes type 2	49 (29.2)	18 (33.3)	31 (27.2)	0.413
Hyperlipidemia	59 (51.8)	33 (61.1)	92 (54.8)	0.255
Obstructive Sleep Apnea	24 (14.3)	10 (18.5)	14 (12.3)	0.281
Osteoporosis	21 (12.5)	2 (3.7)	19 (16.7)	0.018
Cancer	21 (12.5)	7 (13.0)	14 (12.3)	0.901
Depression	22 (13.1)	6 (11.1)	16 (14.0)	0.600
Anxiety Disorder	8 (4.8)	1 (1.9)	7 (6.1)	0.223
Comorbidities ≥ 1	149 (88.7)	48 (88.9)	101 (88.6)	0.955

Data are presented as N (%) for categorical variables and mean values ± SD or median (25th–75th percentile) for continuous variables; BMI: Body Mass Index; CVD: cardiovascular diseases.

Table 2 displays the distribution of patients into the GOLD groups based on the CAT categorization. The majority of participants (52.4%) were classified in the GOLD group B, whereas group E accounted for less than 17%, according to the GOLD 2023 classification. In the 12-month period prior to the study, the majority (85%) of patients did not suffer from COPD exacerbations or had just one, whereas 14.9% experienced two or more exacerbations and 4.8% required hospitalization. The mMRC scores are also presented in Table 2.

Regarding social support, the mean (SD) values of the MSPSS are presented in Table 3. The highest score was observed in the domain of family support, followed closely by the "significant other" domain. The three subscales are highly correlated to each other and to the total social support scale. The highest correlation was observed between the "significant other" subscale and the "family" subscale (rho = 0.887, $p < 0.001$) and the lowest between the "family" and the "friends" subscale (rho = 0.685, $p < 0.001$). Also, the correlations with the total scale were strong and highly significant, ranging from 0.898 for the "friends" subscale to 0.921 for the "significant other subscale" (all *p*-values < 0.001). The "significant other" and the "family" subscales accounted for 86% of the variance in the total social support scale, and this percentage for the "friends" subscale was 80%.

Table 2. Patient disease characteristics (n = 168).

Characteristics	Overall	High Support MSPPS > 5	Low Support MSPPS ≤ 5	*p*-Value
	N = 168 (100%)	N = 54 (32.1%)	N = 114 (68.9%)	
CAT score	12.1 ±5.7	9.2 ±5.1	13.4 ±5.4	<0.001
CAT score ≥ 10	112 (66.7)	24 (44.4)	88 (77.2)	<0.001
mMRC *				0.001
0	**28 (16.8)**	**18 (15.8)**	**10 (18.9)**	
1	**101 (60.5)**	**61 (53.5)**	**40 (75.5)**	
2	**37 (22.2)**	**34 (29.8)**	**3 (5.7)**	
3	**1 (0.6)**	**1 (0.9)**	**0 (0.0)**	
Exacerbations in the past year, n(%)				
≤1	143 (85.1)	49 (90.7)	94 (82.5)	0.159
≥2	25 (14.9)	5 (9.3)	20 (17.5)	
≥1 hospitalization	8 (4.8)	2 (3.7)	6 (5.3)	0.658
GOLD groups (n%)				
A	52 (31)	27 (50)	25 (21.9)	
B	88 (52.4)	22 (40.7)	66 (57.9)	<0.001
E	28 (16.7)	5 (9.3)	23 (20.2)	

Data are presented as mean values ± SD or median (25th–75th percentile), unless otherwise indicated; CAT: COPD Assessment Test; GOLD: Global Initiative for Chronic Obstructive Lung Disease (GOLD 2023).* None of the patients had an mMRC score of 4.

Table 3. Descriptive statistics of the MSPSS questionnaire.

	Mean ± SD	High Support MSPPS > 5 N = 54 (32.1%)	Low Support MSPPS ≤ 5 N = 114 (68.9%)	Min–Max	25th–75th Percentile
MSPSS "significant other"	4.6 (0.9)	76 (45.2)	92 (54.8)	1–7	4.3–5
MSPSS "family"	4.7 (0.9)	95 (56.5)	73 (43.5)	1–7	4.3–5
MSPSS "friends"	4.0 (1.3)	59 (35.1)	109 (64.9)	1–7	3–5
MSPSS total	4.4 (1.0)	54 (32.1)	114 (67.9)	1–7	3.8–5

3.2. Differences in Clinical Characteristics of Patients with COPD with High and Low Social Support

The application of an MPSS ≤ 5 cutoff to define low social support led to the identification of 32.1% of patients with high social support and 68.9% of patients with low social support. The clinical variables of the two groups are summarized in Tables 1 and 2. No significant differences were found in the anthropometrics and comorbidities between the groups. However, patients with lower social support had lower educational levels, were slightly older, and had worse COPD health status based on the CAT score and GOLD classification.

3.3. Correlation of Social Support with PROMs

With regard to PROMs, it is important to highlight that a substantial proportion of patients displayed elevated levels of fatigue and nighttime symptoms, as assessed using the AIS and PSQI. Furthermore, patients lacking social support exhibited the most severe functional impairments, with statistical significance observed across nearly all the questionnaires (Table 4). It is evident that individuals who lacked adequate social support experienced heightened levels of fatigue, depression, anxiety, symptoms of insomnia, and a poorer quality of sleep compared to those with high support. The ESS score did not differ between the groups. However, the mean ESS score for the entire sample was relatively low, and most of the patients who reported an ESS score > 10 were in the low social support group. Nevertheless, these differences were not statistically significant.

Table 4. Questionnaire (PROMs) scores of the 168 patients according to their social support status.

Symptoms	Overall	High Support MSPPS > 5	Low Support MSPPS ≤ 5	*p*-Value
	N = 168 (100%)	**N = 54 (32.1%)**	**N = 114 (68.9%)**	
Daytime symptoms				
Fatigue				
FSS	39.5 (27.0, 48.0)	32.0 (18.0, 43.0)	45.0 (27.0, 54.0)	<0.001
FSS ≥ 36	107 (64.5)	26 (49.1)	81 (71.7)	0.005
Daytime sleepiness				
ESS	3.0 (3.0, 9.0)	3.0 (1.5, 8.0)	3.0 (3.0, 9.0)	0.081
ESS ≥ 11	26 (15.8)	7 (13.5)	19 (16.8)	0.583
Depressive symptoms				
PHQ-9	4.0 (2.5, 8.0)	3.0 (1.0, 5.0)	5.0 (3.0, 8.0)	<0.001
PHQ-9 ≥ 10	26 (15.5)	4 (7.4)	22 (19.3)	0.047
Anxiety symptoms				
GAD-7	7.0 (3.3, 8.0)	5.0 (3.0, 7.0)	7.0 (4.0, 9.0)	0.005
GAD-7 ≥ 10	29 (17.3)	5 (9.3)	24 (21.1)	0.059
Nighttime symptoms				
PSQI	7.2 (2.9)	6.1 (2.8)	7.6 (2.8)	0.017
PSQI > 5	80 (69.0)	15 (51.7)	65 (74.7)	0.020
Insomnia symptoms				
Athens Insomnia Scale Score	8.2 (4.1)	6.2 (4.3)	9.2 (3.6)	<0.001
Athens Insomnia Scale Score ≥ 6	123 (75.5)	29 (54.7)	94 (85.5)	<0.001

After adjusting for age, gender, marital status, and level of education, it was observed that not only the total score of the MPSSP but also its individual domains displayed an inverse relationship with the CAT, FSS, PHQ-9, GAD-7, and AIS scores (Table 5). Moreover, the presence of low social support was still found to be independently associated with COPD symptoms (CAT score ≥ 10) (OR = 3.97, 95% CI 1.86–8.44; $p < 0.01$), fatigue (FSS ≥ 36) (OR = 2.74, 95% CI 1.31–5.74; $p = 0.01$), and insomnia symptoms (AIS ≥ 6) (OR = 5.17 (2.23, 12.01, 95% CI 2.23–12.01; $p < 0.01$) (Table 6). The association between low social support and the presence of depressive symptoms was close to being statistically significant (OR = 3.1, 95% CI 0.93–10.36; $p = 0.07$), possibly due to the low number of patients with a PHQ-9 score ≥10. The same principle applies to the correlation between symptoms of anxiety and a lack of social support (OR = 2.57, 95% CI 0.82–8.12; $p = 0.11$). Further adjustments for obesity and the presence of any other chronic disease resulted in similar results (Tables S1 and S2).

Table 5. Adjusted associations between perceived social support (continuous scales) and PROMs, estimated by linear regression models.

Symptoms	N [a]	MSPSS "Significant Other" (Range 1–7)		MSPSS "Family" (Range 1–7)		MSPSS "Friends" (Range 1–7)		MSPSS Total (Range 1–7)	
		Beta (95%CI)	*p*-Value	Beta (95%CI)	*p*-Value	Beta (95%CI)	*p*-Value	Beta (95%CI)	*p*-Value
CAT score	163	−0.03 (−0.06, −0.01)	0.01	−0.03 (−0.05, −0.01)	0.01	−0.03 (−0.06, 0.01)	0.10	−0.03 (−0.06, −0.01)	0.02
CAT score ≥ 10	163	−0.33 (−0.63, −0.03)	0.03	−0.32 (−0.61, −0.02)	0.04	−0.23 (−0.65, 0.2)	0.29	−0.29 (−0.6, 0.01)	0.06
mMRC	162								
1 vs. 0		0.14 (−0.26, 0.53)	0.496	0.07 (−0.32, 0.46)	0.738	0.18 (−0.36, 0.73)	0.507	0.13 (−0.27, 0.53)	0.526
2 or 3 vs. 0		−0.20 (−0.66, 0.26)	0.397	−0.11 (−0.56, 0.35)	0.644	−0.18 (−0.82, 0.47)	0.590	−0.16 (−0.63, 0.31)	0.501
Daytime symptoms									
Fatigue									
FSS (range 9–63)	161	−0.01 (−0.02, 0,00)	0.02	−0.01 (−0.02, 0,00)	0.02	−0.02 (−0.03, 0.00)	0.03	−0.01 (−0.02, 0,00)	0.01
FSS ≥ 36	161	−0.12 (−0.41, 0.18)	0.43	−0.19 (−0.48, 0.11)	0.21	−0.11 (−0.52, 0.30)	0.60	−0.14 (−0.44, 0.16)	0.37
Daytime sleepiness									
ESS (range 0–24)	160	−0.02 (−0.05, 0.01)	0.24	−0.02 (−0.05, 0.01)	0.19	−0.04 (−0.08, 0.01)	0.1	−0.03 (−0.06, 0.01)	0.12
ESS ≥ 11	160	−0.17 (−0.58, 0.24)	0.41	−0.23 (−0.63, 0.17)	0.26	−0.36 (−0.92, 0.21)	0.22	−0.25 (−0.67, 0.16)	0.23
Depressive symptoms									
PHQ-9 (range 0–27)	163	−0.05 (−0.08, −0.02)	<0.01	−0.06 (−0.09, −0.03)	<0.01	−0.07 (−0.12, −0.02)	<0.01	−0.06 (−0.09, −0.03)	<0.01
PHQ-9 ≥ 10	163	−0.52 (−0.9, −0.15)	0.01	−0.78 (−1.13, −0.42)	<0.01	−0.67 (−1.19, −0.15)	0.01	−0.66 (−1.03, −0.28)	<0.01
Anxiety symptoms									
GAD-7 (range 0–21)	163	−0.05 (−0.09, −0.02)	<0.01	−0.06 (−0.09, −0.02)	<0.01	−0.07 (−0.12, −0.02)	0.01	−0.06 (−0.1, −0.02)	<0.01
GAD-7 ≥ 10	163	−0.44 (−0.83, −0.05)	0.03	−0.4 (−0.78, −0.02)	0.04	−0.6 (−1.14, −0.06)	0.03	−0.48 (−0.87, −0.09)	0.02
Nighttime symptoms									
PSQI (range 0–21)	112	−0.01 (−0.07, 0.05)	0.78	−0.03 (−0.09, 0.04)	0.37	−0.02 (−0.11, 0.06)	0.59	−0.02 (−0.09, 0.04)	0.52
PSQI > 5	112	−0.09 (−0.5, 0.32)	0.67	−0.17 (−0.59, 0.25)	0.42	0.04 (−0.51, 0.59)	0.88	−0.07 (−0.48, 0.34)	0.73
Insomnia symptoms									
Athens Insomnia Scale Score (range 0–24)	158	−0.05 (−0.08, −0.01)	0.01	−0.05 (−0.08, −0.01)	0.01	−0.07 (−0.11, −0.02)	0.01	−0.05 (−0.09, −0.02)	<0.01
Athens Insomnia Scale Score ≥ 6	158	−0.53 (−0.85, −0.2)	<0.01	−0.47 (−0.8, −0.15)	<0.01	−0.74 (−1.2, −0.29)	<0.01	−0.58 (−0.91, −0.25)	<0.01

Effect estimates are expressed for a 1-unit increase in each of the continuous scales. All models were adjusted for the participants' age, sex, education, and marital status. [a] N represents the number of participants that had available PROM data and were included in each model.

Table 6. Adjusted associations between perceived low social support (binary variable, high support was set as the referent category) and PROMs, estimated by logistic regression models.

Symptoms	N [a]	MSPSS "Significant Other" ≤ 5 N = 92 (54.8%)		MSPSS "Family" ≤ 5 N = 73 (43.5%)		MSPSS "Friends" ≤ 5 N = 109 (64.9%)		MSPSS Total ≤ 5 N = 114 (67.9%)	
		OR (95%CI)	*p*-Value	OR (95%CI)	*p*-Value	OR (95%CI)	*p*-Value	OR (95%CI)	*p*-Value
CAT score	163	1.15 (1.07, 1.23)	<0.01	1.08 (1.02, 1.15)	<0.01	1.11 (1.04, 1.2)	0.01	1.17 (1.08, 1.27)	<0.01
CAT score ≥ 10	163	3.88 (1.86, 8.08)	<0.01	3.44 (1.55, 7.61)	<0.01	2.96 (1.4, 6.26)	0.01	3.97 (1.86, 8.44)	<0.01
mMRC	162								
1 vs. 0		1.05 (0.43, 2.59)	0.912	0.70 (0.27, 1.77)	0.449	0.80 (0.31, 2.11)		0.80 (0.31, 2.09)	0.651
2 or 3 vs. 0		2.53 (0.85, 7.54)	0.095	0.96 (0.32, 2.82)	0.935	2.58 (0.73, 9.09)	0.141	5.61 (1.28, 24.6)	0.022
Daytime symptoms									
Fatigue									
FSS (range 9–63)	161	1.04 (1.01, 1.06)	0.01	1.04 (1.01, 1.07)	0.01	1.06 (1.03, 1.09)	<0.01	1.06 (1.03, 1.09)	<0.01
FSS ≥ 36	161	1.66 (0.84, 3.27)	0.15	2.05 (0.98, 4.26)	0.06	2.4 (1.15, 5.02)	0.02	2.74 (1.31, 5.74)	0.01
Daytime sleepiness									
ESS (range 0–24)	160	1.07 (0.99, 1.16)	0.07	1.11 (1.02, 1.2)	0.01	1.12 (1.02, 1.22)	0.01	1.08 (0.99, 1.17)	0.08
ESS ≥ 11	160	1.71 (0.65, 4.46)	0.28	2.68 (1.01, 7.12)	0.05	2.57 (0.82, 8.09)	0.11	1.94 (0.64, 5.84)	0.24
Depressive symptoms									
PHQ-9 (range 0–27)	163	1.11 (1.02, 1.21)	0.02	1.15 (1.05, 1.26)	<0.01	1.17 (1.05, 1.3)	<0.01	1.19 (1.07, 1.34)	<0.01
PHQ-9 ≥ 10	163	1.64 (0.66, 4.1)	0.29	3.00 (1.18, 7.6)	0.02	1.92 (0.66, 5.61)	0.23	3.1 (0.93, 10.36)	0.07
Anxiety symptoms									
GAD-7 (range 0–21)	163	1.1 (1.01, 1.21)	0.03	1.13 (1.03, 1.23)	0.01	1.13 (1.03, 1.25)	0.01	1.12 (1.02, 1.23)	0.02
GAD-7 ≥ 10	163	1.7 (0.67, 4.34)	0.26	2.5 (0.99, 6.31)	0.05	3.09 (0.96, 9.94)	0.06	2.57 (0.82, 8.12)	0.11
Nighttime symptoms									
PSQI (range 0–21)	112	1.08 (0.93, 1.25)	0.31	1.1 (0.95, 1.27)	0.21	1.2 (1, 1.45)	0.05	1.19 (1, 1.43)	0.06
PSQI > 5	112	1.42 (0.58, 3.51)	0.45	1.18 (0.47, 2.92)	0.73	1.94 (0.71, 5.26)	0.19	2.09 (0.78, 5.64)	0.14
Insomnia symptoms									
Athens Insomnia Scale Score (range 0–24)	158	1.18 (1.07, 1.29)	<0.01	1.14 (1.04, 1.25)	<0.01	1.21 (1.09, 1.34)	<0.01	1.22 (1.1, 1.36)	<0.01
Athens Insomnia Scale Score ≥ 6	158	4.72 (2.04, 10.93)	<0.01	5.39 (2, 14.51)	<0.01	4.81 (2.06, 11.25)	<0.01	5.17 (2.23, 12.01)	<0.01

Effect estimates are expressed for a 1-unit increase in each of the continuous scales. All models were adjusted for the participants' age, sex, education, and marital status. [a] N represents the number of participants that had available PROM data and were included in each model.

4. Discussion

In the present study, we explored the link between social support and various PROMs among patients with COPD in primary care settings. Our findings indicated that a significant proportion of patients with COPD exhibited low levels of social support. Furthermore, lower levels of social support were positively associated with worse health status, increased fatigue, depression, anxiety, and symptoms of insomnia in these patients, independently of participants' age, sex, obesity, presence of chronic diseases, education, and marital status.

The average level of social support within our population, as measured by MSPSS, was 4.4, indicating a relatively lower level of support compared to the average of 5.1–5.7 among mixed COPD populations including patients with COPD [71,72] or populations with COPD and with comorbid heart failure [73] and/or other diseases [74,75]. On the other hand, our findings were similar (4.2) to a recent study focusing on COPD populations [76]. In our study, the majority of the patients with COPD lacked sufficient social support. This supports previous research showing that among those with COPD, roughly one in six patients underwent social isolation and one in five experienced feelings of loneliness [77]. Fear of being judged and experiencing social stigmatization due to visible symptoms of their disease, such as coughing and the presence of phlegm, are potential contributing factors [78]. Another important point to consider is the findings of a previous study that highlighted that patients with COPD are less likely to have a partner than non-COPD subjects [79]. Furthermore, even among COPD patients who do have a partner, they are less likely to feel "very satisfied" with the daily support provided by their partner [79]. In contrast, our analysis revealed that perceived social support from family members, the domain of family support, received the highest rating score, indicating a higher level of familial support, which is a common trait in interpersonal relationships within Greek society, particularly within Greek families [80]. After all, the Greek family is known for its strong bonds and often serves as the primary source of support and feedback, as well as acting as a protective shield during challenging times [80].

Research has indicated that social support has a significant positive effect on health-related PROMs in individuals with COPD [33]. This was also the case in our study, wherein social support exhibited a notable influence on PROMs encompassing COPD-specific health status, fatigue, mental health, and sleep health. The COPD health status of our population was characterized by a mean CAT score of 12.1, indicating a moderate impact of COPD on health. Additionally, individuals with less social support exhibited a poorer health status related to COPD, as indicated by their higher CAT scores and a greater proportion of individuals falling into GOLD classification groups B and E. These results are in line with previous studies indicating that patients with COPD with high CAT scores (worse health status) had significantly lower scores on social support scales, as evaluated by the Social Provision Scale (SPS) [81] and Social/Family Well-Being domain of the self-reported Functional Assessment of Chronic Illness Therapy-Fatigue questionnaire [82]. This is further corroborated by a recent study conducted in primary care settings, which revealed a positive correlation between CAT scores and low social support [83]. One possible explanation for this finding could be that social support might influence the psychological and physiological mechanisms related to health outcomes [84–87]. For example, it has been suggested that higher levels of social support in conjunction with the presence of the neuropeptide oxytocin could increase the cortisol levels of patients with COPD in stressful situations, such as exacerbations [84–86]. On the other hand, by reducing cortisol levels, these factors may contribute to heightened feelings of calmness and decreased anxiety during stressful situations related to COPD [84–86]. Therefore, our results indicate that respiratory-specific quality of life (as measured by the CAT) is positively linked to perceived social support.

Another crucial clinical indicator of health status among patients with COPD is fatigue, which is a complex symptom [88], influencing both physical and mental functioning, quality of life, and perceived control over life [89]. This symptom is highly prevalent, as in a previous study, it was found in nearly half of the patients diagnosed with stable, moderate-to-severe COPD [90], with a range of 17–95% in a recent review [91]. Our study's participants also exhibited a high prevalence of fatigue, with 65% of participants reporting this symptom. Moreover, individuals who reported symptoms of fatigue were 2.74 times more likely to have low social support. Although the literature does not provide sufficient evidence, previous studies have indicated that patients who have a partner experience less fatigue, whereas widowed individuals tend to experience more severe fatigue than both married and unmarried individuals [92,93]. However, fatigue is linked to more than just social support; it also affects social functioning, leading to social isolation, loneliness, and increased mental burden [89]. This finding could be explained through the social exchange theory [94]. This theory suggests that social interactions can have both positive and negative outcomes, including health-related ones [95–98]. In this case, patients with COPD could experience some of their symptoms (such as fatigue, depression, and anxiety) more intensely as a result of negative social interactions and possibly a lack of social support [82,96,99]. Therefore, more consideration should be given to social support in future research and clinical practice.

Our study found a relatively lower prevalence of depressive (15.5%) and anxiety symptoms (17.7%), thus highlighting the possibility of mental disorders being overlooked in these individuals. It is well known that individuals with COPD often experience mental health issues such as anxiety and depression, which greatly affect their overall well-being [100–102]. It is estimated that approximately 30% of people diagnosed with COPD also experience depression, and between 10% and 50% have coexisting anxiety [100,101]. More importantly, the prevalence of depression (19.3%) and anxiety (21.1%) symptoms was higher in participants with lower social support. Additionally, the higher PHQ-9 and GAD-7 scores (indicating more depressive and anxiety symptoms) showed a significant positive correlation with the presence of low social support. A possible explanation for these findings could be that social support may have the potential to augment the coping skills of patients with COPD by strengthening their ability to solve problems, stimulating greater motivation to take appropriate actions [103], and promoting their adherence to medication [24]. Consequently, our findings suggest that higher levels of social support could have a beneficial effect on mental health, particularly in patients with COPD, by helping them to better cope with their symptoms and aspects of the disease [24,103], and thus reducing the symptoms of depression and anxiety and improving their overall psychological well-being [82,104–109].

Research on the association between social support and sleep disturbances in patients with COPD is lacking, despite the extensive research conducted on the prevalence of poor sleep quality in these patients [9,14,110]. Sleep disturbances are prevalent in these patients and have been found to be associated with unfavorable clinical outcomes and reduced quality of life [14]. The results of our study indicated a high prevalence of poor sleep quality (69%) and symptoms of insomnia (75.5%), mirroring findings from prior studies [9,13,111–114]. Our study also revealed a higher prevalence of poor sleep quality and insomnia symptoms in patients with lower social support. The presence of low social support was strongly associated with insomnia symptoms, with a significant odds ratio of 5.17, even after accounting for potential confounders. However, this was not the case for sleep quality, although there was a borderline association between PSQI and MSPSS scores. Unfortunately, there is a scarcity of relevant studies supporting these results, with only one previous study demonstrating an association between being married and poor sleep quality, as assessed by PSQI [115]. Nevertheless, considering the potential importance of sleep patterns in managing COPD and overall well-being [116], there is a need for more targeted research on how social support affects sleep quality and insomnia symptoms in individuals with COPD. Conversely, our study also found a low prevalence of sleepiness in our sample, which is consistent with previous research [117–119]. In addition, we did not find any association between social support and daytime sleepiness; however, this could be explained by the small number of patients who reported sleepiness. Moreover, these findings suggest the need for further research to determine the role of social support in daytime sleepiness among these patients.

Our findings could help improve the management of patients with COPD and the development of interventions for these patients. Based on our analyses, it is evident that insufficient social support is associated with worse health outcomes, as explored using various PROMs. This could have a significant impact on the overall quality of life and well-being of patients with COPD. Especially in primary care settings where healthcare professionals have greater face-to-face interaction with patients, they have the opportunity to utilize PROMs and implement interventions that improve social support.

To the best of our knowledge, this is the first study in Greece that examines the link between social support and different PROMs, including sleep health. Moreover, to date, this study is the first to simultaneously assess all these PROMs and their relationship with the perceived social support of patients with COPD in primary care. However, our study had a few limitations. First, we utilized a cross-sectional research approach, which prevented us from establishing causal relationships between social support and PROMs. Despite the limitations in providing conclusive evidence, cross-sectional studies provide important insights into the relationships between different variables and could aid in the design of future prospective studies. Therefore, future research should employ a longitudinal approach that includes additional important measures, such as mortality rates and hospitalizations resulting from exacerbations, and overall quality of life. Second, the findings cannot be generalized due to the limited study sample, which consisted of only patients with COPD from six primary healthcare centers in Southern Greece, Crete. Third, it is difficult to compare our results with other studies that have used different methods to assess social support. Finally, the majority of the patients included in our study fell into categories A and B of the GOLD classification, while only a small number belonged to group E. This limited the applicability of our findings to populations with more severe COPD populations.

5. Conclusions

In conclusion, lower levels of social support were positively linked with several PROMs, such as worse health status, increased fatigue, depression, anxiety, and insomnia symptoms. Therefore, lower levels or a lack of social support could contribute to lower overall health among these patients. Policymakers and healthcare professionals could utilize our findings by implementing the evaluation of social support and not only the various PROMs to everyday clinical practice. Implementing this holistic approach to evaluate and improve COPD management has the potential to enhance the overall health of patients, especially in primary care settings.

Supplementary Materials: The following supporting information can be downloaded at https://www.mdpi.com/article/10.3390/healthcare12050544/s1, Table S1. Adjusted associations between perceived social support (continuous scales) and PROMs, estimated by linear regression models. Table S2. Adjusted associations between perceived low social support (binary variable, high support was set as the referent category) and PROMs, estimated by logistic regression models.

Author Contributions: Conceptualization, I.B., A.C., K.M., A.A.K. and I.T.; methodology, I.B., A.C., K.M., A.A.K. and I.T.; formal analysis, I.B. and K.M.; resources, I.B., A.C., K.M. and I.T.; writing—original draft preparation, I.B., A.C., K.M., A.A.K. and I.T.; writing—review and editing, I.B., A.C., K.M., A.A.K. and I.T.; supervision, I.T. All authors have read and agreed to the published version of the manuscript.

Funding: This research received no external funding.

Institutional Review Board Statement: The study adhered to the guidelines specified in the Declaration of Helsinki and received approval from the University of Crete Research Ethics Committee (Protocol Number: 183/13.12.2022).

Informed Consent Statement: Informed consent was obtained from all subjects involved in the study.

Data Availability Statement: The data presented in this study are available on request from the corresponding author. The data are not publicly available due to privacy restrictions.

Acknowledgments: We would like to thank all the patients with COPD for their voluntary participation.

Conflicts of Interest: The authors declare no conflicts of interest.

References

1. Soriano, J.B.; Abajobir, A.A.; Abate, K.H.; Abera, S.F.; Agrawal, A.; Ahmed, M.B.; Aichour, A.N.; Aichour, I.; Aichour, M.T.E.; Alam, K.; et al. Global, regional, and national deaths, prevalence, disability-adjusted life years, and years lived with disability for chronic obstructive pulmonary disease and asthma, 1990–2015: A systematic analysis for the Global Burden of Disease Study 2015. *Lancet Respir. Med.* **2017**, *5*, 691–706. [CrossRef] [PubMed]
2. GOLD Report. Global Strategy for Prevention, Diagnosis and Management of COPD: 2023 Report. Available online: https://goldcopd.org/2023-gold-report-2/ (accessed on 20 December 2023).
3. Lozano, R.; Naghavi, M.; Foreman, K.; Lim, S.; Shibuya, K.; Aboyans, V.; Abraham, J.; Adair, T.; Aggarwal, R.; Ahn, S.Y.; et al. Global and regional mortality from 235 causes of death for 20 age groups in 1990 and 2010: A systematic analysis for the Global Burden of Disease Study 2010. *Lancet* **2012**, *380*, 2095–2128. [CrossRef] [PubMed]
4. GOLD Report. Global Strategy for Prevention, Diagnosis and Management of COPD: 2024 Report. Available online: https://goldcopd.org/2024-gold-report/ (accessed on 24 December 2023).
5. Tzanakis, N.; Anagnostopoulou, U.; Filaditaki, V.; Christaki, P.; Siafakas, N. Prevalence of COPD in Greece. *Chest* **2004**, *125*, 892–900. [CrossRef] [PubMed]
6. Kourlaba, G.; Hillas, G.; Vassilakopoulos, T.; Maniadakis, N. The disease burden of chronic obstructive pulmonary disease in Greece. *Int. J. Chron. Obstruct Pulmon Dis.* **2016**, *11*, 2179–2189. [CrossRef] [PubMed]
7. Christenson, S.A.; Smith, B.M.; Bafadhel, M.; Putcha, N. Chronic obstructive pulmonary disease. *Lancet* **2022**, *399*, 2227–2242. [CrossRef] [PubMed]
8. Williams, V.; Bruton, A.; Ellis-Hill, C.; McPherson, K. What really matters to patients living with chronic obstructive pulmonary disease? An exploratory study. *Chron. Respir. Dis.* **2007**, *4*, 77–85. [CrossRef]
9. Agusti, A.; Hedner, J.; Marin, J.M.; Barbé, F.; Cazzola, M.; Rennard, S. Night-time symptoms: A forgotten dimension of COPD. *Eur. Respir. Rev.* **2011**, *20*, 183–194. [CrossRef]
10. Soler, X.; Siddall, J.; Small, M.; Stiegler, M.; Bogart, M. The Burden of Nocturnal Symptoms in Patients with Chronic Obstructive Pulmonary Disease: Results of a Real-World Survey in the USA. *Pulm. Ther.* **2022**, *8*, 269–282. [CrossRef]
11. Fei, F.; Koffman, J.; Zhang, X.; Gao, W. Chronic Obstructive Pulmonary Disease Symptom Cluster Composition, Associated Factors, and Methodologies: A Systematic Review. *West. J. Nurs. Res.* **2022**, *44*, 395–415. [CrossRef]
12. Ding, B.; Small, M.; Bergström, G.; Holmgren, U. A cross-sectional survey of night-time symptoms and impact of sleep disturbance on symptoms and health status in patients with COPD. *Int. J. Chron. Obstruct. Pulmon. Dis.* **2017**, *12*, 589–599. [CrossRef]
13. Budhiraja, R.; Parthasarathy, S.; Budhiraja, P.; Habib, M.P.; Wendel, C.; Quan, S.F. Insomnia in patients with COPD. *Sleep* **2012**, *35*, 369–375. [CrossRef] [PubMed]
14. Sunwoo, B.Y.; Owens, R.L. Sleep Deficiency, Sleep Apnea, and Chronic Lung Disease. *Clin. Chest Med.* **2022**, *43*, 337–352. [CrossRef]
15. van der Molen, T.; Willemse, B.W.; Schokker, S.; ten Hacken, N.H.; Postma, D.S.; Juniper, E.F. Development, validity and responsiveness of the Clinical COPD Questionnaire. *Health Qual. Life Outcomes* **2003**, *1*, 13. [CrossRef]
16. Jones, P.W.; Harding, G.; Berry, P.; Wiklund, I.; Chen, W.H.; Kline Leidy, N. Development and first validation of the COPD Assessment Test. *Eur. Respir. J.* **2009**, *34*, 648–654. [CrossRef]
17. Jones, P.W.; Quirk, F.H.; Baveystock, C.M. The St George's Respiratory Questionnaire. *Respir. Med.* **1991**, *85* Suppl. B, 25–31, discussion 33–27. [CrossRef] [PubMed]
18. Cave, A.J.; Atkinson, L.; Tsiligianni, I.G.; Kaplan, A.G. Assessment of COPD wellness tools for use in primary care: An IPCRG initiative. *Int. J. Chron. Obstruct Pulmon Dis.* **2012**, *7*, 447–456. [CrossRef] [PubMed]
19. van der Molen, T.; Diamant, Z.; Kocks, J.W.; Tsiligianni, I.G. The use of health status questionnaires in the management of chronic obstructive pulmonary disease patients in clinical practice. *Expert. Rev. Respir. Med.* **2014**, *8*, 479–491. [CrossRef]
20. Black, N. Patient reported outcome measures could help transform healthcare. *BMJ* **2013**, *346*, f167. [CrossRef]
21. Bandurska, E. The Voice of Patients Really Matters: Using Patient-Reported Outcomes and Experiences Measures to Assess Effectiveness of Home-Based Integrated Care-A Scoping Review of Practice. *Healthcare* **2022**, *11*, 98. [CrossRef]
22. Drageset, J. Social Support. In *Health Promotion in Health Care—Vital Theories and Research*; Haugan, G., Eriksson, M., Eds.; Springer International Publishing: Cham, Switzerland, 2021; pp. 137–144.
23. Rausa, B.A. Social Support. In *Encyclopedia of Aging and Public Health*; Loue, S.J.D., Sajatovic, M., Eds.; Springer US: Boston, MA, USA, 2008; pp. 751–754.
24. Shahin, W.; Kennedy, G.A.; Stupans, I. The association between social support and medication adherence in patients with hypertension: A systematic review. *Pharm. Pract.* **2021**, *19*, 2300. [CrossRef]
25. Roehrle, B.; Strouse, J. Influence of social support on success of therapeutic interventions: A meta-analytic review. *Psychotherapy* **2008**, *45*, 464–476. [CrossRef] [PubMed]

26. Bélanger, E.; Ahmed, T.; Vafaei, A.; Curcio, C.L.; Phillips, S.P.; Zunzunegui, M.V. Sources of social support associated with health and quality of life: A cross-sectional study among Canadian and Latin American older adults. *BMJ Open* **2016**, *6*, e011503. [CrossRef] [PubMed]
27. Siedlecki, K.L.; Salthouse, T.A.; Oishi, S.; Jeswani, S. The Relationship Between Social Support and Subjective Well-Being Across Age. *Soc. Indic. Res.* **2014**, *117*, 561–576. [CrossRef] [PubMed]
28. Kara Kaşikçi, M.; Alberto, J. Family support, perceived self-efficacy and self-care behaviour of Turkish patients with chronic obstructive pulmonary disease. *J. Clin. Nurs.* **2007**, *16*, 1468–1478. [CrossRef]
29. Chen, Z.; Fan, V.S.; Belza, B.; Pike, K.; Nguyen, H.Q. Association between Social Support and Self-Care Behaviors in Adults with Chronic Obstructive Pulmonary Disease. *Ann. Am. Thorac. Soc.* **2017**, *14*, 1419–1427. [CrossRef] [PubMed]
30. Lenferink, A.; van der Palen, J.; Effing, T. The role of social support in improving chronic obstructive pulmonary disease self-management. *Expert. Rev. Respir. Med.* **2018**, *12*, 623–626. [CrossRef] [PubMed]
31. Sarwar, M.R.; McDonald, V.M.; Abramson, M.J.; Paul, E.; George, J. Treatable traits in an English cohort: Prevalence and predictors of future decline in lung function and quality of life in COPD. *ERJ Open Res.* **2021**, *7*, 00934-2020. [CrossRef] [PubMed]
32. Jun, H.S.; Kang, Y. Factors contributing to chronic obstructive pulmonary disease patients' functional performance: Structural equation modelling based on theory of unpleasant symptoms. *Nurs. Open* **2023**, *10*, 3132–3144. [CrossRef]
33. Aravantinou-Karlatou, A.; Bouloukaki, I.; Christodoulakis, A.; Tsiligianni, I. The Influence of Social Support in PROMs of Patients with COPD in Primary Care: A Scoping Review. *Healthcare* **2023**, *11*, 3141. [CrossRef]
34. Zimet, G.; Dahlem, N.; Zimet, S.; Farley, G. The Multidimensional Scale of Perceived Social Support. *J. Personal. Assess.* **1988**, *52*, 30–41. [CrossRef]
35. Procedures Online. Multidimensional Scale of Percieved Social Support—Scoring Options. Available online: https://proceduresonline.com/trixcms2/media/11962/multi-dimensional-scale-of-perceived-social-support.pdf (accessed on 31 January 2024).
36. Dambi, J.M.; Corten, L.; Chiwaridzo, M.; Jack, H.; Mlambo, T.; Jelsma, J. A systematic review of the psychometric properties of the cross-cultural translations and adaptations of the Multidimensional Perceived Social Support Scale (MSPSS). *Health Qual. Life Outcomes* **2018**, *16*, 80. [CrossRef]
37. Tsilika, E.; Galanos, A.; Polykandriotis, T.; Parpa, E.; Mystakidou, K. Psychometric Properties of the Multidimensional Scale of Perceived Social Support in Greek Nurses. *Can. J. Nurs. Res.* **2019**, *51*, 23–30. [CrossRef]
38. Tsiligianni, I.G.; van der Molen, T.; Moraitaki, D.; Lopez, I.; Kocks, J.W.; Karagiannis, K.; Siafakas, N.; Tzanakis, N. Assessing health status in COPD. A head-to-head comparison between the COPD assessment test (CAT) and the clinical COPD questionnaire (CCQ). *BMC Pulm. Med.* **2012**, *12*, 20. [CrossRef]
39. Kroenke, K.; Spitzer, R.L.; Williams, J.B. The PHQ-9: Validity of a brief depression severity measure. *J. Gen. Intern. Med.* **2001**, *16*, 606–613. [CrossRef] [PubMed]
40. Spitzer, R.L.; Kroenke, K. Test Review: Patient Health Questionnaire–9 (PHQ-9). *Rehabil. Couns. Bull.* **2014**, *57*, 246–248. [CrossRef]
41. Beard, C.; Hsu, K.J.; Rifkin, L.S.; Busch, A.B.; Björgvinsson, T. Validation of the PHQ-9 in a psychiatric sample. *J. Affect. Disord.* **2016**, *193*, 267–273. [CrossRef]
42. Petersen, J.J.; Paulitsch, M.A.; Hartig, J.; Mergenthal, K.; Gerlach, F.M.; Gensichen, J. Factor structure and measurement invariance of the Patient Health Questionnaire-9 for female and male primary care patients with major depression in Germany. *J. Affect. Disord.* **2015**, *170*, 138–142. [CrossRef] [PubMed]
43. de Jonge, P.; Mangano, D.; Whooley, M.A. Differential association of cognitive and somatic depressive symptoms with heart rate variability in patients with stable coronary heart disease: Findings from the Heart and Soul Study. *Psychosom. Med.* **2007**, *69*, 735–739. [CrossRef]
44. Krause, J.S.; Reed, K.S.; McArdle, J.J. Factor structure and predictive validity of somatic and nonsomatic symptoms from the patient health questionnaire-9: A longitudinal study after spinal cord injury. *Arch. Phys. Med. Rehabil.* **2010**, *91*, 1218–1224. [CrossRef]
45. Liu, S.I.; Yeh, Z.T.; Huang, H.C.; Sun, F.J.; Tjung, J.J.; Hwang, L.C.; Shih, Y.H.; Yeh, A.W. Validation of Patient Health Questionnaire for depression screening among primary care patients in Taiwan. *Compr. Psychiatry* **2011**, *52*, 96–101. [CrossRef]
46. Yu, X.; Tam, W.W.; Wong, P.T.; Lam, T.H.; Stewart, S.M. The Patient Health Questionnaire-9 for measuring depressive symptoms among the general population in Hong Kong. *Compr. Psychiatry* **2012**, *53*, 95–102. [CrossRef]
47. Hyphantis, T.; Kotsis, K.; Voulgari, P.V.; Tsifetaki, N.; Creed, F.; Drosos, A.A. Diagnostic accuracy, internal consistency, and convergent validity of the Greek version of the patient health questionnaire 9 in diagnosing depression in rheumatologic disorders. *Arthritis Care Res.* **2011**, *63*, 1313–1321. [CrossRef]
48. Spitzer, R.L.; Kroenke, K.; Williams, J.B.; Löwe, B. A brief measure for assessing generalized anxiety disorder: The GAD-7. *Arch. Intern. Med.* **2006**, *166*, 1092–1097. [CrossRef]
49. Byrd-Bredbenner, C.; Eck, K.; Quick, V. Psychometric Properties of the Generalized Anxiety Disorder-7 and Generalized Anxiety Disorder-Mini in United States University Students. *Front. Psychol.* **2020**, *11*, 550533. [CrossRef]
50. Dhira, T.A.; Rahman, M.A.; Sarker, A.R.; Mehareen, J. Validity and reliability of the Generalized Anxiety Disorder-7 (GAD-7) among university students of Bangladesh. *PLoS ONE* **2021**, *16*, e0261590. [CrossRef]

51. Fattah, A.; Ebadi, A.; Borumand, N.; Saeedi, A.; Darbani, M.; Setayesh, S.; Mohammadi, G.; Babakhanian, M. Generalized Anxiety Disorder 7-Item Scale and Templer's Death Anxiety Scale in Iranian Inpatients with COVID-19: Evaluation of Psychometric Properties and Diagnostic Accuracy. *Middle East. J. Rehabil. Health Stud.* **2021**, *8*, e111377. [CrossRef]
52. Johnson, S.U.; Ulvenes, P.G.; Øktedalen, T.; Hoffart, A. Psychometric Properties of the General Anxiety Disorder 7-Item (GAD-7) Scale in a Heterogeneous Psychiatric Sample. *Front. Psychol.* **2019**, *10*, 1713. [CrossRef]
53. Kertz, S.; Bigda-Peyton, J.; Bjorgvinsson, T. Validity of the Generalized Anxiety Disorder-7 scale in an acute psychiatric sample. *Clin. Psychol. Psychother.* **2013**, *20*, 456–464. [CrossRef] [PubMed]
54. Lee, B.; Kim, Y.E. The psychometric properties of the Generalized Anxiety Disorder scale (GAD-7) among Korean university students. *Psychiatry Clin. Psychopharmacol.* **2019**, *29*, 864–871. [CrossRef]
55. Tiirikainen, K.; Haravuori, H.; Ranta, K.; Kaltiala-Heino, R.; Marttunen, M. Psychometric properties of the 7-item Generalized Anxiety Disorder Scale (GAD-7) in a large representative sample of Finnish adolescents. *Psychiatry Res.* **2019**, *272*, 30–35. [CrossRef] [PubMed]
56. The Patient Health Questionnaire (PHQ). Screeners Greek Version of GAD-7. Available online: https://www.phqscreeners.com/images/sites/g/files/g10060481/f/201412/GAD7_Greek%20for%20Greece.pdf (accessed on 12 December 2023).
57. Buysse, D.J.; Reynolds, C.F., 3rd; Monk, T.H.; Berman, S.R.; Kupfer, D.J. The Pittsburgh Sleep Quality Index: A new instrument for psychiatric practice and research. *Psychiatry Res.* **1989**, *28*, 193–213. [CrossRef]
58. Mystakidou, K.; Parpa, E.; Tsilika, E.; Gennatas, C.; Galanos, A.; Vlahos, L. How is sleep quality affected by the psychological and symptom distress of advanced cancer patients? *Palliat. Med.* **2009**, *23*, 46–53. [CrossRef]
59. Kotronoulas, G.C.; Papadopoulou, C.N.; Papapetrou, A.; Patiraki, E. Psychometric evaluation and feasibility of the Greek Pittsburgh Sleep Quality Index (GR-PSQI) in patients with cancer receiving chemotherapy. *Support. Care Cancer* **2011**, *19*, 1831–1840. [CrossRef]
60. Beck, S.L.; Schwartz, A.L.; Towsley, G.; Dudley, W.; Barsevick, A. Psychometric evaluation of the Pittsburgh Sleep Quality Index in cancer patients. *J. Pain. Symptom Manag.* **2004**, *27*, 140–148. [CrossRef]
61. Backhaus, J.; Junghanns, K.; Broocks, A.; Riemann, D.; Hohagen, F. Test-retest reliability and validity of the Pittsburgh Sleep Quality Index in primary insomnia. *J. Psychosom. Res.* **2002**, *53*, 737–740. [CrossRef]
62. Barbero, E.M.; Carpenter, D.M.; Maier, J.; Tseng, D.S. Healthcare Encounters for Pokemon Go: Risks and Benefits of Playing. *Games Health J.* **2018**, *7*, 157–163. [CrossRef]
63. Carpenter, J.S.; Andrykowski, M.A. Psychometric evaluation of the Pittsburgh Sleep Quality Index. *J. Psychosom. Res.* **1998**, *45*, 5–13. [CrossRef]
64. Tavakol, M.; Dennick, R. Making sense of Cronbach's alpha. *Int. J. Med. Educ.* **2011**, *2*, 53–55. [CrossRef] [PubMed]
65. Soldatos, C.R.; Dikeos, D.G.; Paparrigopoulos, T.J. Athens Insomnia Scale: Validation of an instrument based on ICD-10 criteria. *J. Psychosom. Res.* **2000**, *48*, 555–560. [CrossRef] [PubMed]
66. Jahrami, H.; Trabelsi, K.; Saif, Z.; Manzar, M.D.; BaHammam, A.S.; Vitiello, M.V. Reliability generalization meta-analysis of the Athens Insomnia Scale and its translations: Examining internal consistency and test-retest validity. *Sleep Med.* **2023**, *111*, 133–145. [CrossRef] [PubMed]
67. Johns, M.W. A new method for measuring daytime sleepiness: The Epworth sleepiness scale. *Sleep* **1991**, *14*, 540–545. [CrossRef]
68. Tsara, V.; Serasli, E.; Amfilochiou, A.; Constantinidis, T.; Christaki, P. Greek version of the Epworth Sleepiness Scale. *Sleep Breath.* **2004**, *8*, 91–95. [CrossRef]
69. Hjollund, N.H.; Andersen, J.H.; Bech, P. Assessment of fatigue in chronic disease: A bibliographic study of fatigue measurement scales. *Health Qual. Life Outcomes* **2007**, *5*, 12. [CrossRef]
70. Ferentinos, P.; Kontaxakis, V.; Havaki-Kontaxaki, B.; Dikeos, D.; Lykouras, L. Psychometric evaluation of the Fatigue Severity Scale in patients with major depression. *Qual. Life Res.* **2011**, *20*, 457–465. [CrossRef] [PubMed]
71. De Maria, M.; Vellone, E.; Durante, A.; Biagioli, V.; Matarese, M. Psychometric evaluation of the Multidimensional Scale of Perceived Social Support (MSPSS) in people with chronic diseases. *Ann. Ist. Super. Sanita* **2018**, *54*, 308–315. [CrossRef] [PubMed]
72. Bos-Touwen, I.; Schuurmans, M.; Monninkhof, E.M.; Korpershoek, Y.; Spruit-Bentvelzen, L.; Ertugrul-van der Graaf, I.; de Wit, N.; Trappenburg, J. Patient and disease characteristics associated with activation for self-management in patients with diabetes, chronic obstructive pulmonary disease, chronic heart failure and chronic renal disease: A cross-sectional survey study. *PLoS ONE* **2015**, *10*, e0126400. [CrossRef] [PubMed]
73. Bugajski, A.; Frazier, S.K.; Moser, D.K.; Lennie, T.A.; Chung, M. Psychometric testing of the Multidimensional Scale of Perceived Social Support in patients with comorbid COPD and heart failure. *Heart Lung* **2019**, *48*, 193–197. [CrossRef] [PubMed]
74. Korpershoek, Y.; Bos-Touwen, I.D.; de Man-van Ginkel, J.M.; Lammers, J.W.; Schuurmans, M.J.; Trappenburg, J. Determinants of activation for self-management in patients with COPD. *Int. J. Chron. Obstruct. Pulmon. Dis.* **2016**, *11*, 1757–1766. [CrossRef] [PubMed]
75. Moy, M.L.; Wayne, P.M.; Litrownik, D.; Beach, D.; Klings, E.S.; Davis, R.B.; Pinheiro, A.; Yeh, G.Y. Long-term Exercise After Pulmonary Rehabilitation (LEAP): A pilot randomised controlled trial of Tai Chi in COPD. *ERJ Open Res.* **2021**, *7*. [CrossRef] [PubMed]
76. Zhao, H.; Wu, B.; Kong, L.; Fan, J.; Wang, Q.; Li, J.; Mao, J. Personal Growth and Associated Factors Among Patients with Chronic Obstructive Pulmonary Disease in China: A Cross-Sectional Study. *Int. J. Chron. Obstruct. Pulmon. Dis.* **2020**, *15*, 2977–2983. [CrossRef] [PubMed]

77. Suen, A.O.; Iyer, A.S.; Cenzer, I.; Farrand, E.; White, D.B.; Singer, J.; Sudore, R.; Kotwal, A. National Prevalence of Social Isolation and Loneliness in Adults with Chronic Obstructive Pulmonary Disease. *Ann. Am. Thorac. Soc.* **2023**, *20*, 1709–1717. [CrossRef]
78. Disler, R.T.; Gallagher, R.D.; Davidson, P.M. Factors influencing self-management in chronic obstructive pulmonary disease: An integrative review. *Int. J. Nurs. Stud.* **2012**, *49*, 230–242. [CrossRef]
79. Franssen, F.M.E.; Smid, D.E.; Deeg, D.J.H.; Huisman, M.; Poppelaars, J.; Wouters, E.F.M.; Spruit, M.A. The physical, mental, and social impact of COPD in a population-based sample: Results from the Longitudinal Aging Study Amsterdam. *NPJ Prim. Care Respir. Med.* **2018**, *28*, 30. [CrossRef]
80. Tselebis, A.; Anagnostopoulou, T.; Bratis, D.; Moulou, A.; Maria, A.; Sikaras, C.; Ilias, I.; Karkanias, A.; Moussas, G.; Tzanakis, N. The 13 item Family Support Scale: Reliability and validity of the Greek translation in a sample of Greek health care professionals. *Asia Pac. Fam. Med.* **2011**, *10*, 3. [CrossRef]
81. Halding, A.G.; Grov, E.K. Self-rated health aspects among persons living with chronic obstructive pulmonary disease. *Int. J. Chron. Obstruct. Pulmon. Dis.* **2017**, *12*, 1163–1172. [CrossRef] [PubMed]
82. Turnier, L.; Eakin, M.; Woo, H.; Dransfield, M.; Parekh, T.; Krishnan, J.A.; Kanner, R.; Cooper, C.B.; Woodruff, P.G.; Wise, R.; et al. The influence of social support on COPD outcomes mediated by depression. *PLoS ONE* **2021**, *16*, e0245478. [CrossRef]
83. Nkhoma, K.B.; Farrant, L.; Mzimkulu, O.; Hunter, J.; Higginson, I.; Gao, W.; Maddocks, M.; Gwyther, L.; Harding, R. High Prevalence and Burden of Physical and Psychological Symptoms in a Chronic Obstructive Pulmonary Disease Population in Primary Care Settings in South Africa. *Int. J. Chron. Obstruct. Pulmon. Dis.* **2023**, *18*, 1665–1679. [CrossRef] [PubMed]
84. Roberts, M.H.; Klatzkin, R.R.; Mechlin, B. Social Support Attenuates Physiological Stress Responses and Experimental Pain Sensitivity to Cold Pressor Pain. *Ann. Behav. Med.* **2015**, *49*, 557–569. [CrossRef] [PubMed]
85. Ozbay, F.; Johnson, D.C.; Dimoulas, E.; Morgan, C.A.; Charney, D.; Southwick, S. Social support and resilience to stress: From neurobiology to clinical practice. *Psychiatry* **2007**, *4*, 35–40.
86. Heinrichs, M.; Baumgartner, T.; Kirschbaum, C.; Ehlert, U. Social support and oxytocin interact to suppress cortisol and subjective responses to psychosocial stress. *Biol. Psychiatry* **2003**, *54*, 1389–1398. [CrossRef]
87. Gryksa, K.; Neumann, I.D. Consequences of pandemic-associated social restrictions: Role of social support and the oxytocin system. *Psychoneuroendocrinology* **2022**, *135*, 105601. [CrossRef]
88. Lee, J.E.; Nguyen, H.Q.; Fan, V.S. Inflammatory Markers and Fatigue in Individuals With Moderate to Severe Chronic Obstructive Pulmonary Disease. *Nurs. Res.* **2024**, *73*, 54–61. [CrossRef]
89. Kouijzer, M.; Brusse-Keizer, M.; Bode, C. COPD-related fatigue: Impact on daily life and treatment opportunities from the patient's perspective. *Respir. Med.* **2018**, *141*, 47–51. [CrossRef]
90. Peters, J.B.; Heijdra, Y.F.; Daudey, L.; Boer, L.M.; Molema, J.; Dekhuijzen, P.N.; Schermer, T.R.; Vercoulen, J.H. Course of normal and abnormal fatigue in patients with chronic obstructive pulmonary disease, and its relationship with domains of health status. *Patient Educ. Couns.* **2011**, *85*, 281–285. [CrossRef]
91. Ebadi, Z.; Goërtz, Y.M.J.; Van Herck, M.; Janssen, D.J.A.; Spruit, M.A.; Burtin, C.; Thong, M.S.Y.; Muris, J.; Otker, J.; Looijmans, M.; et al. The prevalence and related factors of fatigue in patients with COPD: A systematic review. *Eur. Respir. Rev.* **2021**, *30*, 200298. [CrossRef]
92. Goërtz, Y.M.J.; Spruit, M.A.; Van't Hul, A.J.; Peters, J.B.; Van Herck, M.; Nakken, N.; Djamin, R.S.; Burtin, C.; Thong, M.S.Y.; Coors, A.; et al. Fatigue is highly prevalent in patients with COPD and correlates poorly with the degree of airflow limitation. *Ther. Adv. Respir. Dis.* **2019**, *13*, 1753466619878128. [CrossRef]
93. Karakurt, P.; Ünsal, A. Fatigue, anxiety and depression levels, activities of daily living of patients with chronic obstructive pulmonary disease. *Int. J. Nurs. Pract.* **2013**, *19*, 221–231. [CrossRef]
94. Homans, G.C. Social behavior as exchange. *Am. J. Sociol.* **1958**, *63*, 597–606. [CrossRef]
95. Ahmad, R.; Nawaz, M.R.; Ishaq, M.I.; Khan, M.M.; Ashraf, H.A. Social exchange theory: Systematic review and future directions. *Front. Psychol.* **2022**, *13*, 1015921. [CrossRef] [PubMed]
96. Eidelman, P.; Jensen, A.; Rappaport, L.M. Social support, negative social exchange, and response to case formulation-based cognitive behavior therapy. *Cogn. Behav. Ther.* **2019**, *48*, 146–161. [CrossRef] [PubMed]
97. Cropanzano, R.; Mitchell, M.S. Social Exchange Theory: An Interdisciplinary Review. *J. Manag.* **2005**, *31*, 874–900. [CrossRef]
98. Umberson, D.; Montez, J.K. Social relationships and health: A flashpoint for health policy. *J. Health Soc. Behav.* **2010**, *51*, S54–S66. [CrossRef] [PubMed]
99. Grey, I.; Arora, T.; Thomas, J.; Saneh, A.; Tohme, P.; Abi-Habib, R. The role of perceived social support on depression and sleep during the COVID-19 pandemic. *Psychiatry Res.* **2020**, *293*, 113452. [CrossRef] [PubMed]
100. Pollok, J.; van Agteren, J.E.; Esterman, A.J.; Carson-Chahhoud, K.V. Psychological therapies for the treatment of depression in chronic obstructive pulmonary disease. *Cochrane Database Syst. Rev.* **2019**, *3*, Cd012347. [CrossRef] [PubMed]
101. Yohannes, A.M.; Alexopoulos, G.S. Depression and anxiety in patients with COPD. *Eur. Respir. Rev.* **2014**, 23, 345–349. [CrossRef] [PubMed]
102. Pollok, J.; van Agteren, J.E.; Carson-Chahhoud, K.V. Pharmacological interventions for the treatment of depression in chronic obstructive pulmonary disease. *Cochrane Database Syst. Rev.* **2018**, *12*, Cd012346. [CrossRef] [PubMed]
103. Paek, S.; Lee, K.; Um, Y.-J.; Koo, H.-Y.; Park, S.-Y.; Ryou, I. Influence of Social Support and Patient Activation Measure, Perceived by Chronic Patients Over Age 65 in Medical Center, to Quality of Life. *Korean J. Fam. Pract.* **2018**, *8*, 493–498. [CrossRef]

104. Ghaemi Kerahrodi, J.; Brähler, E.; Wiltink, J.; Michal, M.; Schulz, A.; Wild, P.S.; Münzel, T.; Toenges, G.; Lackner, K.J.; Pfeiffer, N.; et al. Association between medicated obstructive pulmonary disease, depression and subjective health: Results from the population-based Gutenberg Health Study. *Sci. Rep.* **2019**, *9*, 20252. [CrossRef]
105. Arabyat, R.M.; Raisch, D.W. Relationships Between Social/Emotional Support and Quality of Life, Depression and Disability in Patients With Chronic Obstructive Pulmonary Disease: An Analysis Based on Propensity Score Matching. *Ann. Behav. Med.* **2019**, *53*, 918–927. [CrossRef]
106. Keil, D.C.; Vaske, I.; Kenn, K.; Rief, W.; Stenzel, N.M. With the strength to carry on. *Chron. Respir. Dis.* **2017**, *14*, 11–21. [CrossRef]
107. Fuller-Thomson, E.; Lacombe-Duncan, A. Understanding the Association Between Chronic Obstructive Pulmonary Disease and Current Anxiety: A Population-Based Study. *Copd* **2016**, *13*, 622–631. [CrossRef] [PubMed]
108. Dinicola, G.; Julian, L.; Gregorich, S.E.; Blanc, P.D.; Katz, P.P. The role of social support in anxiety for persons with COPD. *J. Psychosom. Res.* **2013**, *74*, 110–115. [CrossRef] [PubMed]
109. Lee, H.; Yoon, J.Y.; Kim, I.; Jeong, Y.H. The effects of personal resources and coping strategies on depression and anxiety in patients with chronic obstructive pulmonary disease. *Heart Lung* **2013**, *42*, 473–479. [CrossRef]
110. Omachi, T.A.; Blanc, P.D.; Claman, D.M.; Chen, H.; Yelin, E.H.; Julian, L.; Katz, P.P. Disturbed sleep among COPD patients is longitudinally associated with mortality and adverse COPD outcomes. *Sleep Med.* **2012**, *13*, 476–483. [CrossRef]
111. Sampol, J.; Miravitlles, M.; Sáez, M.; Pallero, M.; Sampol, G.; Ferrer, J. Poor sleep quality, COPD severity and survival according to CASIS and Pittsburgh questionnaires. *Sci. Rep.* **2023**, *13*, 18656. [CrossRef] [PubMed]
112. Sowho, M.O.; Koch, A.L.; Putcha, N.; Woo, H.; Gassett, A.; Paulin, L.M.; Koehler, K.; Barr, R.G.; Comellas, A.P.; Cooper, C.B.; et al. Ambient Air Pollution Exposure and Sleep Quality in COPD. *Chronic Obstr. Pulm. Dis.* **2023**, *10*, 102–111. [CrossRef]
113. Baugh, A.; Buhr, R.G.; Quibrera, P.; Barjaktarevic, I.; Barr, R.G.; Bowler, R.; Han, M.K.; Kaufman, J.D.; Koch, A.L.; Krishnan, J.; et al. Risk of COPD exacerbation is increased by poor sleep quality and modified by social adversity. *Sleep* **2022**, *45*, zsac107. [CrossRef]
114. Kauffman, K.S.; Doede, M.; Diaz-Abad, M.; Scharf, S.M.; Bell-Farrell, W.; Rogers, V.E.; Geiger-Brown, J. Experience of insomnia, symptom attribution and treatment preferences in individuals with moderate to severe COPD: A qualitative study. *Patient Prefer. Adherence* **2014**, *8*, 1699–1704. [CrossRef]
115. Aldabayan, Y.S. Mental health and sleep quality among patients with asthma and COPD. *Front Med.* **2023**, *10*, 1181742. [CrossRef]
116. Lewthwaite, H.; Effing, T.W.; Olds, T.; Williams, M.T. Physical activity, sedentary behaviour and sleep in COPD guidelines: A systematic review. *Chron. Respir. Dis.* **2017**, *14*, 231–244. [CrossRef]
117. Enz, C.; Brighenti-Zogg, S.; Steveling-Klein, E.H.; Dürr, S.; Maier, S.; Miedinger, D.; Leuppi, J.D. Predictors of Increased Daytime Sleepiness in Patients with Chronic Obstructive Pulmonary Disease: A Cross-Sectional Study. *Sleep Disord.* **2016**, *2016*, 1089196. [CrossRef] [PubMed]
118. Chen, R.; Tian, J.W.; Zhou, L.Q.; Chen, X.; Yan, H.Y.; Zeng, B.; Zhang, M.S. The relationship between sleep quality and functional exercise capacity in COPD. *Clin. Respir. J.* **2016**, *10*, 477–485. [CrossRef] [PubMed]
119. Zohal, M.A.; Yazdi, Z.; Kazemifar, A.M.; Mahjoob, P.; Ziaeeha, M. Sleep Quality and Quality of Life in COPD Patients with and without Suspected Obstructive Sleep Apnea. *Sleep Disord.* **2014**, *2014*, 508372. [CrossRef] [PubMed]

healthcare

MDPI

Article

A Cross-Sectional, Multicentric, Disease-Specific, Health-Related Quality of Life Study in Greek Transfusion Dependent Thalassemia Patients

Philippos Klonizakis [1,*], Noémi Roy [2], Ioanna Papatsouma [3], Maria Mainou [1], Ioanna Christodoulou [1], Despina Pantelidou [4], Smaro Kokkota [4], Michael Diamantidis [5], Alexandra Kourakli [6], Vasileios Lazaris [6], Dimitrios Andriopoulos [7], Apostolos Tsapas [8], Robert J. Klaassen [9] and Efthymia Vlachaki [1]

1 Adults Thalassemia Unit—2nd Department of Internal Medicine, Aristotle University, Hippokration General Hospital Thessaloniki, 54642 Thessaloniki, Greece; mfcmary@hotmail.com (M.M.); ioannchrist@auth.gr (I.C.); efivlachaki@yahoo.gr (E.V.)
2 Department of Haematology, Oxford University Hospitals, NHS Foundation Trust, Oxford OX3 0AG, UK; noemi.roy@ouh.nhs.uk
3 Department of Mathematics, Imperial College London, London SW7 2BP, UK; i.papatsouma@imperial.ac.uk
4 Thalassemia Unit, AHEPA General Hospital of Thessaloniki, 54636 Thessaloniki, Greece; dpantelidou@yahoo.gr (D.P.); smaro_kokkota@hotmail.com (S.K.)
5 Thalassemia and Sickle Cell Disease Unit, General Hospital of Larissa, 41110 Larissa, Greece; diamantidis76@gmail.com
6 Thalassemia and Hemoglobinopathies Center, University Hospital of Patras, 26504 Patras, Greece; akourakli@gmail.com (A.K.); vlazaris@gmail.com (V.L.)
7 Haemato-Oncology Department, Royal Marsden Hospital NHS Foundation Trust, London SW3 6JJ, UK; dimitrios.andriopoulos@rmh.nhs.uk
8 2nd Department of Internal Medicine, Aristotle University, Hippokration General Hospital of Thessaloniki, 54642 Thessaloniki, Greece
9 Department of Pediatrics, Division of Hematology/Oncology, University of Ottawa, Children's Hospital of Eastern Ontario, Ottawa, ON K1H 8L1, Canada; rklaassen@cheo.on.ca
* Correspondence: philklon@gmail.com; Tel.: +30-2310892003

Abstract: The assessment of health-related quality of life (HRQoL) in thalassemia offers a holistic approach to the disease and facilitates better communication between physicians and patients. This study aimed to evaluate the HRQoL of transfusion-dependent thalassemia (TDT) patients in Greece. This was a multicentric, cross-sectional study conducted in 2017 involving 283 adult TDT patients. All participants completed a set of two QoL questionnaires, the generic SF-36v2 and the disease-specific TranQol. Demographic and clinical characteristics were used to predefine patient subgroups. Significant factors identified in the univariate analysis were entered into a multivariate analysis to assess their effect on HRQoL. The SF-36 scores of TDT patients were consistently lower compared to the general population in Greece. The mean summary score of TranQol was relatively high (71 ± 14%), exceeding levels observed in national surveys in other countries. Employment emerged as the most significant independent factor associated with better HRQoL, whereas age had the most significant negative effect. This study represents the first comprehensive QoL assessment of a representative sample of the TDT population in Greece. The implementation of TranQol allowed for the quantification of HRQoL in Greece, establishing a baseline for future follow-up, and identifying more vulnerable patient subgroups.

Keywords: Transfusion-Dependent Thalassemia; health-related quality of life; patient reported outcomes; disease-specific TranQol questionnaire; healthcare policy; Thalassemia infrastructure

1. Introduction

Transfusion-dependent β-thalassemia (TDT) is a congenital disease characterized by reduced or no production of hemoglobin, leading to chronic anemia and necessitating lifelong blood transfusions [1]. During the last decades, TDT has gradually transformed from a life-threatening disorder into a chronic disease. The significant increase in survival rates has been attributed to the implementation of safe and systematic blood transfusions, the development of three effective iron chelators, and the guided follow-up of patients in well-organized thalassemia units. Nevertheless, the patients still confront the burden of the disease, which affects their functional status and health-related quality of life (HRQoL).

There is still an unmet need for a more holistic approach to assessing and managing health in thalassemia, aligning with the World Health Organization's definition, which emphasizes that "health is a state of complete physical, mental, and social well-being and not merely the absence of disease". The concept of HRQoL encompasses dimensions of life beyond traditional health indicators and can be delineated as "those aspects of self-perceived well-being that are related to or affected by the presence of disease or treatment" [2]. By measuring HRQoL in thalassemia, a comprehensive understanding of the disease burden emerges, facilitating improved communication among healthcare providers, patients, and their families [3]. Emerging research indicates that psychological well-being may serve as a protective factor against chronic physical ailments and promote longevity [4,5]. Consequently, the assessment of HRQoL has become a pivotal endpoint in the majority of clinical trials involving evolving treatments or interventions [6–9]. Especially in countries with a high prevalence of thalassemia, evaluating HRQoL status can inform and enhance social and healthcare policies, fostering better support for affected populations.

HRQoL can be assessed with quality of life (QoL) questionnaires completed by the patients themselves, constituting a prevalent form of patient reported outcome (PRO) [10]. Globally, very few reports have adequately addressed the HRQoL of adult thalassemia patients, with the majority utilizing the generic SF-36 questionnaire [11–15]. While generic QoL questionnaires facilitate comparisons with the general population, they may lack sensitivity for discerning QoL disparities among patient subgroups or evaluating intervention outcomes. In 2014, Klaassen et al. developed the TranQol, a disease-specific QoL questionnaire for TDT patients [16]. The conceptual framework for this new measure aims to comprehensively capture HRQoL dimensions in TDT patients, including social, emotional, and physical well-being domains [17]. The translated versions of TranQol, including the Greek adaptation, are actively utilized in international thalassemia clinical trials, such as the recently published phase 3 BELIEVE trial of Luspatercept [18]. However, real-world data regarding TranQol implementation beyond clinical trial settings remains limited.

Greece is among the countries with a high prevalence of TDT, with 19.4 cases per 100,000 individuals recorded from 2010 to 2015 [19]. However, there remains a dearth of evidence concerning disease-specific QoL among representative samples of the TDT patient population. In 2012, Lyrakos et al. developed and evaluated the psychometric properties of the Specific Thalassemia Quality of Life Instrument (STQOLI) to assess HRQoL in TDT patients [20]. Nevertheless, this instrument saw limited utilization in subsequent QoL studies, both within Greece and internationally. In all other studies involving Greek TDT patients, only generic questionnaires were employed among small patient cohorts, focusing on restricted domains of HRQoL, such as mental health and satisfaction with iron chelation therapy [12,21]. However, in 2017, the successful validation of the Greek version of TranQol offered the potential for a comprehensive and disease-specific assessment of HRQoL in TDT patients [22].

In this cross-sectional, multicentric study, our primary endpoint was to evaluate HRQoL in a representative cohort of Greek patients with TDT. This assessment involved employing both the generic SF-36v2 and the disease-specific TranQol questionnaire. The secondary endpoint was to investigate disparities in HRQoL among predefined patient subgroups, utilizing the high sensitivity of the disease-specific TranQol questionnaire. We hypothesized that various sociodemographic and clinical factors would exert an influence on the HRQoL of TDT patients in Greece. This research represents the inaugural examination of HRQoL, utilizing a combination of a generic and Thalassemia-specific questionnaire within a representative sample of TDT patients in Greece. The outcomes of this study are anticipated to establish a foundational benchmark for HRQoL, which can inform ongoing and forthcoming clinical trials involving TDT patients. Furthermore, our findings have the potential to highlight particularly vulnerable subgroups within the TDT patient population and contribute significantly to understanding the impact of the disease and available interventions on HRQoL.

2. Materials and Methods

2.1. Study Design and Setting

This was a cross-sectional, multicentric study in a population of adult TDT patients that took place from October to December 2017. All patients were systematically transfused and closely monitored at four well-organized thalassemia units in Greece. The study sites were all located in urban areas of Greece and involved the adult Thalassemia Unit of the Second Department of Internal Medicine, Aristotle University, Hippokration General Hospital of Thessaloniki, the Thalassemia Unit of the AHEPA General Hospital of Thessaloniki, the Thalassemia and Sickle Cell Disease Unit of the General Hospital of Larissa, and the Thalassemia Unit of the University Hospital of Patras. We evaluated HRQoL using a comprehensive approach that combined two distinct quality-of-life assessment tools. Firstly, we utilized the generic Greek SF-36v2 [23], which measures both physical and mental QoL domains. This allowed for comparisons of HRQoL between our study TDT patients and the general population. Secondly, we employed the validated Greek version of the disease-specific TranQol questionnaire [22]. This instrument is more sensitive in revealing differences among patient subgroups and offers a detailed evaluation of overall HRQoL and its five subdomains: physical health (PH), emotional health (EH), sexual health (SH), family functioning (FF), and school and career functioning (SCF).

2.2. Inclusion and Exclusion Criterion

The participants were selected according to predefined and specific inclusion and exclusion criteria. Briefly, the participants were aged 18 years and older, had a confirmed diagnosis of transfusion-dependent beta-thalassemia, and had efficient reading and writing skills without significant intellectual or sensory disorders. We excluded patients who were participating in a clinical trial, were pregnant, or had been recently hospitalized on the grounds of avoiding factors that could cause any transient change in the participants' QoL.

2.3. Sampling and Sample Size

To reflect real life and avoid selection bias, all TDT patients from each thalassemia unit were invited consecutively. During their routine transfusion visit, we asked the participants to complete the two quality-of-life questionnaires, SF-36v2 and TranQol. In terms of the study's secondary endpoint, we prespecified patient subgroups that might have different QoL according to clinical, demographic, and socioeconomic status. Thus, we looked for differences between age groups, gender, family structures, educational backgrounds, working status, comorbidities, types of iron chelation therapy, and hemosiderosis status. We used the MRI T_2* examination, a standard of care for all the participating thalassemia units, to assess iron overload status and define patients with no heart or no hepatic iron overload (heart $T_2^* > 20$ ms and liver iron concentration (LIC) ≤ 3 mg Fe/g dry weight, respectively) [1,24]. All data were retrieved from the patients' medical records, and the variables collected are listed in Table 1.

We determined the study population sample size according to the study's primary aim, which was to evaluate HRQoL in the Greek TDT patient population. A representative sample was estimated to be 242 patients for the total 2099 TDT population in Greece [19], with a 90% confidence interval and a 5% margin of error [25]. The total study population was set to be at least 403 patients, taking into account a 40% nonresponse rate and a minimum 60% response rate (RR), respectively (definition proposed by the American Association of Public Opinion Research, AAPOR RR6) [26,27]. We set the power to 0.8 (80%) and a 5% significance level to have a high probability of detecting a minimal clinically important difference (MCID) between patient subgroups in terms of the secondary endpoint of the study. The minimal sample size was estimated to be 64 patients for each subgroup [25]. A minimal clinically important difference (MCID) in SF-36v2 and TranQol scores was defined according to Norman et al. [28], who suggested that the value of half a standard deviation (0.5 × SD) of baseline scores can serve as a default value for important patient-perceived change on QoL measures used with patients with chronic diseases. In this study, the MCID was calculated from the half a standard deviation (0.5 × SD) of previously published SF-36v2 and TranQol scores, in a survey of 94 Greek TDT patients (Table 2) [22].

Table 1. Sociodemographic and clinical characteristics of the study population.

Characteristics	Parameter Value
Sex, N (%)	
Male	110 (39)
Female	165 (58)
NA	11 (4)
Age, mean ± SD (range) years	39 ± 9 (18–68)
Age Groups N (%)	
Under 25 yrs	20 (8)
26–35 yrs	70 (27)
36–45 yrs	115 (44)
46–55 yrs	41 (16)
Above 56	14 (5)
NA	26 (9)
Marital status	
Single	143 (54)
Married	124 (46)
NA	19 (7)
Offsprings, N (%)	
Yes	114 (42)
No	156 (58)
NA	15 (5)
Educational Level, N (%)	
Basic	38 (23)
Higher	127 (77)
NA	121 (42)
Employment Status, N (%)	
Unemployed	110 (41)
Employed	158 (59)
NA	18 (6)
Co-Morbidities, Yes N (%)	
No	89 (31)
Yes	191 (68)
Splenectomy	82 (29)
Osteoporosis	112 (39)
Hypothyroidism	74 (26)
Hypogonadism	76 (27)
Diabetes	19 (7)
NA	6 (2)
Type of Chelator N (%)	
Deferasirox	90 (35)
Deferoxamine	52 (20)
Deferiprone	15 (6)
Deferoxamine/Deferiprone	99 (39)
Abnormal Liver MRI T_2 * N (%)	101 (39)
Abnormal Heart MRI T_2 * N (%)	20 (7)

Abbreviations: MRI T_2*; T_2 Star Magnetic Resonance Imaging pulse sequence.

Table 2. TranQol and SF-36v2 scores in transfusion-dependent thalassemia patients and Minimal Clinically Important Difference values.

Quality of Life Questionnaires		Scores% (Mean ± SD)	MCID (0.5 × SD *) [2]
SF-36v2 [1]	Physical Functioning	50 ± 7	≥8
	Role-Physical	50 ± 9	≥11
	Bodily Pain	52 ± 10	≥10
	General Health	46 ± 10	≥12
	Vitality	54 ± 9	≥11
	Social Functioning	50 ± 8	≥9
	Role Emotional	47 ± 10	≥11
	Mental Health	48 ± 9	≥9
	Physical Component Summary	51 ± 8	≥5
	Mental Component Summary	49 ± 9	≥5
TranQol [1]	Physical Health	71 ± 15	≥7
	Emotional Health	68 ± 17	≥8
	Sexual Health	78 ± 21	≥16
	Family Functioning	75 ± 17	≥10
	School and Career	76 ± 21	≥12
	Summary	71 ± 14	≥6

The table reports the TranQol and SF-36v2 summary and subdomain scores in the study population and the corresponding minimal clinically important difference values. TranQol©: Transfusion-dependent quality of life (Children's Hospital of Eastern Ontario, Laurentian University, and The Hospital for Sick Children, 2013); SF-36®: Short-Form Health Survey 36 version 2 (Medical Outcomes Trust). [1] The TranQol and SF-36 questionnaires are scored on a 0 (poor) to 100 (good health) scale. MCID: Minimal clinically important difference, defined according to Norman et al. [28], who suggested that the value of half a standard deviation (0.5 × SD) of baseline scores can serve as a default value for important patient-perceived change on QoL measures used with patients with chronic diseases. [2] (0.5 × SD *): calculated 0.5 × SD on previously published TranQol and SF-36v2 scores in TDT patients.

2.4. Statistical Tools

We analyzed qualitative and quantitative variables descriptively, with qualitative data presented as frequencies and quantitative data as mean ± standard deviation (SD). We calculated TranQol scores from a mathematical equation provided by the developers [16] and the SF-36 scores from the QualityMetric Health Outcomes™ Scoring Software 4.5 [29]. Higher scores on both questionnaires indicate better QoL (0 indicates the worst possible health state, and 100 indicates the best health state). The TranQol and SF-36 were considered complete if ≥75% and ≥50% of the questionnaire items were answered, respectively [16,30] We used the "$\frac{1}{2}$ SD method", a distribution-based approach that has been developed to define clinically meaningful differences in each QoL questionnaire score [28]. Any differences of 0.5 × SD on previously published TranQol and SF-36v2 scores were considered clinically significant [22]. We performed univariate linear regression analysis to assess the association between independent variables (age, gender, working status, educational status, marital status, offspring, heart and liver MRI T_2* status, co-morbidities, and type of chelation therapy) and TranQol summary and subdomain scores. We used a less-restrictive α-level of 0.2 in univariate linear regression analysis to identify a broad range of factors that would be retained as candidate variables in the next step of multivariate analysis. We conducted stepwise regression to select the most parsimonious models of independent explanatory factors that may be associated with overall and subdomain QoL status, after adjusting for confounding factors. We employed a less restrictive alpha level of 0.1 to identify a broader range of independent factors, indicating statistical trends for values where $0.05 < p < 0.10$. The multivariate analysis data were checked and met the assumptions of homogeneity of variance and linearity, and the residuals were approximately normally distributed. For each of the significant predictors, we estimated the regression coefficients (B) and their 95% confidence intervals. The data were analyzed using IBM SPSS version 27.0 (IBM Corp., Armonk, NY, USA).

2.5. Ethical Considerations

The study was approved by the Ethics Committee, and written informed consent was obtained from each patient.

3. Results

3.1. Sociodemographic and Clinical Characteristics of Study Participants

A total of 474 adult TDT patients were screened from four thalassemia units, of which 286 (60%) met eligibility criteria and consented to participate in the study. The primary reason for exclusion was patient refusal, accounting for 22% of those screened. Additionally, 10% of patients were excluded for not meeting the study's inclusion/exclusion criteria, whereas no reason was recorded for the remaining 8% of patients who were not recruited. The response rates of the patients who completed the SF-36v2 ($\geq$50% items) and the TranQol ($\geq$75% items) questionnaires were 61% (n = 227) and 66% (n = 283), respectively (Figure 1 flow diagram). The sociodemographic and clinical characteristics of the study population are summarized in Table 1. The participants' mean $\pm$ SD age was 39 $\pm$ 9 years (range:18–68), and 58% were female. Almost half of the study population were married (46%) and had offspring (42%). Most participants had a higher educational level (77%), and 59% were employed. Among the participants with a history of co-morbidity (68%), the most frequent disorder was osteoporosis (39%). Regarding chelation therapy, Deferasirox monotherapy (35%) or the combination of Deferoxamine/Deferiprone (39%) were the two most frequently used iron chelating regimens. Only 7% of the participants had an abnormal heart MRI T_2*, whereas 39% of the participants had an abnormal liver MRI T_2*.

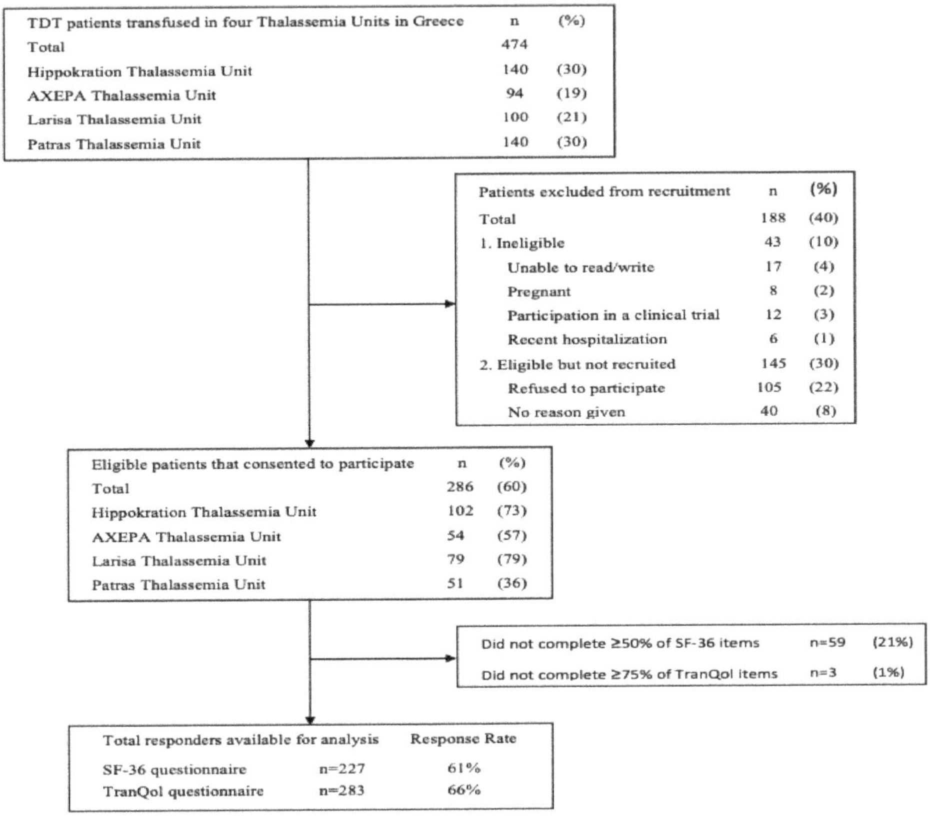

Figure 1. Flow diagram of participants and response rate.

The Response Rate 6 definition proposed by the American Association of Public Opinion Research (AAPOR) was used to calculate response rates.

3.2. Health-Related Quality of Life in Transfusion-Dependent Thalassemia Patients

The TranQol and SF-36 summary and subdomain scores in the study population are reported in Table 2. The overall mean ± SD TranQol summary score was 71 ± 14%, and the overall mean ± SD of SF-36v2 PCS and MCS scores were 51 ± 8% and 49 ± 9%, respectively. In the same table, we report the SF-36v2 and TranQol MCID values that represent a threshold for meaningful changes in each questionnaire's score. In Figure 2, we present the comparison of HRQoL between TDT patients and the general population. The SF-36 subdomain scores from our survey of TDT patients were substantially lower compared to the only available data on SF-36 scores in the general Greek population, published in 2005 [23], and the differences were clinically important (>MCID). On the other hand, the TranQol scores from our survey were higher compared to national surveys in the United Kingdom [31], Canada [16], and Peshawar, Pakistan [32], and the differences in TranQol summary and most subdomain scores were clinically important (Figure 3).

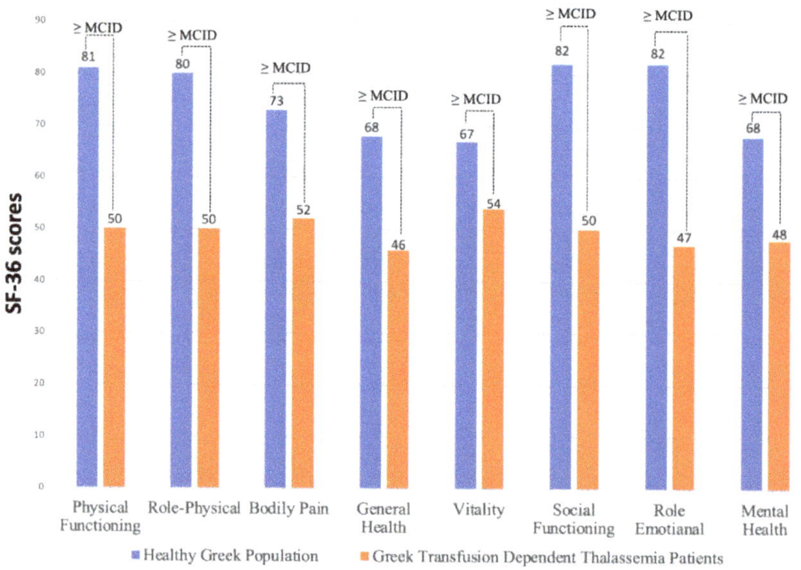

MCID: Minimal Clinically Important Difference; SF-36®: Short-Form Health Survey 36 (Medical Outcomes Trust).

Figure 2. Comparison of the SF-36 scores between the present study and the study in the general Greek population provided by Pappa et al. The bar charts depict the differences in the mean scores between the two studies. The minimal clinical important difference (MCID), defined as the 0.5 × SD on previously reported SF-36v2 scores in TDT patients, was used as a threshold value to demonstrate clinically meaningful differences in QoL between the general population and TDT patients.

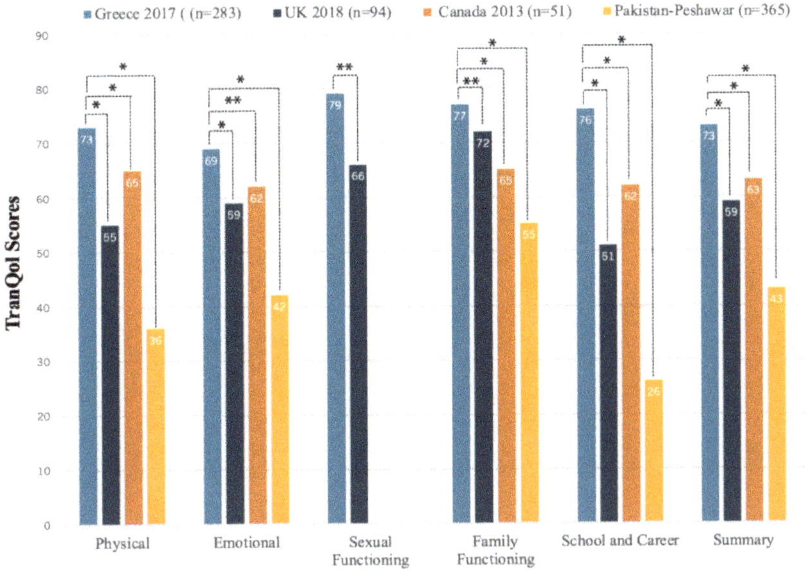

*: Clinically important difference. **: Not clinically important difference. TranQol©: Transfusion-dependent quality of life (Children's Hospital of Eastern Ontario, Laurentian University and The Hospital for Sick Children, 2013).

Figure 3. The TranQol summary and subdomain scores from national surveys conducted in different countries are compared and visually represented using different colored bars. We used the minimal clini-cal important difference (MCID), defined as the 0.5 × SD on previously reported TranQol scores in TDT pa-tients, as a threshold value to demonstrate clinically meaningful differences in HRQoL between national surveys in different countries.

3.3. Factors That Influence Health-Related Quality of Life among TDT Patients

In terms of statistical trends, the factors that were associated with summary TranQol scores in univariate regression analysis included age (B = −0.3, 95% CI −0.5,−0.2), marriage (B = −3.2, 95% CI −6.5,0.2), employment (B = 7.5, 95% CI 4.2,10.7), higher education (B = 4.2, 95% CI 0.4,7.9), comorbidities (B = −5.1, 95% CI −8.6,1.6), iron chelation with Deferasirox compared to Deferoxamine monotherapy (B = 4.1, 95% CI −0.4,8.5), and abnormal liver MRI T2* (B = 3.2, 95% CI −0.3,6.7) (Table 3). Abnormal heart MRI T2* (B = −2.6, 95% CI −8.4,3.3) was negatively associated only with the physical subdomain. Female gender exhibited a significant association with higher scores in family functioning (B = 4.5, 95% CI 0.2,8.6) and school and career (B = 7.2, 95% CI 1.9,12.5) subdomains. In multivariate regression analysis (Table 4), age, female gender, employment, and iron chelation with Deferasirox compared to Deferoxamine monotherapy were the independent factors that significantly influenced HRQoL, after adjusting for confounding factors. Based on the multivariate model, there was on average a decrease of 0.3 units in TranQol summary scores for every 1-year increase in age (B = −0.3, 95%CI 0.5,−0.02), corresponding to a 20-year increase in age for a TranQol MCID of 6 units (clinically important increase in age = 6/0.3). Employment was associated with a significant average increase in TranQol summary, physical, emotional, and family functioning scores, and the levels of increase were greater than the MCID reported in Table 2, reflecting clinically meaningful changes. Female gender was associated with a significant increase in the TranQol family functioning (B = 7.4, 95% 1.5,13.4), and school and career (B = 10.8, 95% 3.3,18.2) subdomain scores, and the change was clinically important (B > MCID, Table 2). Deferasirox compared to Deferoxamine monotherapy was only associated with an average increase in the TranQol physical subdomain score (B = 5.8, 95%CI 0.01,11.6), and the change was marginally clinically important (MCID = 6, Table 2).

Table 3. Univariate analysis of covariates associated with TranQol Summary and subdomain scores.

Variables	* TranQol Summary and Subdomains																	
	Summary			Physical Health			Emotional Health			Sexual Health			Family Functioning			School and Career		
	B	S.E	95%CI	B	S.E	95%CI	B	S.E	95%CI	B	S.E	95%CI	B	S.E	95%CI	B	S.E	95%CI
Age (yrs)	**−0.3 ***	0.1	(−0.5, −0.2)	**−0.4 ***	0.1	(−0.6, −0.2)	**−0.3 ***	0.1	(−0.5, −0.03)	**−0.3 ***	0.2	(−0.7, −0.01)	**−0.5 ***	0.1	(−0.7, −0.3)	−0.1	0.2	(−0.5, 0.2)
Marital Status																		
Married Ref:Unmarried	−3.2 **	1.7	(−6.5, 0.2)	−3.2 **	1.8	(−6.8, 0.4)	−3.8 **	2.0	(−7.8, 0.1)	0.5	2.8	(−4.9, 5.9)	−1.8	2.1	(−5.9, 2.3)	−0.1	2.7	(−5.4, 5.3)
Employment																		
Yes Ref:No	**7.5 ***	1.7	(4.2, 10.7)	**6.6 ***	1.8	(3.0, 10.2)	**6.4 ***	2.0	(3.0, 10.2)	**6.4 ***	2.8	(0.8, 12.0)	**8.6 ***	2.1	(4.5, 12.7)	**8.3 ***	2.8	(2.9, 13.8)
Educational Status																		
Higher Ref:Not Higher	**4.2 ***	1.9	(0.4, 7.3)	**5.5 ***	2.1	(1.5, 9.5)	1.5	2.3	(−3.0, 5.9)	−5.6 **	3.3	(−11.9, 0.8)	4.5 **	2.4	(−0.2, 9.1)	**7.5 ***	3.2	(1.3, 13.7)
Comorbidities																		
Yes Ref:No	**−5.1 ***	1.8	(−8.6, −1.6)	−3.7 **	1.9	(−7.5, 0.2)	**−4.9 ***	2.1	(−9.1, 0.8)	**−8.8 ***	2.9	(−14.5, −3.1)	**−8.2 ***	2.2	(−12.5, −3.8)	−3.1	2.9	(−8.7, 2.6)
Iron Chelator																		
DFX Ref:DFO	4.1 **	2.2	(−0.4, 8.5)	**6.9 ***	2.5	(2.0, 11.9)	3.4 **	2.6	(2.0, 11.9)	6.6 **	3.9	(−1.2, 14.3)	4.3 **	3.1	(−1.7, 10.3)	−6.1 **	3.6	(−13.3, 1.0)
DFX Ref:DFO + DFP	0.9	2.0	(−3.0, 4.9)	3.0 **	2.1	(−1.2, 7.2)	1.4	2.4	(−1.2, 7.2)	3.3	3.3	(−3.2, 9.8)	−2.5	2.5	(−7.3, 2.4)	−4.8 **	3.1	(−11.0, 1.3)
Liver MRI T2 *																		
Abnormall Ref:Normal	3.2 **	1.8	(−0.3, 6.7)	2.9 **	1.9	(−0.9, 6.7)	3.9 **	2.1	(−0.2, 8.0)	1.3	2.9	(−4.5, 7.0)	1.5	2.2	(−2.8, 5.8)	−0.1	2.8	(−5.5, 5.4)
Heart MRI T2 *																		
Abnormal Ref:Normal	−2.6	3.0	(−8.4, 3.3)	−3.9 **	3.2	(−10.2, 2.5)	−1.7	3.5	(−8.7, 5.2)	−2.4	4.9	(−12.1, 7.3)	−0.9	3.7	(−8.1, 6.4)	−0.9	4.8	(−10.5, 8.5)
Gender																		
Female Ref:Male	1.6	1.7	(−1.8, 5.0)	−0.6	1.4	(4.1, 3.3)	−0.4	1.5	(−4.3, 3.8)	1.9	2.1	(−2.1, 8.9)	**4.4 ***	2.1	(0.2, 8.6)	**7.2 ***	2.7	(1.9, 12.5)
Offsprings																		
Yes Ref:No	−1.7	1.6	(−4.8, 1.3)	−2.9 **	1.7	(−6.2, 0.4)	−1.3	1.9	(−4.9, 2.4)	−0.1	2.8	(−5.3, 5.6)	−0.9	1.9	(−4.8, 2.8)	0.9	2.7	(−4.5, 6.2)

A negative correlation coefficient indicates that a patient subgroup has worse QoL compared to the reference subgroup. Highlighted effects are statistically significant. A less restrictive *a*-level of 0.2 was used to identify factors that would be retained as candidate variables in multivariate analysis. Ref: Reference; *: *p*-value < 0.05; **: *p*-value < 0.2; B: Standardized beta coefficient; CI: Confidence interval; DFX: Deferasirox; DFO: Deferoxamine; DFP: Deferiprone.

Table 4. Multivariate model of significant factors ($p < 0.05$) associated with HRQoL.

TranQol	Age			Female Gender			Employed			DFX (Ref:DFO)		
	B	S.E	95%CI	B	S.E	95%CI	B	S.E	95%CI	B	S.E	95%CI
Summary	−0.3	0.1	(−0.5, −0.02)	-		-	**7.5**	2.4	(2.8, 12.2)	-		-
Physical Health	−0.3	0.1	(−0.6, −0.01)	-		-	**5.8**	2.8	(0.2, 11.4)	5.8	2.9	(0.01, 11.6)
Emotional Health	−0.3	0.1	(−0.6, −0.01)	-		-	**8.1**	2.8	(2.5, 13.6)			
Sexual Health	-	-	-	-		-	-		-	-		-
Family Functioning	−0.6	0.2	(−0.9, −0.3)	**7.4**	3.0	(1.5,13.4)	**8.2**	3.0	(2.2, 14.2)	-		-
School and Career	-	-		**10.8**	3.8	(3.3,18.2)	-		-	-		-

Stepwise linear regression was conducted to select the most parsimonious models of independent explanatory factors that may be associated with overall and subdomain QoL status, after adjusting for confounding factors. A less-restrictive a-level of 0.1, in terms of statistical trends ($0.05 < p < 0.10$), was used to identify a broader range of independent factors. The multivariate analysis data were checked and met the assumptions of homogeneity of variance and linearity, and the residuals were approximately normally distributed. For each of the significant predictors, we estimated the regression coefficients (B), standard error and the 95% confidence intervals. Highlighted Beta coefficients imply a clinically meaningful change in TranQol score according to predefined Minimal Clinically Important Difference. B: standardized beta coefficient; S.E: Standard Error; CI: Confidence Interval; Ref: Reference; DFX: Deferasirox; DFO: Deferoxamine.

4. Discussion

This survey marks a significant milestone as the first comprehensive assessment of QoL in a representative sample of the adult TDT population in Greece. Employing a combination of the generic SF-36v2 and the thalassemia-specific TranQol questionnaires, our study sheds light on the nuanced aspects of HRQoL in this patient cohort. Our findings reveal a concerning trend: adult TDT patients exhibit significantly lower HRQoL compared to the general Greek population, with notable differences observed in both physical and mental health domains. Despite considerable advancements in the clinical management and treatment of TDT patients, our results underscore a critical need for further optimization of QoL (Figure 2). Our findings align with existing literature, which reports a significant negative impact of TDT on the physical and mental health status of adult patients [11,13,32–35]. Similarly, studies focusing on pediatric TDT patients generally agree that HRQoL falls below population norms, with a more pronounced difference observed in adolescents compared to children [36–39]

Intriguingly, our study also reveals relatively high TranQol scores in Greece, indicative of a comparatively good level of HRQoL among TDT patients (Figure 3). Specifically, the TranQol summary score in our survey was 73%, a clinically important higher score compared to the TranQol summary score of 54% in a recently published Global Longitudinal Study of HRQoL in adult TDT patients (preliminary results) in the U.S.A., United Kingdom, France, Italy, and Germany [40]. Moreover, while the Summary and TranQol subdomain scores in our study were marginally higher compared to the TranQol results from the phase 3 BELIEVE trial of luspatercept across 15 countries (Australia and countries across Europe, the Middle East, North Africa, North America, and Southeast Asia), these differences were not clinically important [18]. The relatively high TranQol scores in Greece may be attributed to the established special infrastructure, including well-organized medical centers, access to medical resources, and the availability of blood units and iron chelators, coupled with social, educational, and professional benefits. It is important to note that such a supportive social and healthcare environment may not be available in all countries, as healthcare policies and services for TDT patients vary considerably [41]. The notable disparity in HRQoL between Greece and Pakistan (TranQol Summary: 73% vs. 43%, Figure 3) addresses the need to promote health equity in thalassemia across the world, especially in light of emerging novel drugs and therapeutic strategies.

After controlling for possible confounding sociodemographic and clinical variables, as demonstrated in the multivariate analysis presented in Table 3, we identified older age and unemployment as the two most significant factors associated with lower HRQoL. The absence of higher education, comorbidities, and iron chelation with Deferoxamine monotherapy were additional factors that negatively affected certain subdomains of HRQoL.

Our results are in alignment with previous studies reporting that age is independently associated with reduced QoL in TDT [14,15,31,42]. However, it is noteworthy that most researchers agree that in the general population, older adults exhibit social and emotional functioning that is equal to or superior to that of younger adults [4,43]. Sobota et al. compared the HRQoL in TDT with the US norms and showed that HRQoL is lower in older TDT patients than would be expected in the general population [15]. The impact of age on HRQoL in TDT patients should be interpreted cautiously, considering that older TDT patients may have grown up in less favourable healthcare environments, lacking access to oral iron chelators and the improved thalassemia infrastructure available today. Conversely, TDT, being a chronic disease, may have a cumulative negative effect on HRQoL, akin to other individuals with disabilities [44]. Further investigation, particularly through close follow-up of younger TDT patients, may provide insights into the effect of age on HRQoL.

Employed TDT patients exhibited both significantly and clinically higher TranQol summary and subdomain scores (physical health, emotional health, and family functioning). Existing literature suggests a positive relationship between employment and HRQoL among persons with disabilities [44]. However, there is limited published data on the effect of employment on HRQoL in TDT. Most studies have utilized generic QoL questionnaires, which may not be as sensitive as TranQol in detecting the impact of employment on HRQoL. A recent survey in Saudi Arabia was among the few studies reporting that TDT participants holding professional jobs had better mental HRQoL scores compared to those engaged in clerical or manual occupations [45]. Similarly, another survey in Bangladesh demonstrated that lower income was associated with a deterioration of HRQoL [46]. It is important to note that employment rates for TDT patients vary across countries. In our study population, 59% of patients were employed, while a study in the Middle East reported an employment rate of 54% [47]. Conversely, preliminary data from the Global Survey conducted in the U.S.A., United Kingdom, France, Italy, and Germany indicated that only 34% of TDT patients were employed [40]. Our findings underscore the significance of established employment policies for TDT patients in Greece, which provide job opportunities in the public sector and the potential for earlier retirement with a fully paid pension. Nevertheless, creating an accessible and suitable working environment for TDT patients remains a challenge for policymakers, especially considering recent findings by Shah et al., which indicated that the mean working productivity impairment for TDT patients was 42% compared to a typical working week [31].

Gender and choice of iron chelator were significantly associated only with certain domains of HRQoL. As shown in Table 4, female patients exhibited significantly higher TranQol scores in the family functioning and school and career subdomains. There is no consensus in the literature regarding the effect of gender on HRQoL in TDT. Sobota et al. reported that female patients in the USA had worse HRQoL [15], whereas studies in Iran and Bangladesh demonstrated that female patients had a better quality of life [39,46,48]. It could be speculated that the differences in cultural and social environments between countries may explain the contradictory effect of gender on HRQoL.

Regarding comparisons between different iron chelators, Deferasirox was positively associated only with the physical health subdomain compared with Deferoxamine monotherapy, with no difference in HRQoL compared to patients treated with Deferoxamine combined with oral Deferiprone. The published data regarding the effect of iron chelators on HRQoL are heterogeneous in the literature. Sobota et al., in one of the largest studies of TDT patients, concluded that the type of chelator was not associated with HRQoL and suggested that this may be due to patients typically being free to choose their chelation therapy [15]. Goulas et al., in a study of quality of life and iron chelation treatment satisfaction, showed that TDT patients receiving Deferoxamine, alone or in combination with an oral iron chelator, perceived higher treatment efficacy, comparable HRQoL, and comparable satisfaction with the iron chelator compared to patients receiving Deferoxamine, alone or in combination with an oral iron chelator [12]. In clinical practice, physicians may utilize our findings to inform patients about the choice of iron chelator and address any concerns about their impact on everyday life.

This study had some limitations. The cross-sectional design of the study may be less informative in detecting differences in HRQoL between patient subgroups compared to a longitudinal prospective design. Additionally, all participants were recruited from reference thalassemia centers in urban areas of Greece, so our results may not fully reflect HRQoL among TDT patients residing in rural areas and treated in less organized thalassemia institutions. Nevertheless, the study had a high participation rate and a high probability of detecting significant differences between almost all patient subgroups (power = 0.8, significance level = 5%), representing real-world clinical practice in a routine care environment.

The assessment of HRQoL status among TDT patients in Greece has been an unmet need until now. In this multicentric study, we have successfully measured HRQoL using the combination of the generic SF-36v2 and the disease-specific TranQol questionnaires, with an adequate response rate from the participants in a representative sample of the Greek TDT population. We have demonstrated that both social-demographic and clinical factors may impact the HRQoL of TDT patients. The implementation of the disease-specific

TranQol offers the potential for future re-evaluation of HRQoL and the identification of emerging factors affecting HRQoL in the era of novel treatments and interventions in TDT.

5. Conclusions

The integration of TranQol, an internationally recognized disease-specific QoL questionnaire, has provided us with a robust framework to assess the HRQoL of TDT patients in Greece. This approach not only enabled us to quantify HRQoL levels but also established a baseline for future monitoring and comparison with other countries. The identification of vulnerable patient subgroups, particularly older individuals and those who were unemployed, underscores the need for targeted interventions to enhance their QoL. Overall, the HRQoL status in TDT is relatively high in Greece, possibly due to the healthcare environment and social support. Other countries with high incidence rates of TDT may adopt the "paradigm of Greece" and improve the HRQoL of TDT patients.

Author Contributions: Conceptualization, P.K.; methodology, P.K., M.M. and I.P.; software, V.L., D.A. and R.J.K.; validation, P.K., I.P. and M.M.; formal analysis, P.K.; investigation, P.K.; resources, P.K., I.C., S.K., D.P., M.D., A.K. and V.L.; data curation, I.P. and M.M.; writing—original draft preparation, P.K.; writing—review and editing, P.K., N.R., M.M., I.P., D.P., M.D., R.J.K. and A.K.; visualization, P.K.; supervision, A.T. and E.V.; project administration, P.K., D.P., S.K., M.D., A.K. and V.L. All authors have read and agreed to the published version of the manuscript.

Funding: This research received no external funding.

Institutional Review Board Statement: The study was conducted in accordance with the Declaration of Helsinki, and approved by the Ethics Committee of Hippokration General Hospital of Thessaloniki, Greece on 4 May 2015 (213/4-5-2015).

Informed Consent Statement: Informed consent was obtained from all subjects involved in the study. Written informed consent has been obtained from the patient(s) to publish this paper.

Data Availability Statement: The authors confirm that the data supporting the findings of this study are available within the article.

Conflicts of Interest: The authors declare no conflicts of interest.

References

1. Taher, A.T.; Musallam, K.M.; Cappellini, M.D. β-Thalassemias. *N. Engl. J. Med.* **2021**, *384*, 727–743. [CrossRef]
2. Ebrahim, S. Clinical and public health perspectives and applications of health-related quality of life measurement. *Soc. Sci. Med.* **1995**, *41*, 1383–1394. [CrossRef] [PubMed]
3. Rotenstein, L.S.; Huckman, R.S.; Wagle, N.W. Making Patients and Doctors Happier—The Potential of Patient-Reported Outcomes. *N. Engl. J. Med.* **2017**, *377*, 1309–1312. [CrossRef] [PubMed]
4. Steptoe, A.; Deaton, A.; Stone, A. Subjective wellbeing, health, and ageing. *Lancet* **2014**, *385*, 640–648. [CrossRef] [PubMed]
5. Trachtenberg, F.L.; Gerstenberger, E.; Xu, Y.; Mednick, L.; Sobota, A.; Ware, H.; Thompson, A.A.; Neufeld, E.J.; Yamashita, R. Relationship among chelator adherence, change in chelators, and quality of life in Thalassemia. *Qual. Life Res.* **2014**, *23*, 2277–2288. [CrossRef] [PubMed]
6. Basch, E. Patient-Reported Outcomes—Harnessing Patients' Voices to Improve Clinical Care. *N. Engl. J. Med.* **2017**, *376*, 105–108. [CrossRef] [PubMed]
7. Gebski, V.; Obermair, A.; Janda, M. Toward Incorporating Health-Related Quality of Life as Coprimary End Points in Clinical Trials: Time to Achieve Clinical Important Differences and QoL Profiles. *J. Clin. Oncol.* **2022**, *40*, 2378–2388. [CrossRef] [PubMed]
8. Miguel, R.S.; López-González, A.M.; Sanchez-Iriso, E.; Mar, J.; Cabasés, J.M. Measuring health-related quality of life in drug clinical trials: Is it given due importance? *Pharm. Weekbl.* **2007**, *30*, 154–160. [CrossRef]
9. Chassany, O.; Sagnier, P.; Marquis, P.; Fullerton, S.; Aaronson, N. Patient-Reported Outcomes: The Example of Health-Related Quality of Life—A European Guidance Document for the Improved Integration of Health-Related Quality of Life Assessment in the Drug Regulatory Process. *Drug Inf. J.* **2002**, *36*, 209–238. [CrossRef]
10. Higgins, T.J.; Chandler, J.; Cumpston, M.; Li, T.; Page, M.J.; Welch, V.A. *Cochrane Handbook for Systematic Reviews of Interventions*, 2nd ed.; John Wiley & Sons: Chichester, UK, 2019.
11. Rodigari, F.; Brugnera, G.; Colombatti, R. Health-related quality of life in hemoglobinopathies: A systematic review from a global perspective. *Front. Pediatr.* **2022**, *10*, 886674. [CrossRef]

12. Goulas, V.; Kouraklis-Symeonidis, A.; Manousou, K.; Lazaris, V.; Pairas, G.; Katsaouni, P.; Verigou, E.; Labropoulou, V.; Pesli, V.; Kaiafas, P.; et al. A multicenter cross-sectional study of the quality of life and iron chelation treatment satisfaction of patients with transfusion-dependent β-thalassemia, in routine care settings in Western Greece. *Qual. Life Res.* **2020**, *30*, 467–477. [CrossRef]
13. Arian, M.; Mirmohammadkhani, M.; Ghorbani, R.; Soleimani, M. Health-related quality of life (HRQoL) in beta-thalassemia major (β-TM) patients assessed by 36-item short form health survey (SF-36): A meta-analysis. *Qual. Life Res.* **2018**, *28*, 321–334. [CrossRef] [PubMed]
14. Amid, A.; Leroux, R.; Merelles-Pulcini, M.M.; Yassobi, S.; Saliba, A.N.; Ward, R.; Karimi, M.; Taher, A.T.; Klaassen, R.J.; Kirby-Allen, M. Factors Impacting Quality of Life in Thalassemia Patients; Results from the Intercontinenthal Collaborative Study. *Blood* **2016**, *128*, 3633. [CrossRef]
15. Sobota, A.; Yamashita, R.; Xu, Y.; Trachtenberg, F.; Kohlbry, P.; Kleinert, D.; Giardina, P.; Kwiatkowski, J.; Foote, D.; Thayalasuthan, V.; et al. Quality of life in thalassemia: A comparison of SF-36 results from the thalassemia longitudinal cohort to reported literature and the US norms. *Am. J. Hematol.* **2010**, *86*, 92–95. [CrossRef] [PubMed]
16. Klaassen, R.J.; Barrowman, N.; Merelles-Pulcini, M.; Vichinsky, E.P.; Sweeters, N.; Kirby-Allen, M.; Neufeld, E.J.; Kwiatkowski, J.L.; Wu, J.; Vickars, L.; et al. Validation and reliability of a disease-specific quality of life measure (the TranQol) in adults and children with thalassaemia major. *Br. J. Haematol.* **2013**, *164*, 431–437. [CrossRef]
17. Klaassen, R.J.; Alibhai, S.; Allen, M.K.; Moreau, K.; Pulcini, M.M.; Forgie, M.; Blanchette, V.; Buckstein, R.; Odame, I.; Quirt, I.; et al. Introducing the Tran Qol: A New Disease-Specific Quality of Life Measure for Children and Adults with Thalassemia Major. *J. Blood Disord. Transfus.* **2013**, *4*. [CrossRef]
18. Cappellini, M.D.; Taher, A.T.; Piga, A.; Shah, F.; Voskaridou, E.; Viprakasit, V.; Porter, J.B.; Hermine, O.; Neufeld, E.J.; Thompson, A.A.; et al. Health-related quality of life in patients with β-thalassemia: Data from the phase 3 BELIEVE trial of luspatercept. *Eur. J. Haematol.* **2023**, *111*, 113–124. [CrossRef]
19. Voskaridou, E.; Kattamis, A.; Fragodimitri, C.; Kourakli, A.; Chalkia, P.; Diamantidis, M.; Vlachaki, E.; Drosou, M.; Lafioniatis, S.; Maragkos, K.; et al. National registry of hemoglobinopathies in Greece: Updated demographics, current trends in affected births, and causes of mortality. *Ann. Hematol.* **2018**, *98*, 55–66. [CrossRef]
20. Lyrakos, G.; Vini, D.; Aslani, H.; Drosou-Servou, M. Psychometric properties of the Specific Thalassemia Quality of Life Instrument for adults. *Patient Prefer. Adherence* **2012**, *6*, 477–497. [CrossRef]
21. Vlachaki, E.; Neokleous, N.; Paspali, D.; Vetsiou, E.; Onoufriadis, E.; Sousos, N.; Hissan, S.; Vakalopoulou, S.; Garypidou, V.; Boura, P. Evaluation of Mental Health and Physical Pain in Patients with β-Thalassemia Major in Northern Greece. *Hemoglobin* **2015**, *39*, 169–172. [CrossRef]
22. Klonizakis, P.; Klaassen, R.; Sousos, N.; Liakos, A.; Tsapas, A.; Vlachaki, E. Evaluation of the Greek TranQol: A novel questionnaire for measuring quality of life in transfusion-dependent thalassemia patients. *Ann. Hematol.* **2017**, *96*, 1937–1944. [CrossRef]
23. Pappa, E.; Kontodimopoulos, N.; Niakas, D. Validating and norming of the Greek SF-36 Health Survey. *Qual. Life Res.* **2005**, *14*, 1433–1438. [CrossRef]
24. Kattamis, A.; Aydinok, Y.; Taher, A. Optimising management of deferasirox therapy for patients with transfusion-dependent thalassaemia and lower-risk myelodysplastic syndromes. *Eur. J. Haematol.* **2018**, *101*, 272–282. [CrossRef]
25. Walters, S.J. *Qulatiy of Life Outcomes in Clinical Trials and Health-Care Evaluation: A Practical Guide to Analysis and Interpretation*; John Wiley & Sons. Ltd.: Hoboken, NJ, USA, 2009.
26. The American Association for Public Opinion Research. *Standard Definitions: Final Dispositions of Case Codes and Outcome Rates for Surveys*, 9th ed.; The American Association for Public Opinion Research: Alexandria, VA, USA, 2016.
27. Bennett, C.; Khangura, S.; Brehaut, J.C.; Graham, I.D.; Moher, D.; Potter, B.K.; Grimshaw, J.M. Reporting Guidelines for Survey Research: An Analysis of Published Guidance and Reporting Practices. *PLoS Med.* **2011**, *8*, e1001069. [CrossRef]
28. Norman, G.R.; Sloan, J.A.; Wyrwich, K.W. Interpretation of Changes in Health-related Quality of Life. *Med. Care* **2003**, *41*, 582–592. [CrossRef]
29. Short-Form Health Survey 36 Version 2. Available online: https://www.qualitymetric.com/health-surveys/the-sf-36v2-health-survey/ (accessed on 25 March 2015).
30. Maruish, M.E. *User's Manual for the sf-36v2 Health Survey*; Quality Metric Inc.: Johnston, RI, USA, 2011.
31. Shah, F.; Telfer, P.; Velangi, M.; Pancham, S.; Wynn, R.; Pollard, S.; Chalmers, E.; Kell, J.; Carter, A.M.; Hickey, J.; et al. Routine management, healthcare resource use and patient and carer-reported outcomes of patients with transfusion-dependent β-thalassaemia in the United Kingdom: A mixed methods observational study. *eJHaem* **2021**, *2*, 738–749. [CrossRef]
32. Yousafzai, Y.M.; Roghani, S.; Khan, N.; Shah, I.; Khan, S.; Taj, A.S. Quality of life and its determinants in transfusion dependent thalassemia. *Pak. J. Physiol.* **2018**, *14*, 64–67.
33. Cappellini, M.D.; Kattamis, A.; Viprakasit, V.; Sutcharitchan, P.; Pariseau, J.; Laadem, A.; Jessent-Ciaravino, V.; Taher, A. Quality of life in patients with β-thalassemia: A prospective study of transfusion-dependent and non-transfusion-dependent patients in Greece, Italy, Lebanon, and Thailand. *Am. J. Hematol.* **2019**, *94*, E261–E264. [CrossRef] [PubMed]
34. Floris, F.; Comitini, F.; Leoni, G.; Moi, P.; Morittu, M.; Orecchia, V.; Perra, M.; Pilia, M.P.; Zappu, A.; Casini, M.R.; et al. Quality of life in Sardinian patients with transfusion-dependent Thalassemia: A cross-sectional study. *Qual. Life Res.* **2018**, *27*, 2533–2539. [CrossRef] [PubMed]
35. Bazi, A.; Sargazi-Aval, O.; Safa, A.; Miri-Moghaddam, E. Health-related Quality of Life and Associated Factors among Thalassemia Major Patients, Southeast of Iran. *J. Pediatr. Hematol.* **2017**, *39*, 513–517. [CrossRef] [PubMed]

36. Hakeem, G.L.A.; Mousa, S.O.; Moustafa, A.N.; Mahgoob, M.H.; Hassan, E.E. Health-related quality of life in pediatric and adolescent patients with transfusion-dependent β-thalassemia in upper egypt (single center study). *Health Qual. Life Outcomes* **2018**, *16*, 59. [CrossRef] [PubMed]
37. Clarke, S.A.; Skinner, R.; Guest, J.; Darbyshire, P.; Cooper, J.; Shah, F.; Roberts, I.; Eiser, C. Health-related quality of life and financial impact of caring for a child with Thalassaemia Major in the UK. *Child Care Health Dev.* **2009**, *36*, 118–122. [CrossRef]
38. Bukhari, G.J. Quality of life among beta-thalassemic major children presented at Federal Government Hospital Islamabad, Pakistan. *J. Pak. Med. Assoc.* **2022**, *72*, 2241–2244. [CrossRef] [PubMed]
39. Etemad, K.; Mohseni, P.; Aghighi, M.; Bahadorimonfared, A.; Hantooshzadeh, R.; Taherpour, N.; Piri, N.; Ghorbani, S.S.; Malek, F.; Kheiry, F.; et al. Quality of Life and Related Factors in β-Thalassemia Patients. *Hemoglobin* **2021**, *45*, 245–249. [CrossRef]
40. Li, N.; Drahos, J.; Boateng-Kuffour, A.; Calvert, M.; Levine, L.; Dongha, N.; Pakbaz, Z.; Oran, F.K.; Iqbal, K.; Shah, F.; et al. Health-Related Quality of Life and Disease Impacts in Adults with Transfusion-Dependent β-Thalassemia: Preliminary Results from the Global Longitudinal Survey. *Blood* **2022**, *140*, 10869–10870. [CrossRef]
41. Bellis, G.; Parant, A. Beta-thalassemia in Mediterranean countries. Findings and outlook. *Investig. Geogr.* **2022**, 129–138. [CrossRef]
42. Panepinto, J.A. Health-related quality of life in patients with hemoglobinopathies. *Hematology* **2012**, *2012*, 284–289. [CrossRef] [PubMed]
43. Charles, S.T.; Carstensen, L.L. Social and Emotional Aging. *Annu. Rev. Psychol.* **2010**, *61*, 383–409. [CrossRef]
44. Ra, Y.-A.; Kim, W.H. Impact of Employment and Age on Quality of Life of Individuals with Disabilities. *Rehabilit. Couns. Bull.* **2015**, *59*, 112–120. [CrossRef]
45. Adam, S. Quality of life outcomes in thalassaemia patients in Saudi Arabia: A cross-sectional study. *East. Mediterr. Health J.* **2019**, *25*, 887–895. [CrossRef]
46. Hossain, J.; Islam, W.; Munni, U.R.; Gulshan, R.; Mukta, S.A.; Miah, S.; Sultana, S.; Karmakar, M.; Ferdous, J.; Islam, M.A. Health-related quality of life among thalassemia patients in Bangladesh using the SF-36 questionnaire. *Sci. Rep.* **2023**, *13*, 7734. [CrossRef] [PubMed]
47. Bou-Fakhredin, R.; Ghanem, N.N.; Kreidieh, F.; Tabbikha, R.; Daadaa, H.; Ajouz, J.; Koussa, S.; Taher, A.T. A Report on the Education, Employment and Marital Status of Thalassemia Patients from a Tertiary Care Center in the Middle East. *Hemoglobin* **2020**, *44*, 278–283. [CrossRef] [PubMed]
48. Ansari, S.; Baghersalimi, A.; Azarkeivan, A.; Nojomi, M.; Rad, A.H. Quality of life in patients with thalassemia major. *Iran. J. Ped. Hematol. Oncol.* **2014**, *4*, 57–63. [PubMed]

healthcare

MDPI

Article

Ageing with Parkinson's: Identification of Personal Needs in the Northern Spanish Context

Patricia Solís García [1,*], María Souto Serrano [2], Mª Ángeles Alcedo Rodríguez [3], Elsa Peña Suárez [4], Ignacio Pedrosa [5] and Antonio León Aguado Diaz [3]

1 Faculty of Education, Universidad Internacional de La Rioja, 26006 Logroño, Spain
2 Asturian Society of Rehabilitation Psychology, 33001 Oviedo, Spain; mariasouto83@hotmail.com
3 Faculty of Psychology, Universidad de Oviedo, 33009 Oviedo, Spain; malcedo@uniovi.es (M.Á.A.R.); aaguado17@gmail.com (A.L.A.D.)
4 Department of Education of the Government of the Principality of Asturias, 33007 Oviedo, Spain; elsaps@educastur.org
5 Information and Communication Technology Center, 33203 Gijón, Spain; npedrosa@cop.es
* Correspondence: patricia.solis@unir.net

Abstract: As individuals diagnosed with Parkinson's disease enter older age, the myriad challenges and complications associated with this condition tend to escalate. Hence, there is a critical necessity to comprehensively discern the perceived needs of these individuals, along with their proposed remedies and essential support requisites. Additionally, understanding the perspectives of their families becomes imperative to formulate tailored interventions aimed at enhancing their overall development, progression, and quality of life. The study's main objective is to assess the perceived needs of individuals with PD and their family members, propose necessary solutions, and suggest future perspectives. The study encompassed a cohort of 268 participants, comprising 179 individuals diagnosed with Parkinson's disease and 89 of their relatives. A meticulously designed structured interview instrument consisting of 93 items was employed to assess various domains encompassing perceived needs, institutional support mechanisms, essential solutions, and future anticipations. Results: Statistically significant differences were found in health resources, social services resources, obstacles, solutions, and future outlook, with higher mean values from the relatives. Conclusions: The results highlight the most concerning needs in this context. Specifically, those needs related to health resources, social services resources, and future outlook present the greatest differences between the two subsamples, with the family members perceiving more needs. This alignment extended to both the categorization of unmet needs and the requisite solutions envisioned to address them. Suggested improvements include a sociosanitary strategy, stakeholder involvement, and prioritizing flexible home assistance to support older individuals with PD and their families.

Keywords: clinical health psychology; health care; elder; quality of life; Parkinson's disease

1. Introduction

Parkinson's disease (PD) presents a prevalent neurological disorder with a crude prevalence between 100 and 200 per 100,000 persons, expected to rise due to aging populations and increased life expectancy [1,2]. PD ranks as the second-most common progressive neurodegenerative disorder, often leading to substantial disability, discrimination, and stigma, impacting the overall quality of life (QoL) [3].

As individuals affected by PD age, the challenges posed by this illness also grow [4]. The lower prevalence and wide geographical dispersion can result in isolation and hinder social interaction among those affected [5].

Motor complications related to walking and posture control, fatigue, pain, psychiatric issues, sleep disturbances, and mood disorders significantly affect the lives of those with PD, highlighting multiple unmet needs [6–12]. In this regard, the perceived and unmet needs related to the motor profile in people with PD have not varied significantly since the 1980s [13]. On the other hand, researchers have also focused their interest on individuals who experienced a significant symptom burden and concerns at the early to middle disease stage [14], highlighting how relatively common non-motor neuropsychiatric features such as anxiety and depression can also lead to social isolation [15]. Other needs, including those of families, pertain to training and information related to health care associated with the disease, symptoms, how to recognize them, coping strategies, and necessary lifestyle changes [16]. Identifying and addressing these needs are closely tied to enhancing quality of life, where meeting all requirements determines a good quality of life [17–19].

Unfortunately, these needs often receive inadequate attention, and information on this subject is relatively scarce [20,21]. Therefore, there is a critical need to identify the perceived needs, propose solutions, and determine necessary measures and support, including those perceived by family members. Understanding the needs of individuals with PD is crucial for providing essential services and enhancing their progress and quality of life [22,23].

The repercussions of this disease extend beyond the affected individuals to impact their families significantly. The symptomatology's dependency often positions families as the primary caregivers, experiencing their own substantial support needs [24]. However, if families lack the necessary assistance and professional services for patient care, they themselves may suffer considerably [25].

Projections suggest that families will increasingly struggle to meet these needs [26]. The burden on families, associated with halting work, loss of social connections, and increased caregiving time, restricts the possibility of keeping individuals within their familiar environments. Therefore, a reevaluation of efforts between families, private sectors, and the state becomes imperative to establish an effective care model. Furthermore, there is a pressing need for developing therapies and care plans that can address the multifaceted needs of PD, ultimately improving the lives of those affected and their families. Finally, tailored support plans must be designed to offer appropriate services and assistance according to specific needs [27].

Given this context and the lack of conclusive data [28], the study's main objective is to assess the perceived needs of individuals with PD and their family members, propose necessary solutions, and suggest future perspectives. From this overall objective, the following research questions arise: (I) What are the most prominent perceived needs of individuals diagnosed with PD and their family members, according to the assessment results? (II) What solutions are proposed as necessary to address the identified needs during the evaluation of individuals with PD and their family members? (III) What future perspectives are suggested by the participants regarding the needs and proposed solutions in the context of PD?

The following initial hypotheses are proposed: (I) Perceived needs of individuals with PD will mainly be related to health, economic and healthcare resources, dependence, home assistance, and the existence of barriers. (II) Proposed solutions, in relation to this first hypothesis, are directly related to health, lack of or difficulty with economic resources, the development of dependence in terms of care, specialization of home assistance, and the control of barriers. (III) Support will be needed, to be developed in the institutional, economic, healthcare, family, and social domains. (IV) There will be no significant differences in perceived needs between individuals with PD and their family members.

By gathering this information, the study aims to pinpoint the most crucial areas and differences between individuals with PD and their relatives regarding identifying these needs. This study aims to provide a valuable contribution by delving into a comprehensive understanding of the perceived needs of individuals diagnosed with PD and their families as they face the challenges associated with aging. This alignment underscores the importance of considering both perspectives in order to formulate tailored interventions to enhance overall development, progression, and quality of life for those affected by PD in older age. To achieve this, the study assesses the needs of the primary stakeholders in this disease—the aging individuals with PD and their families. Only by understanding their needs can resources be effectively planned to enhance individual autonomy and quality of life for both individuals with PD and their families.

2. Materials and Methods

2.1. Participants

The study included 268 participants categorized into two groups: individuals diagnosed with PD and their respective relatives. All participants resided in Spain, with the majority (82.68%) hailing from the Principality of Asturias.

The PD group consisted of 179 participants, aged between 45 and 92 years (M = 72.40; SD = 9.40), with 54.75% being female. Among them, 65.37% lived in family settings, 15.08% in supportive living facilities, and 16.2% lived alone.

The group of relatives reporting on the needs of PD individuals comprised 89 participants (53.93% women). Predominantly, they were identified as sons/daughters (38.20%) or spouses (37.80%), with ages ranging from 46 to 91 years (M = 72.01; SD = 9.96). Note that there is a smaller number of individuals in the sample of family members compared to individuals with PD because many did not have a close relative willing to complete the interview.

2.2. Instrument

Needs evaluation was conducted using the Interview for Needs Assessment of Ageing People with Disabilities (INEAD), a well-established interview consisting of 93 items; this scale has been used in previous studies and has estimated reliability coefficient (alpha coefficient of 0.85) [20]. The personal interview is a semi-structured interview that combines closed-ended questions with multiple-choice alternatives, with a final open-ended interview. It gathers comprehensive information on descriptive variables related to disability and sociodemographic and environmental variables (personal data, interview completion data, clinical data, and information about living arrangements). Additionally, it assesses eight categories of needs: personal health, economic resources, health resources and social services resources, physical and social barriers, social support measures and networks, solutions required, and future outlook. Finally, an open-ended question is included for "other considerations to add". On the other hand, the family interview is formally integrated into the final part of the personal interview and consists of 6 questions regarding the family members' opinions about concerns and needs, solutions, institutional measures and support, and thoughts about the future of the person with Parkinson's.

2.3. Data Analysis

Initially, normality was assessed using the Kolmogorov–Smirnov (K–S) test. Subsequently, non-parametric tests were employed to analyze perceived needs, solutions required, and future outlook. The effect size was estimated using Cohen's (1988) criteria (η^2) with values categorized as low ($\leq$0.02), moderate (between 0.03 and 0.14), and large (>0.14). Independence tests (X^2) were applied, and the phi coefficient measured associations between variables. IBM SPSS 20 for Windows facilitated all analyses, conducted at a CL = 95%.

2.4. Procedure

To gather sample data, we proceeded to contact all public and private services that cater to individuals with PD in the northern region of Spain. First, a list of potential candidate centers was developed, and the necessary institutional contacts were established with the entities involved to inform them about the study and coordinate meetings with the individuals concerned. This included more than 100 associations, residential centers, healthcare facilities, support services, and rehabilitation services. Professionals and representatives from these centers and institutions disseminated information about the research among their associates through letters or phone calls. In all cases, prior consent was requested for participation. Once individuals expressed their willingness to collaborate, personal interviews were scheduled. All participants received information about the study and its objectives, and confidentiality and anonymous use of the information for research purposes were guaranteed. The recruitment of the sample was carried out in compliance with the regulations governing the protection of personal data (LOPD 15/1999).

Given the mobility and accessibility challenges faced by this group, the interviews were conducted individually in accessible premises of the associations or by visiting the home or residence of the evaluated person. The completion of each interview took approximately 60–75 min. The interviews were administered individually to individuals with Parkinson's disease and their families by the interviewing team, which had received prior information and training. In cases where participants faced communication or understanding limitations, family members or caregivers familiar with the individual's needs provided assistance. In those cases where the interview could not be completed or data were missing, the entire interview was discarded.

Ethical considerations: The principles for conducting research contained in the Declaration of Helsinki were respected. Although the study involves the participation of human subjects, no experimentation has been conducted on them and confidentiality and voluntariness of data have been ensured, complying with articles 40 and 45 of the Deontological Code of Psychology in Spain, which can be cited as national legislation safeguarding the rights and duties of assessment within the field of Psychology, as well as with the guidelines of the international document 'Guide for the Assessment Process'. All participants were informed of the research and its objectives. Permission and informed consent were collected from all participants. Removing names and using identifying codes that the researchers did not know guaranteed confidentiality and anonymity.

3. Results

As the data did not fit a normal distribution, the Mann–Whitney U test was used to examine the statistical differences between both subsamples. Statistically significant differences were found in health resources, social services resources, obstacles, solutions, and future outlook, with higher mean values from the relatives (Table 1). In order to avoid possible sample size influences on these results, the effect size ($p < 0.05$) was estimated, giving overall large results (ranging from 0.24 to 0.90).

Table 1. Results of the Mann–Whitney U test on perceived needs, solutions required, and future outlook.

	Subsample	Mean Rank	χ^2 (df)	Asymp. Sig.	η^2
Personal health	PDP	132.65	0.33 (1)	>0.05	-
	Relatives	138.23			
Economic resources	PDP	129.35	2.87 (1)	>0.05	-
	Relatives	144.87			
Health resources	PDP	127.99	3.96 (1)	<0.05	0.24
	Relatives	147.59			
Social services resources	PDP	122.07	14.80 (1)	<0.05	0.90
	Relatives	159.49			
Physical and social barriers	PDP	127.65	4.56 (1)	<0.05	0.28
	Relatives	148.28			
Social support measures and network	PDP	129.85	2.12 (1)	>0.05	-
	Relatives	143.85			
Solutions required	PDP	122.20	13.63 (1)	<0.05	0.83
	Relatives	159.23			
Future outlook	PDP	128.10	3.97 (1)	<0.05	0.24
	Relatives	147.37			

Note. PDP: people with Parkinson's disease; df = degrees of freedom; η^2 = estimated effect size.

The factor of "personal health" encompasses concerns related to overall health status, dependence, the presence of pain, daily personal care, and difficulties in medication management, among others. The "economic resources" factor aggregates concerns related to pensions, family economic situation, economic independence, grants, and work disability. The "health resources" area encompasses concerns related to treatment and physiotherapy, improved healthcare facilities, hospital healthcare, quality of healthcare, and lack of information about these resources, among others. Concerns related to "social services resources" address home assistance, improved social facilities, lack of information about these resources, support services, and leisure time, among others. The "physical and social barriers" area addresses concerns about architectural barriers, transportation ease, accessibility to public buildings, social barriers, societal acceptance, etc. In the "social support and network" area, support from municipalities, equal opportunities, training activities, and environmental support, among others, are addressed. Regarding "solutions required", all those related to previous needs are addressed, and as for "future outlook", thoughts regarding living with quality of life, personal autonomy, loneliness, boredom, etc., are considered.

Pearson Chi-squared tests were then performed between the areas and categories that were statistically significant in the previous analysis in order to specify in which items the differences were found.

For the existence of physical and social obstacles, there were only significant differences in "technical assistance which aids mobility and access". However, this difference disappeared once Yates' correction ($p > 0.05$) was applied.

In terms of factors related to health and social services resources and future outlook, which demonstrated statistically significant differences, all of the items except "rely on physiotherapy treatment" suggested more concern on the part of the families (Table 2).

Table 2. Statistically significant types of health resources, social services resources, and future outlook.

			Yes (%)	χ^2 (df)	φ	Asymp. Sig.
Health Resources	Difficulties in attending treatment	PDP	10.6	10.62 (1)	−0.210	<0.01
		Relatives	27.0			
	Have support appliances and prosthetics	PDP	10.6	30.64 (1)	−0.348	<0.01
		Relatives	40.4			
	Have physiotherapeutic treatment	PDP	33.5	5.35 (1)	0.150	<0.05
		Relatives	19.1			
	Information on health and care resources	PDP	16.2	6.36 (1)	−0.164	<0.05
		Relatives	30.3			
	Quality of healthcare	PDP	25.1	4.27 (1)	−0.135	<0.05
		Relatives	38.2			
Social services resources	Have help in the home	PDP	33.5	4.89 (1)	−0.143	<0.05
		Relatives	48.3			
	Appropriate quality of social services attendance	PDP	16.2	12.09 (1)	−0.222	<0.01
		Relatives	36.0			
Future outlook	Face a solitary future	PDP	10.1	40.63 (1)	−0.399	<0.01
		Relatives	44.9			
	A future living independently	PDP	10.1	59.31 (1)	−0.480	<0.01
		Relatives	53.9			
	Face an uncertain, worrying future	PDP	17.3	11.70 (1)	−0.218	<0.01
		Relatives	37.1			
	Face the future with no problems	PDP	9.5	44.75 (1)	−0.418	<0.01
		Relatives	46.1			
	Face the future with personal autonomy	PDP	19.0	14.42 (1)	−0.241	<0.01
		Relatives	41.6			
	Have assurance about the future	PDP	19.0	11.81 (1)	−0.219	<0.01
		Relatives	39.3			

Note. Yes % = percentage of people with Parkinson's disease (PDP) and relatives who mention this indicator; df = degrees of freedom; φ = phi coefficient.

Similar results were found with respect to the types of solutions needed (Table 3). Again, there were statistically significant differences between the two subsamples, with the family members requiring more solutions, except for the availability of help for personal daily care, having more and better health facilities, having more specialist health professionals, more transport facilities, promotion of adapted living spaces, and increased resources from patient associations and community support.

Table 3. Statistically significant solutions are required.

		Yes (%)	χ^2 (df)	φ	Asymp. Sig.
Availability of help for personal daily care	PDP	27.9	6.19 (1)	0.161	<0.05
	Relatives	13.5			
Increased family help	PDP	12.8	54.15 (1)	−0.458	<0.01
	Relatives	56.2			
Have more and better health installations	PDP	33.5	4.47 (1)	0.138	<0.05
	Relatives	20.2			
Retire earlier	PDP	5.6	17.13 (1)	−0.265	<0.01
	Relatives	23.6			
Have more specialized professionals	PDP	29.6	7.56 (1)	0.177	<0.01
	Relatives	13.5			
Improved prosthetics support	PDP	10.6	13.42 (1)	−0.234	<0.01
	Relatives	29.2			
Have more and better information about health	PDP	21.8	11.69 (1)	−0.218	<0.01
	Relatives	42.7			
Availability of legal and administrative support	PDP	11.7	7.63 (1)	−0.179	<0.01
	Relatives	25.8			
Better quality of health care	PDP	19.6	11.04 (1)	−0.212	<0.01
	Relatives	39.3			
Availability of support services for leisure and free time	PDP	19.6	22.46 (1)	−0.298	<0.01
	Relatives	48.3			
Societal acceptance	PDP	12.8	21.33 (1)	−0.292	<0.01
	Relatives	38.2			
Acceptance by the family	PDP	8.4	29.38 (1)	−0.342	<0.01
	Relatives	36.0			
More transport facilities	PDP	30.7	16.21 (1)	0.255	<.01
	Relatives	7.9			
Promote adapted living arrangements	PDP	21.8	8.58 (1)	0.190	<0.01
	Relatives	6.7			
Support for informal carers	PDP	23.5	4.04 (1)	−0.132	<0.05
	Relatives	36.0			
Coordination between different administrations	PDP	25.7	11.50 (1)	−0.216	<0.01
	Relatives	47.2			
Increased resources for associations	PDP	42.5	39.12 (1)	0.391	<0.01
	Relatives	4.5			
Community support	PDP	22.9	15.14 (1)	0.248	<0.01
	Relatives	3.4			

Note. Yes % = percentage of people with Parkinson's disease (PDP) and relatives who mention this indicator; df = degrees of freedom; φ = phi coefficient.

Looking at the Phi coefficient, it is worth mentioning the concern shown by the relatives regarding the difficulty the person with PD has in achieving an independent future with no problems, which is related to those solutions linked to increased family support and the need for those people with PD to have more resources from patient associations.

4. Discussion

The study's main objective is to assess the perceived needs of individuals with PD and their family members, propose necessary solutions, and suggest future perspectives, since any proposed course of action must stem from a thorough study and analysis of the reality characterizing this aging process. In general, the profile of older individuals with PD who participated in this research is quite heterogeneous.

The evaluation instrument used to discover the needs of ageing people with PD incorporates a view of systems which encompasses the multiple settings that have an impact on the person (e.g., the family) while at the same time including the participation of the subject with PD themselves in the evaluation of their needs. The results are in line with previous research, confirming that more than half of the population with PD live with their family, who are the main caregivers, combining that care with their support needs [29,30]. For that reason, it is crucial to include these carers' perspectives in this study, as it should never be forgotten that a person's quality of life cannot be isolated from the care they receive or the people who manage that care [31].

The results highlight the most concerning needs in this context. Specifically, those needs related to health resources, social services resources, and future outlook present the greatest differences between the two subsamples, with the family members perceiving more needs. The main concerns about health resources revolve around the quality of the health care itself and treatment. These results are not surprising, given the frequent motor complications in PD, which have a marked impact on these people's quality of life [32]. Faced with this, it seems necessary to reinforce strategic health plans to make the necessary support available and to achieve the best outcomes possible [33].

Regarding social services resources, the participants demonstrated particular concern about having help in the home and having good quality social help. The family members more often indicated these issues. These results suggest that, despite the undeniable preventive and family-supporting nature of social services, current access to professional care is insufficient [34]. A possible explanation for this, it should be noted, is that these types of services are provided by public administrations to a small number of homes, making it extremely expensive for many families in the current socioeconomic situation. When developing interventions, the development of this type of resource would reduce the burden on carers, making it possible for people with PD to stay in the family environment, as families are not capable of providing total care for those with PD, especially in the later stages of the illness.

When considering the future, the biggest worries are about autonomy, loneliness and independence of those with PD. Staying within their individual, family and social environment is a facilitating factor in satisfaction and quality of life [30]. However, from the carer's perspective, there are more needs in this category. This is logical, as most of the care this kind of health problem requires can bring with it rather negative effects; one notable example is high stress [20,35]. The only way to alleviate these needs and prevent future problems is to make resources available to those caregivers, which compensate for lack of functioning, avoid total dependency on another person, and facilitate social contact [36]. Nonetheless, research suggests a lack of resources and support for families, who will find that their capacity to respond to the needs of those with DP diminishes as they get older [37].

The results demonstrate a significant requirement for solutions for a similar number of perceived needs. Chief among the solutions required by those with PD are increased patient association resources (42.50%) and the need to have more and better health facilities (33.50%). The care and services provided to those with PD and their families by these various associations are fundamental, bearing the brunt of specialist care, which is not simple as it is not managed by public health and social care systems [38]. In the face of this problem, some solutions should be geared towards those approaches that the older adults suggest, such as having more specialized professionals (29.60%), and availability of daily personal care (27.90%), ensuring the maintenance of their quality of life [39].

The relatives requested more solutions to respond to their perceived needs. They proposed things such as increased family support (56.20%), having more and better information about the health of the person with PD (42.70%), leisure and free time services (48.30%), and coordination between various administrations (47.20%). It is important to highlight the need for these services because if the right level of family involvement is not achieved, it could lead to serious pathologies such as anxiety, stress [35], or burnout syndrome. These issues, which put the emotional well-being of carers at risk, require there to be quality social support networks which provide the families with the support they need [40].

In summary, this research provides a holistic view of needs evaluation in the area of PD thanks to the participation of the two principal agents involved: the ageing person with PD and the family [23]. Regarding the coincidences and discrepancies observed in the comparative analysis regarding perceived needs and concerns in general, there is a certain harmony between individuals and families. Both groups prioritize personal health issues, and it is worth noting that PD presents a sequence of health problems that manifest as a consequence of the progression of the disease and disability [34]. To such an extent, both groups identify assistance for daily personal care and support for informal caregivers as a solution.

Although the family members tended to indicate more needs, they agree with the people with PD in terms of the type of needs which are not being met and the solutions they require, sharing the demand for more and better services in which quality is the prime factor. It indicates a call for the implementation of activities and solutions appropriate to these unmet needs so that those with PD can enjoy a sufficient quality of life following diagnosis [41]. To that end, it is crucial to provide good quality services, as that is the best guarantee of respecting these people's rights and meeting their needs [42]. Firstly, the study is based on the perception of needs from the two fundamental agents, but it should be noted that the sample size is limited, and the study focuses on a specific geographical area. Additionally, there has not been an in-depth analysis regarding the influence of sociodemographic variables on the perception of needs in individuals with PD. It is important to acknowledge these limitations to ensure a nuanced interpretation of the findings. Furthermore, a more comprehensive view of the subject could be achieved by including the opinions of professionals working in this field. Secondly, it would be interesting to design a longitudinal study to provide a detailed view of the development of needs as a person ages, allowing the definition of intervention measures appropriate to individual characteristics.

Considering the discussed data, some improvement proposals are suggested, encompassing various areas, and outlined in the following intervention guidelines. Firstly, there should be an encouragement for the implementation of a sociosanitary strategy involving all relevant stakeholders to integrate the available resources in addressing the needs of older individuals with PD and their families. Additionally, there should be a prioritization of home assistance tailored to the needs of users and the family unit, thus being flexible in terms of schedules and tasks, thereby promoting the continued residence of the older person with PD within their family environment.

5. Conclusions

Key findings included concerns regarding health resources, social services resources, and future outlook, with family members expressing more significant needs. Health resource concerns pertained to the quality of healthcare and treatment, while social services resource concerns focused on in-home assistance and the quality of social help. For the future outlook, the main worries were related to autonomy, loneliness, and independence, particularly from the perspective of family members.

Solutions required included a need for increased patient association resources and better health facilities from the perspective of individuals with PD. Family members sought more solutions, such as enhanced family support, better health information, increased leisure and free time services, and improved coordination between administrations.

In conclusion, this comprehensive study emphasized the importance of considering the needs of both individuals with PD and their family members to enhance the quality of life and wellbeing of those affected. While family members expressed more concerns and sought more solutions, their alignment on unmet needs highlights the necessity for increased and higher-quality services to support individuals with PD as well as their caregivers. These results underscore the importance of respecting patients' rights and addressing their needs. The findings provide valuable insights for developing targeted intervention measures and warrant further research, potentially involving professionals in the field, to gain a more comprehensive understanding of the needs and experiences of those living with PD and their families. Additionally, a longitudinal study could shed light on the evolution of needs as individuals age, guiding the development of personalized intervention strategies.

Author Contributions: Conceptualization, P.S.G., M.S.S., M.Á.A.R. and A.L.A.D.; methodology, E.P.S. and I.P.; software, E.P.S. and I.P.; validation, P.S.G., E.P.S. and I.P.; formal analysis, E.P.S. and I.P.; investigation, P.S.G., M.S.S., M.Á.A.R. and AA.; resources, P.S.G., M.S.S., M.Á.A.R. and A.L.A.D.; data curation, E.P.S. and I.P.; writing—original draft preparation, P.S.G., M.S.S. and M.Á.A.R.; writing—review and editing, P.S.G. and M.Á.A.R.; visualization, P.S.G., M.S.S. and M.Á.A.R.; supervision, A.L.A.D. All authors have read and agreed to the published version of the manuscript.

Funding: This research received no external funding.

Institutional Review Board Statement: This study has been conducted in accordance with the ethical guidelines established in the Deontological Code of Psychology in Spain, which governs the rights and duties within the field of Psychology. Adherence to these guidelines ensures the protection and respect of research participants and upholds the ethical integrity of this study. https://www.cop.es/pdf/CodigoDeontologicodelPsicologo-vigente.pdf. Accessed on 11 November 2022.

Informed Consent Statement: Informed consent was obtained from all subjects involved in the study.

Data Availability Statement: The data presented in this study are available on request from the corresponding author. The data are not publicly available due to privacy considerations.

Conflicts of Interest: The authors declare no conflicts of interest.

References

1. Ponte, C.; Almeida, V.; Fernandes, L. Suicidal Ideation, Depression and Quality of Life in the Elderly: Study in a Gerontopsychiatric Consultation. *Span. J. Psychol.* **2014**, *17*, E14. [CrossRef]
2. Tysnes, O.B.; Storstein, A. Epidemiology of Parkinson's disease. *J. Neural Transm.* **2017**, *124*, 901–905. [CrossRef] [PubMed]
3. Jiang, J.-L.; Chen, S.-Y.; Tsai, S.-T.; Ma, Y.-C.; Wang, J.-H. Long-Term Effects of Subthalamic Stimulation on Motor Symptoms and Quality of Life in Patients with Parkinson's Disease. *Healthcare* **2023**, *11*, 920. [CrossRef] [PubMed]
4. Leonardi, M.; Raggi, A.; Pagani, M.; Carella, F.; Soliveri, P.; Albanese, A.; Romito, L. Relationships between disability, quality of life and prevalence of nonmotor symptoms in Parkinson's disease. *Park. Relat. Disord.* **2012**, *18*, 35–39. [CrossRef] [PubMed]
5. Sánchez-Herrera-Baeza, P.; Rodríguez-Pérez, M.ª.P.; Fernández-Gómez, G.; Bustamante-Palomo, N.; Serrada-Tejeda, S.; Obeso-Benítez, P.; Morales-Cabezas, M.; Martínez-Piédrola, R.M.; Pérez-de-Heredia-Torres, M. The Impact of Social Distancing Due to COVID-19 on Activities of Daily Living in Parkinson's Disease. *Healthcare* **2023**, *11*, 1688. [CrossRef] [PubMed]
6. Gazibara, T.; Pekmezovic, T.; Tepavcevic, D.K.; Svetel, M.; Tomic, A.; Stankovic, I.; Kostic, V.S. Health-related quality of life in patients with Parkinson's disease: Implications for falling. *Park. Relat. Disord.* **2015**, *21*, 573–576. [CrossRef] [PubMed]
7. Estrada-Bellmann, I.; Camara-Lemarroy, C.R.; Calderon-Hernandez, H.J.; Rocha-Anaya, J.J.; Villareal-Velazquez, H.J. Non-motor symptoms and quality of life in patients with Parkinson's disease in Northeastern Mexico. *Acta Neurol. Belg.* **2016**, *116*, 157–161. [CrossRef] [PubMed]
8. Rada, D.; Seco, J.; Echevarría, E.; Tijero, B.; Abecia, L.C.; Gómez-Esteban, J.C. Dysautonomia Differentially Influences the Effect of Affective Pain Perception on Quality of Life in Parkinson's Disease Patients. *Park. Dis.* **2016**, *2016*, 3067426. [CrossRef] [PubMed]
9. Watanabe, K.; Hirano, T.; Katsumi, K.; Ohashi, M.; Ishikawa, A.; Koike, R.; Endo, N.; Nishizawa, M.; Shimohata, T. Characteristics and exacerbating factors of chronic low back pain in Parkinson's disease. *Int. Orthop.* **2015**, *39*, 2433–2438. [CrossRef]
10. Rieu, I.; Houeto, J.L.; Pereira, B.; De Chazeron, I.; Bichon, A.; Chéreau, I.; Ulla, M.; Brefel-Courbon, C.; Ory-Magne, F.; Dujardin, K.; et al. Impact of Mood and Behavioral Disorders on Quality of Life in Parkinson's disease. *J. Park. Dis.* **2016**, *6*, 267–277. [CrossRef]
11. Ylikoski, A.; Martikainen, K.; Sieminski, M.; Partinen, M. Sleeping difficulties and health-related quality of life in Parkinson's disease. *Acta Neurol. Scand.* **2017**, *135*, 459–468. [CrossRef]
12. Perrin, A.J.; Nosova, E.; Co, K.; Book, A.; Iu, O.; Silva, V.; Thompson, C.; McKeown, M.J.; Stoessl, A.J.; Farrer, M.J.; et al. Gender differences in Parkinson's disease depression. *Park. Relat. Disord.* **2017**, *36*, 93–97. [CrossRef]
13. LeWitt, P.A.; Chaudhuri, K.R. Unmet needs in Parkinson disease: Motor and non-motor. *Park. Relat. Disord.* **2020**, *80*, S7–S12. [CrossRef]

14. Kwok, J.Y.Y.; Huang, T.W.; Tretriluxana, J.; Auyeung, M.; Chau, P.H.; Lin, C.C.; Chan, H.Y.L. Symptom burden and unmet support needs of patients with Parkinson's disease: A cross-sectional study in Asia-Pacific regions. *J. Am. Med. Dir. Assoc.* **2021**, *22*, 1255–1264. [CrossRef] [PubMed]
15. Andrejack, J.; Mathur, S. What people with Parkinson's disease want. *J. Park. Dis.* **2020**, *10*, S5–S10. [CrossRef] [PubMed]
16. Uebelacker, L.A.; Epstein-Lubow, G.; Lewis, T.; Broughton, M.K.; Friedman, J.H. A survey of Parkinson's disease patients: Most bothersome symptoms and coping preferences. *J. Park. Dis.* **2014**, *4*, 717–723. [CrossRef]
17. Phillips, C.R. Quality of life in the contemporary politics of healthcare: ... but what is a life? *J. Aging Stud.* **2018**, *44*, 9–14. [CrossRef]
18. Rosqvist, K.; Hagell, P.; Odin, P.; Ekström, H.; Iwarsson, S.; Nilsson, M.H. Factors associated with life satisfaction in Parkinson's disease. *Acta Neurol. Scand.* **2017**, *136*, 64–71. [CrossRef]
19. Lehto, V.; Jolanki, O.; Valvanne, J.; Seinelä, L.; Jylhä, M. Understanding functional ability: Perspectives of nurses and older people living in long-term care. *J. Aging Stud.* **2017**, *43*, 15–22. [CrossRef]
20. Alcedo, M.A.; Fontanil, Y.; Solís, P.; Pedrosa, I.; Aguado, A.L. People with intellectual disability who are ageing. Perceived needs assessment. *Int. J. Clin. Health Psychol.* **2017**, *17*, 38–45. [CrossRef]
21. WHO. *World Report on Ageing and Health*; World Health Organization: Geneva, Switzerland, 2015. Available online: http://www.who.int/ageing/events/world-report-2015-launch/en/ (accessed on 20 January 2021).
22. Abendroth, M.; Lutz, B.J.; Young, M.E. Family caregivers' decision process to institutionalise persons with Parkinson's disease: A grounded theory study. *Int. J. Nurs. Stud.* **2012**, *49*, 445–454. [CrossRef]
23. Kyzar, K.B.; Turnbull, A.P.; Summers, J.A.; Gómez, V.A. The relationship of family support to family outcomes: A synthesis of key findings from research on severe disability. *Res. Pract. Pers. Sev. Disabl.* **2012**, *37*, 31–44. [CrossRef]
24. Takahashi, K.; Kamide, N.; Suzuki, M.; Fukuda, M. Quality of life in people with Parkinson's disease: The relevance of social relationships and communication. *J. Phys. Ther. Sci.* **2016**, *28*, 541–546. [CrossRef]
25. Monin, L.; Doyle, S.; Kershaw, T. The impact of both spousal caregivers' and care recipients' health on relationship satisfaction in the Caregiver Health Effects Study. *J. Health Psychol.* **2017**, *24*, 1744–1755. [CrossRef]
26. Pringsheim, T.; Jette, N.; Frolkis, A.; Steeves, T.D. The prevalence of Parkinson's disease: A systematic review and meta-analysis. *Mov. Disord.* **2014**, *29*, 1583–1590. [CrossRef]
27. Sugarhood, P.; Eakin, P.; Summerfield-Mann, L. Participation in advanced age: Enacting values, an adaptive process. *Ageing Soc.* **2017**, *37*, 1654–1680. [CrossRef]
28. Aguado, A.L.; Alcedo, M.A. La calidad de vida de las personas con discapacidad que envejecen. In *Cómo Mejorar la Calidad de Vida de Las Personas Con Discapacidad. Instrumentos y Estrategias de Evaluación*; Verdugo, M.A., Ed.; Amarú: Salamanca, Spain, 2006; pp. 341–363.
29. Gruijters, R.J. Family care-giving and living arrangements of functionally impaired elders in rural China. *Ageing Soc.* **2017**, *37*, 633–655. [CrossRef]
30. Navarta-Sanchez, M.V.; Garcia, J.M.S.; Riverol, M.; Ursúa Sesma, M.E.; Díaz de Cerio Ayesa, S.; Anaut Bravo, S.; Caparrós Civera, N.; Portillo, M.C. Factors influencing psychosocial adjustment and quality of life in Parkinson patients and informal caregivers. *Qual. Life Res.* **2016**, *25*, 1959–1968. [CrossRef]
31. Womack, J.L.; Lilja, M.; Isaksson, G. Crossing a Line: A narrative of risk-taking by older women serving as caregivers. *J. Aging Stud.* **2017**, *41*, 60–66. [CrossRef]
32. Post, B.; Muslimovic, D.; van Geloven, N.; Speelman, H.; Schamand, B.; de Haan, R. Progression and prognostic factors of motor impairment, disability and quality of life in newly diagnosed Parkinson's disease. *Mov. Disord.* **2011**, *26*, 449–456. [CrossRef]
33. Leturia, F.J.; Díaz, O.; Sannino, C.; Martínez, R. La atención sanitaria a las personas con discapacidad. *REDIS* **2014**, *2*, 151–164. [CrossRef]
34. WHO. *Informe Mundial Sobre la Discapacidad*; World Health Organization: Geneva, Switzerland, 2011; Available online: http://www.who.int/disabilities/world_report/2011/summary_es.pdf (accessed on 20 January 2021).
35. Sánchez, M.A.; Paz, F. Factores de riesgo, severidad y bidireccionalidad de violencia en díadas (cuidador-paciente) en enfermedad de Parkinson (Risk factors, severity and bidirectionality of violence in dyads (caregiver-patient) in Parkinson's disease). *Rev. Argent. Clin. Psicol.* **2013**, *22*, 169–178.
36. Kong, S.T.; Meng-Sang Fang, C.; Weiqun Lou, V. Organizational capacities for 'residential care homes for the elderly' to provide culturally appropriate end-of-life care for Chinese elders and their families. *J. Aging Stud.* **2017**, *40*, 1–7. [CrossRef]
37. Hurt, C.S.; Cleanthous, S.; Newman, S.P. Further explorations of illness uncertainty: Carers' experiences of Parkinson's disease. *Psychol. Health* **2017**, *32*, 549–566. [CrossRef]
38. Désesquelles, A.; Demuru, E.; Salvatore, M.A.; Pappagallo, M.; Frova, L.; Meslé, F.; Egidi, V. Mortality from Alzheimer's Disease, Parkinson's Disease, and Dementias in France and Italy. *J. Aging Health.* **2015**, *26*, 283–315. [CrossRef] [PubMed]
39. Pirhonen, J.; Pietilä, I. Active and non-active agents: Residents' agency in assisted living. *Ageing Soc.* **2018**, *38*, 19. [CrossRef]
40. Risco, E.; Cabrera, E.; Alvira, M.C.; Farré, M.; Miguel, S.; Zabalegui, A. Risk factors related to the admission of people with dementia into a long-term care institution in Spain: An explorative study. *Ageing Soc.* **2018**, *37*, 192–211. [CrossRef]

41. Berridge, C.; Mor, V. Disparities in the Prevalence of Unmet Needs and Their Consequences Among Black and White Older Adults. *J. Aging Health* **2017**, *30*, 1427–1449. [CrossRef] [PubMed]
42. Ferris, R.; Blaum, C.; Kiwak, E.; Austin, J.; Esterson, J.; Harkless, G.; Oftedahl, G.; Parchman, M.; Van Ness, P.H.; Tinetti, M.E. Perspectives of Patients, Clinicians, and Health System Leaders on Changes Needed to Improve the Health Care and Outcomes of Older Adults with Multiple Chronic Conditions. *J. Aging Health* **2017**, *30*, 778–799. [CrossRef] [PubMed]

healthcare

MDPI

Article

Quality of Life for Polish Women with Ovarian Cancer during First-Line Chemotherapy

Grażyna Bączyk [1,*], Anna Pleszewa [2], Dorota Formanowicz [3,4] and Katarzyna A. Kozłowska [1]

[1] Department of Nursing Practices, Poznan University of Medical Sciences, 61-701 Poznan, Poland; kkozlowska@ump.edu.pl
[2] Wielkopolska Oncology Centre Poznan, 61-866 Poznan, Poland; anna.pleszewa@wco.pl
[3] Department of Medical Chemistry and Laboratory Medicine, Poznan University of Medical Sciences, 61-701 Poznan, Poland; doforman@ump.edu.pl
[4] Department of Stem Cells and Regenerative Medicine, Institute of Natural Fibres and Medicinal Plants-National Research, 62-064 Plewiska, Poland
* Correspondence: gbaczyk@ump.edu.pl

Abstract: Ovarian cancer is the worst prognostic gynaecological cancer and represents a grave clinical and social problem. Therefore, the study aimed to assess female patients' emotional, cognitive, physical, and social quality of life. The study included 100 patients diagnosed with ovarian cancer and treated with chemotherapy in a day hospital setting at the Department of Radiotherapy and Gynaecological Oncology at the Wielkopolska Oncology Centre in Poznań. The patients were given a standard treatment regimen: paclitaxel 175 mg/m^2 in a 3 h infusion and carboplatin at an AUC of 6 (5–7) following Calvert as a 1 h infusion for six cycles administered every 21 days. In addition, standardised questionnaires of the Polish version of the EORTC QLQ-C30 and QLQOV28 were used. The analysis of the collected material shows that the patients reported the highest level of general health and quality of life at the study's first stage, i.e., before chemotherapy (mean value of 59.67 points). In contrast, the patients' lowest level of general health and quality of life was observed in the fourth stage of the study (mean value of 45.04 points). The problem of side effects, such as nausea and vomiting, affected the entire study group and was more troublesome in the final stage of treatment for all patients. In the study's first stage, the mean score on the nausea and vomiting symptom scale was 16 points; in the fourth stage, the mean score was 40.07. Of the clinical factors, the symptom of fatigue was the most severe health problem for the subjects. The mean score of the fatigue scale in the study's first stage was 37.11 points, while a score of 70.33 was obtained in the fourth stage of the research. The multivariate linear regression model showed that the lack of professional activity lowers quality of life, especially combined with other side effects of chemotherapy, including hair loss in Stage IV of the study. This study shows that women with ovarian cancer undergoing chemotherapy need exceptional support from psychologists, nurses, dieticians, and physiotherapists.

Keywords: ovarian cancer; quality of life; QLQ-C30 and QLQ-OV28 questionnaire; first-line chemotherapy

1. Introduction

Clinical research of ovarian cancer has evolved significantly in recent years due to the changing perception of ovarian cancer as a single disease to one encompassing several different histotypes, which differ in aetiological origin, risk factors, molecular profiles, therapeutic approaches, and clinical outcomes [1]. Despite significant progress in understanding the aetiological heterogeneity of ovarian cancer and clinical advances, ovarian cancer ranks seventh among malignancies in women. It is ranked eighth as a cause of cancer deaths in women worldwide. It is currently the most significant obstacle to achieving desirable life expectancy in most countries [1,2]. Although ovarian cancer occurs less frequently than breast cancer, it is three times more lethal. Epidemiological projections indicate that ovarian

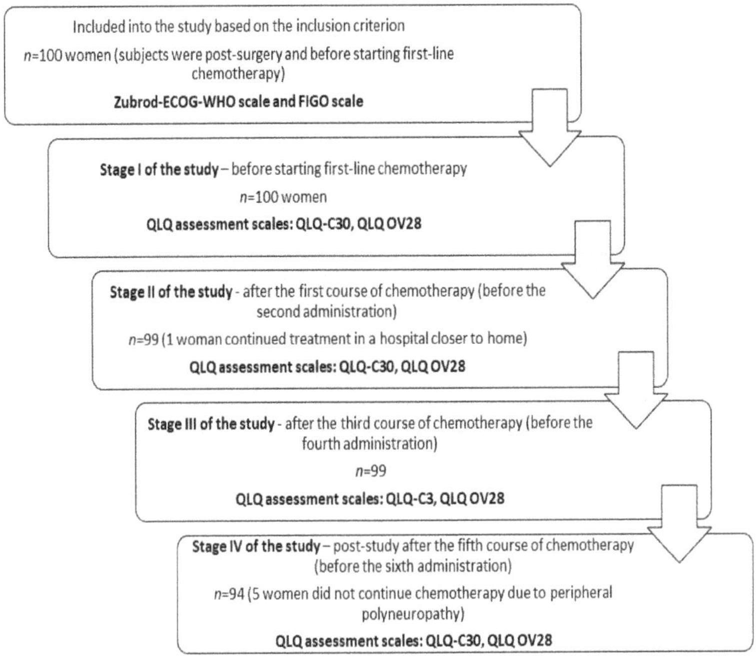

Figure 1. Course of the study.

2. Methodology

Polish versions of the scales were used to assess the quality of life: QLQ-C30 and QLQ OV28.

2.1. Standardised Questionnaires

2.1.1. EORTC QLQ-C30 Version 3.0

The European Organisation for the Research and Treatment of Cancer Quality of Life Questionnaire-Core 30 (EORTC QLQ-C30) was used in this study. The Quality of Life Study Group created the EORTC QLQ-C30 questionnaire in accordance with the European Organisation for the Research and Treatment of Cancer (EORTC). It is a fundamental tool for measuring the quality of life in the cancer patient population; it does not consider the cancer's form, type, or location. It consists of 30 questions using a 4-degree Likert scale. The exceptions are two questions on health status and general quality of life, which use a 7-point scale. The measurement of the patient's functioning includes physical and emotional functioning, functioning in social roles, cognitive and social functioning, and overall quality of life. Assessment of the impact of symptoms on quality of life includes fatigue, nausea and vomiting, dyspnoea, pain, sleep disturbances, constipation, diarrhoea, and loss of appetite. In addition, it is possible to assess the impact of the disease on the patient's financial situation. The QLQ-C30 questionnaire assesses the quality of life in 15 dimensions. In each of these, the quality of life is expressed on a 0–100 scale. The first 6 of these are functional scales, in which a higher score indicates a higher level of functioning, and a higher level of general health means a higher quality of life. The remainder are symptom scales, in which a higher score indicates an intense severity of disease symptoms and, therefore, a lower quality of life.

EORTC approval for the questionnaire was emailed via the European Organisation for Research and Treatment website on 12 February 2019.

2.1.2. EORTC QLQ-OV28

The European Organization for the Research and Treatment of Cancer Quality of Life Questionnaire—Ovarian Cancer Module (EORTC QLQ-OV28) is an ovarian module of the questionnaire, containing questions on physical and psychological symptoms in ovarian cancer patients, taking into account disease state and treatment modality (i.e., surgery, chemotherapy, radiotherapy). The ovarian module should always be completed together with the QLQ-C30 questionnaire.

The questionnaire contains 28 questions grouped into three functional scales assessing self-perception, sexuality, attitude to illness, and treatment. Assessment of the impact of symptoms on quality of life includes gastrointestinal disorders, peripheral neuropathies, menopausal symptoms, and other effects of chemotherapy, as well as the impact of hair loss on quality of life. It consists of 28 questions assessed using a 4-degree Likert scale. The quality of life assessment ranges for each scale from 0–100. For all symptoms and functional scales on the QLQ-OV28, a higher score indicates a higher severity of the problem and, therefore, lower quality of life.

EORTC approval was obtained for using the scales mentioned above, and the key was received by email via the European Organisation for Research and Treatment website on 12 February 2019.

2.2. *Documentation of the Patient's Medical History*

Laboratory results were analysed from each patient's medical history, including haemoglobin, erythrocyte, leukocyte, neurocyte, platelet, and CA125 antigen levels. In addition, comorbidities and stages of disease according to the 2014 FIGO [10] were analysed in the study's first phase. A subsequent article will include laboratory results regarding quality of life analysis.

2.3. *Questionnaire*

A self-administered survey questionnaire comprised five questions concerning age, place of residence, marital status, education, and professional activity.

2.4. *Ethics*

The study was conducted in accordance with the Declaration of Helsinki and was approved by the Ethics Committee of the Poznan University of Medical Sciences and registered under reference numbers 46/16 and 564/16 (all patients gave informed consent, and the Ethics Committee of Poznan University of Medical Sciences approved the study registered as case Nos. 46/16 and 564/16). Participation in the survey was voluntary and anonymous, and all participants in the study gave their informed consent to participate. The informed consent form contained information about the study, its purpose, the method of responding to questions, and the possibility of withdrawing from the study at any time without incurring any consequences.

2.5. *Statistical Methods*

Analysis of the quantitative variables (i.e., expressed in numbers) was carried out by calculating the arithmetic mean, standard deviation, median, and quartiles.

Analysis of the qualitative (i.e., non-numeric) variables was carried out by calculating each value's number and percentage of occurrence.

Qualitative variables were compared across groups using the chi-square test (with Yates correction for 2×2 tables) or Fisher's exact test where low expected counts appeared.

Comparisons of quantitative variables across three or more groups were made using the Kruskal–Wallis test. When statistically significant differences were detected, a post hoc analysis was performed with Dunn's test to identify statistically significantly different groups.

Comparisons of quantitative variables across the four repeated measures were made using the Friedman test. Once statistically significant differences were detected, a post hoc analysis (Wilcoxon paired *t*-tests with Bonferroni correction) was performed to identify statistically significant measurement differences.

Multivariate analysis was used to determine the factors influencing the quality of life and to assess their significance and the amount of variance explained by these factors.

The variables of age, marital status, education, professional activity, comorbidities, and FIGO scale were introduced into the model.

Multivariate analysis was used for the QLQ-OV 28 scale for Stages I and IV.

Statistical analysis was performed in R. version 4.1.0 using the R Core Team (2021) method (R: a language and environment for statistical computing, R Foundation for Statistical Computing, Vienna, Austria. URL https://www.R-project.org/) (accessed on 30 December 2019).

3. Results

3.1. Characteristics of Respondents

One hundred women participated in Stage I of the study. In comparison, 94 respondents participated in Stage IV. Five women did not continue chemotherapy due to the development of peripheral polyneuropathy: three women aged 61 years and over and two women aged 41–50. Moreover, one woman aged 41–50 continued treatment in a hospital closer to home after the first administration.

Almost 38% of the respondents had completed the secondary education level. More than half of the women in the study (64%) were pensioners, and 36% worked professionally. In 68% of the patients, the stage of ovarian cancer was defined as Stage III according to the FIGO classification, with 63% in Stage IV of the study (Table 1).

Table 1. Characteristics of patients upon enrolment in the study.

Variable	Number of Patients (*n*)
Age range (years)	
• ≤50	14
• 51–60	21
• ≥61	65
Marital status	
• Single	12
• Married	54
• Widow	34
Education	
• Elementary	13
• Vocational	30
• Secondary	38
• Higher	19
Professional activity	
• Professionally active	36
• Pension	64
Comorbidities	
• YES	59
• NO	41
FIGO stage	
• II	22
• III	68
• IV	10

3.2. Analysis of the Quality of Life as Based on the QLQ-C30 and QLQ-OV28 Scales of the Subjects in the Different Stages of the Study (Table 2)

The analysis showed statistically significant differences between the different stages of the study for all quality of life scales.

The mean values for general health, physical functioning, role functioning, emotional functioning, cognitive functioning, and social functioning were higher in the first stage of the study compared to the mean values in the subsequent stages of the study. In the fourth stage of the study, the mean values were the lowest, indicating the lowest quality of life of the subjects.

Statistically significant differences were found for all areas of the scale across the stages of the study ($p < 0.001$) (Table 2).

Table 2. Comparison of patients' quality of life by stage of the study based on QLQ-C30 functional scales.

Quality of Life		Stage I	Stage II	Stage III	Stage IV	*p*
General health/QOL	Mean ± SD	59.67 ± 16.31	53.54 ± 14.39	48.65 ± 16.53	45.04 ± 18.59	$p < 0.001$ *
	median	58.33	50	50	41.67	
	quartiles	50–66.67	50–66.67	37.5–58.33	33.33–58.33	I > II > III, IV
Physical functioning	Mean ± SD	74.27 ± 20.19	65.45 ± 19.62	51.11 ± 22.38	45.46 ± 21.99	$p < 0.001$ *
	median	80	66.67	53.33	46.67	
	quartiles	60–93.33	46.67–80	36.66–66.67	26.67–65	I > II > III > IV
Functioning in roles	Mean ± SD	69 ± 24.28	58.08 ± 23.01	46.13 ± 24.38	39.72 ± 26.22	$p < 0.001$ *
	median	66.67	66.67	50	33.33	
	quartiles	50–100	33.33–66.67	33.33–66.67	16.67–66.67	I > II > III.IV
Emotional functioning	Mean ± SD	55.75 ± 18.94	47.47 ± 18.65	37.12 ± 19.06	28.28 ± 22.14	$p < 0.001$ *
	median	58.33	50	33.33	33.33	
	quartiles	41.67–66.67	33.33–66.67	25–50	8.33–47.92	I > II > III > IV
Cognitive functioning	Mean ± SD	77 ± 19.79	71.38 ± 21.57	63.97 ± 21.52	57.98 ± 22.36	$p < 0.001$ *
	median	83.33	66.67	66.67	66.67	
	quartiles	66.67–100	50–83.33	50–83.33	50–66.67	I > II > III > IV
Social functioning	Mean ± SD	63.5 ± 21.54	51.68 ± 22.27	39.39 ± 23.02	35.11 ± 26.04	$p < 0.001$ *
	median	66.67	50	33.33	33.33	
	quartiles	50–66.67	33.33–66.67	25–66.67	16.67–66.67	I > II > III, IV

p—Friedman test + post hoc analysis (Wilcoxon matched pair tests with Bonferroni correction). * statistically significant relationship ($p < 0.05$). QLQ-C30: functional scales—higher value indicates a higher level of functioning/quality of life; range 0–100.

The mean values in the functional and symptom scales increased with the order of the study stage, indicating higher problem severity and lower quality of life for the patients. Statistically significant differences were found for all areas of the symptom scales in the different stages of the study ($p < 0.001$). There was the highest increase in mean values for "hair loss", with a mean value of 8.67 in Stage I, while in Stage IV of the study, the value increased to 65.96 (Table 3).

Table 3. Comparison of patients' quality of life at different study stages based on the QLQ-OV28 functional and symptom scales.

Quality of Life		Stage I	Stage II	Stage III	Stage IV	*p*
Perception of one's own body	Mean ± SD	30.5 ± 23.81	43.1 ± 24.4	54.71 ± 28.87	58.87 ± 31.84	$p < 0.001$ *
	median	33.33	33.33	66.67	66.67	
	quartiles	0–33.33	33.33–66.67	33.33–66.67	33.33–83.33	IV, III > II > I
Sexuality	Mean ± SD	6.43 ± 11.04	2.34 ± 6.64	1.93 ± 6.25	1.23 ± 5.2	$p < 0.001$ *
	median	0	0	0	0	
	quartiles	0–16.67	0–0	0–0	0–0	I > II, III, IV
Approach to disease/treatment	Mean ± SD	63.67 ± 24.46	73.79 ± 19.65	82.27 ± 17.16	86.53 ± 19.27	$p < 0.001$ *
	median	66.67	77.78	77.78	100	
	quartiles	44.44–77.78	55.56–88.89	66.67–100	77.78–100	IV > III > II > I

Table 3. *Cont.*

Quality of Life		Stage I	Stage II	Stage III	Stage IV	p
Gastrointestinal symptoms	Mean ± SD median quartiles	39.52 ± 21.5 38.1 28.57–53.57	41.32 ± 19.02 42.86 28.57–52.38	47.14 ± 18.13 42.86 33.33–57.14	51.32 ± 21.15 47.62 34.52–66.67	$p < 0.001$ * IV > III > II.I
Peripheral neuropathy	Mean ± SD median quartiles	19.44 ± 23.39 11.11 0–33.33	42.54 ± 24.28 33.33 33.33–66.67	59.15 ± 22.04 66.67 33.33–66.67	71.04 ± 21.57 66.67 55.56–97.22	$p < 0.001$ * IV > III > II > I
Hormonal/menopausal symptoms	Mean ± SD median quartiles	15.17 ± 20.25 0 0–33.33	18.18 ± 20.63 16.67 0–33.33	21.38 ± 21.57 16.67 0–33.33	25.53 ± 24.77 33.33 0–33.33	$p < 0.001$ * IV > III > II.I
Other side effects of chemotherapy	Mean ± SD median quartiles	26.53 ± 19.21 20 13.33–40	36.8 ± 17.78 40 26.67–46.67	47.68 ± 17.31 46.67 36.66–60	53.4 ± 16.92 53.33 40–66.67	$p < 0.001$ * IV > III > II > I
Hair loss	Mean ± SD median quartiles	8.67 ± 21.25 0 0–0	44.61 ± 22.57 33.33 33.33–66.67	65.96 ± 26.43 66.67 50–83.33	70.2 ± 21.33 66.67 66.67–83.33	$p < 0.001$ * III > IV > II.I

p—Friedman test + post hoc analysis (Wilcoxon matched pair tests with Bonferroni correction); * statistically significant relationship ($p < 0.05$). QLQ-OV28: functional scales/symptom scales—higher value indicates greater severity of problems/symptoms and lower quality of life; range 0–100.

3.3. Women's Quality of Life According to the QLQ-OV28 Functional and Symptom Scales at Stage I of the Study

1. Perception of One's Own Body Domain—See Table S1 in Supplementary Material.
2. Sexuality Domain—See Table S2 in Supplementary Material.
3. Approach to Disease/Treatment Domain—See Table S3 in Supplementary Material.
4. Gastrointestinal Symptoms Domain—See Table S4 in Supplementary Material.
5. Peripheral Neuropathy Domain—See Table S5 in Supplementary Material.
6. Hormonal/Menopausal Symptoms Domain—See Table S6 in Supplementary Material.
7. Other Side Effects of Chemotherapy Domain—See Table S7 in Supplementary Material.
8. Hair Loss Domain—See Table S8 in Supplementary Material.

3.4. Women's Quality of Life According to the QLQ-OV28 Functional and Symptom Scales at Stage IV of the Study

3.4.1. Perception of One's Own Body Domain

Table 4 presents the results of a multivariate analysis for the QLQ-OV28 scale in the perception of one's own body domain.

The multivariate linear regression model showed that patients aged 61 and over had a perception of one's own body domain score that was, on average, 38.395 points lower than those aged up to 50 years. A lack of professional activity was associated with an increase in the score for the perception of one's own body domain by an average of 34.2 points.

The R^2 coefficient for this model was 13.62%, which means that 13.62% of the variability of the perception of one's own body domain result was explained by the variables included in the model (see Table 4).

Table 4. Women's quality of life according to the QLQ-OV28 in perception of one's own body domain at Stage IV.

Variable		Regression Coefficient	95%CI		*p*
Age	≤50	ref.			
	51–60	−9.722	−35.549	16.104	0.463
	≥61	−38.395	−66.903	−9.887	0.01 *
Marital status	Single	ref.			
	Married	−10.808	−32.485	10.87	0.331
	Widow	−19.17	−42.553	4.212	0.112
Education	Elementary	ref.			
	Vocational	−8.256	−29.952	13.439	0.458
	Secondary	−4.936	−26.961	17.09	0.662
	Higher	0.866	−26.603	28.335	0.951
Professional activity	Professionally active	ref.			
	Pension	34.2	7.019	61.382	0.016 *
Comorbidities	No	ref.			
	Yes	−1.231	−15.145	12.682	0.863
FIGO stage	II	ref.			
	III	0.808	−14.928	16.544	0.92
	IV	0.598	−25.149	26.345	0.964

p—multiple linear regression; * statistically significant ($p < 0.05$).

3.4.2. Sexuality Domain

Table 5 presents the results of a multivariate analysis for the QLQ-OV28 scale in the sexuality domain. The multivariate linear regression model showed that none of the analysed features was a significant independent predictor of the sexuality domain score (all $p > 0.05$).

Table 5. Women's quality of life according to the QLQ-OV28 in the sexuality domain at Stage IV.

Variable		Regression Coefficient	95%CI		*p*
Age	≤50	ref.			
	51–60	−2.055	−6.219	2.109	0.336
	≥61	−3.944	−8.541	0.652	0.096
Marital status	Single	ref.			
	Married	1.845	−1.651	5.34	0.304
	Widow	1.501	−2.269	5.271	0.437
Education	Elementary	ref.			
	Vocational	−0.055	−3.553	3.443	0.975
	Secondary	−0.719	−4.27	2.833	0.693
	Higher	0.963	−3.466	5.392	0.671
Professional activity	Professionally active	ref.			
	Pension	−0.731	−5.114	3.651	0.744
Comorbidities	No	ref.			
	Yes	0.033	−2.21	2.276	0.977
FIGO stage	II	ref.			
	III	0.17	−2.368	2.707	0.896
	IV	−0.458	−4.609	3.693	0.829

p—multiple linear regression.

The R^2 coefficient for this model was 15.71%, which means that 15.71% of the variability of the sexuality domain result was explained by the variables included in the model (see Table 5).

3.4.3. Approach to Disease/Treatment Domain

Table 6 presents the results of a multivariate analysis for the QLQ-OV28 scale in the approach to disease/treatment domain.

Table 6. Women's quality of life according to the QLQ-OV28 in the approach to disease/treatment domain at Stage IV.

Variable		Regression Coefficient	95%CI		*p*
Age	≤50	ref.			
	51–60	2.754	−13.096	18.604	0.734
	≥61	−4.334	−21.83	13.162	0.629
Marital status	Single	ref.			
	Married	−4.036	−17.339	9.268	0.554
	Widow	0.651	−13.699	15.001	0.929
Education	Elementary	ref.			
	Vocational	−9.135	−22.45	4.179	0.182
	Secondary	−2.042	−15.559	11.476	0.768
	Higher	−0.968	−17.826	15.89	0.911
Professional activity	Professionally active	ref.			
	Pension	14.151	−2.531	30.832	0.1
Comorbidities	No	ref.			
	Yes	−4.029	−12.568	4.509	0.358
FIGO stage	II	ref.			
	III	3.802	−5.855	13.459	0.443
	IV	3.993	−11.809	19.794	0.622

p—multiple linear regression.

The multivariate linear regression model showed that none of the analysed features was a significant independent predictor of the disease/treatment domain score (all $p > 0.05$).

The R^2 coefficient for this model was 11.19%, which means that 11.19% of the variability of the disease/treatment domain result was explained by the variables included in the model (see Table 6).

3.4.4. Gastrointestinal Symptoms Domain

Table 7 presents the results of a multivariate analysis for the QLQ-OV28 scale in the gastrointestinal symptoms domain.

The multivariate linear regression model showed the following:

- The status of being married reduces the result on the gastrointestinal symptoms domain by an average of 14.961 points in relation to single and widowed status;
- The lack of professional activity increases the result on the gastrointestinal symptoms domain by an average of 19.389 points.

The R^2 coefficient for this model was 18.17%, which means that 18.17% of the variability of the gastrointestinal symptoms domain result was explained by the variables included in the model (see Table 7).

Table 7. Women's quality of life according to the QLQ-OV28 in the gastrointestinal symptoms domain at Stage IV.

Variable		Regression Coefficient	95%CI		*p*
Age	≤50	ref.			
	51–60	4.447	−12.25	21.143	0.603
	≥61	−3.976	−22.406	14.454	0.674
Marital status	Single	ref.			
	Married	−14.961	−28.976	−0.947	0.039 *
	Widow	−14.078	−29.194	1.039	0.072
Education	Elementary	ref.			
	Vocational	−9.727	−23.752	4.299	0.178
	Secondary	−5.463	−19.702	8.776	0.454
	Higher	−3.348	−21.106	14.41	0.713
Professional activity	Professionally active	ref.			
	Pension	19.389	1.816	36.961	0.033 *
Comorbidities	No	ref.			
	Yes	−1.886	−10.881	7.109	0.682
FIGO stage	II	ref.			
	III	0.476	−9.697	10.65	0.927
	IV	5.285	−11.361	21.93	0.535

p—multiple linear regression; * statistically significant ($p < 0.05$).

3.4.5. Peripheral Neuropathy Domain

Table 8 presents the results of a multivariate analysis for the QLQ-OV28 scale in the peripheral neuropathy domain.

Table 8. Women's quality of life according to the QLQ-OV28 in the peripheral neuropathy domain at Stage IV.

Variable		Regression Coefficient	95%CI		*p*
Age	≤50	ref.			
	51–60	12.852	−2.607	28.31	0.107
	≥61	10.614	−6.45	27.677	0.226
Marital status	Single	ref.			
	Married	−5.969	−18.944	7.006	0.37
	Widow	−5.302	−19.297	8.694	0.46
Education	Elementary	ref.			
	Vocational	−1.427	−14.412	11.559	0.83
	Secondary	0.828	−12.355	14.011	0.902
	Higher	−3.805	−20.246	12.637	0.651
Professional activity	Professionally active	ref.			
	Pension	20.597	4.328	36.867	0.015 *
Comorbidities	No	ref.			
	Yes	−7.103	−15.431	1.224	0.098
FIGO stage	II	ref.			
	III	0.533	−8.886	9.952	0.912
	IV	3.236	−12.175	18.646	0.682

p—multiple linear regression; * statistically significant ($p < 0.05$).

A multivariate linear regression model showed that professional inactivity increases the peripheral neuropathy domain score by an average of 20.597 points.

The R^2 coefficient for this model was 32.57%, which means that 32.57% of the variability of the peripheral neuropathy domain result was explained by the variables included in the model (see Table 8).

3.4.6. Hormonal/Menopausal Symptoms Domain

Table 9 presents the results of a multivariate analysis for the QLQ-OV28 scale in the hormonal/menopausal symptoms domain. The multivariate linear regression model showed the following:

- Being married reduces the score on the hormonal/menopausal symptoms domain by an average of 17.222 points in relation to being single;
- Widowhood reduces the score on the hormonal/menopausal symptoms domain by an average of 22.994 points in relation to being single.

Table 9. Women's quality of life according to the QLQ-OV28 in the hormonal/menopausal symptoms domain at Stage IV.

Variable		Regression Coefficient	95%CI		p
Age	≤50	ref.			
	51–60	−8.082	−28.274	12.109	0.435
	≥61	−20.106	−42.394	2.182	0.081
Marital status	Single	ref.			
	Married	−17.222	−34.169	−0.274	0.05 *
	Widow	−22.994	−41.275	−4.713	0.016 *
Education	Elementary	ref.			
	Vocational	6.841	−10.121	23.803	0.432
	Secondary	1.493	−15.726	18.713	0.865
	Higher	2.829	−18.647	24.305	0.797
Professional activity	Professionally active	ref.			
	Pension	10.269	−10.982	31.52	0.346
Comorbidities	No	ref.			
	Yes	−0.77	−11.648	10.108	0.89
FIGO stage	II	ref.			
	III	−0.009	−12.311	12.294	0.999
	IV	−0.873	−21.003	19.256	0.932

p—multiple linear regression; * statistically significant ($p < 0.05$).

The R^2 coefficient for this model was 12.76%, which means that 12.76% of the variability of the hormonal/menopausal symptoms domain result was explained by the variables included in the model (see Table 9).

3.4.7. Other Side Effects of Chemotherapy Domain

Table 10 presents the results of a multivariate analysis for the QLQ-OV28 scale in the other side effects of chemotherapy domain. The multivariate linear regression model showed the following:

- A lack of professional activity increases the result on the other side effects of chemotherapy domain by an average of 14.401 points.

The R^2 coefficient for this model was 22.34%, which means that 22.34% of the other side effects of chemotherapy domain result was determined by the variables included in the model (see Table 10).

Table 10. Women's quality of life according to the QLQ-OV28 in the other side effects of chemotherapy domain at Stage IV.

Variable		Regression Coefficient	95%CI		p
Age	≤50	ref.			
	51–60	11.071	−1.941	24.084	0.099
	≥61	4.65	−9.714	19.014	0.528
Marital status	Single	ref.			
	Married	−3.607	−14.529	7.315	0.519
	Widow	−0.543	−12.324	11.238	0.928
Education	Elementary	ref.			
	Vocational	−2.964	−13.895	7.967	0.597
	Secondary	−2.055	−13.152	9.043	0.718
	Higher	−3.076	−16.916	10.764	0.664
Professional activity	Professionally active	ref.			
	Pension	14.401	0.706	28.097	0.042 *
Comorbidities	No	ref.			
	Yes	0.25	−6.76	7.26	0.944
FIGO stage	II	ref.			
	III	0.794	−7.134	8.723	0.845
	IV	0.6	−12.373	13.572	0.928

p—multiple linear regression; * statistically significant ($p < 0.05$).

3.4.8. Hair Loss Domain

Table 11 presents the results of a multivariate analysis for the QLQ-OV28 scale in the hair loss domain. The model showed that a lack of professional activity increases the result on the hair loss domain by an average of 21.947 points.

Table 11. Women's quality of life according to the QLQ-OV28 in the hair loss domain at Stage IV.

Variable		Regression Coefficient	95%CI		p
Age	≤50	ref.			
	51–60	−10.947	−31.034	9.141	0.289
	≥61	−16.865	−39.038	5.309	0.14
Marital status	Single	ref.			
	Married	13.815	−3.045	30.675	0.112
	Widow	3.774	−14.412	21.96	0.685
Education	Elementary	ref.			
	Vocational	−14.839	−31.713	2.035	0.089
	Secondary	−1.959	−19.09	15.172	0.823
	Higher	8.203	−13.162	29.568	0.454
Professional activity	Professionally active	ref.			
	Pension	21.947	0.806	43.088	0.045 *
Comorbidities	No	ref.			
	Yes	−10.49	−21.312	0.332	0.061
FIGO stage	II	ref.			
	III	10.296	−1.943	22.535	0.103
	IV	−7.532	−27.558	12.494	0.463

p—multiple linear regression; * statistically significant ($p < 0.05$).

The R^2 coefficient for this model was 24.15%, which means that 24.15% of the variability of the hair loss domain result was explained by the variables included in the model (see Table 11).

4. Discussion

Research on quality of life primarily aims to show how the disease, symptoms or treatment affect patients and how it relates to different life domains/activities. Counterfactually, few research papers analyse the quality of life in women with ovarian cancer treated with chemotherapy. The available scientific papers approach the topic in a general way, cover different types of cancer therapies, and often do not assess the impact of clinical and demographic factors on quality of life, nor do they compare the stages of chemotherapy administration. It should also be noted that in the few studies cited, the methodology, the research tools used, the group sizes, and the determinants analysed differ significantly from our research.

4.1. Quality of Life in Women with Ovarian Cancer during Chemotherapy

In the present study, Polish ovarian cancer patients undergoing first-line chemotherapy had an increasingly poor quality of life assessment with each study stage (four stages). Cytostatics treatment significantly affected overall health, including worsening symptoms/complications and emotional, cognitive, physical, and social functioning.

Statistically significant differences in the assessment of quality of life were observed in areas related to the side effects of chemotherapy. Comparing the results of the first stage of the study with the results of the fourth stage, the following symptoms were observed: nausea and vomiting, loss of appetite, peripheral neuropathy, and hair loss.

Campbell et al. obtained similar results [14] when they investigated the impact of chemotherapy on women with recurrent ovarian cancer and the quality of their lives. They also used the EORTC QLQ-C30 and EORTC QLQ-OV28 questionnaires as well as the MOST-T35 (Measure of Ovarian Symptoms and Treatment Concerns). In their analyses, symptoms originating from the gastrointestinal tract related to symptomatic neuropathy, nausea and vomiting, and psychiatric symptoms negatively affected the quality of life. Also, the patients presented a low quality of life in the functioning and general health questionnaires. In a study conducted by Nho et al. [15], it was found that successive cycles of chemotherapy, where the patients received either platinum or taxane (and, above all, the resultant numerous side effects), worsened their quality of life. Mental stress, fatigue, pain, abdominal discomfort, flu-like symptoms, fluid accumulation, and peripheral neuropathy negatively affected the quality of life of ovarian cancer patients undergoing adjuvant chemotherapy, especially in patients with depression and high anxiety levels, as reported by Hwang et al. [16]. Low quality of life, especially in the area of physical and emotional functioning, and susceptibility to mood disorders, were presented by patients in the study by Shirala et al. [17]. Deterioration of quality of life in women with ovarian cancer was also observed by Chase et al. [18], Tachata et al. [19], Słoniewski et al. (platinum-based chemotherapy) [20], Lee et al. [21], Sarkar et al. [22], Śniadecki et al. (intraperitoneal chemotherapy—IPC) [23], Bhugwandass et al. (chemotherapy type: carboplatin–paclitaxel, cisplatin–paclitaxel, cisplatin–etoposide, and cyclophosphamide–carboplatin) [24], and Perkowska et al. [25] as a result of chemotherapy. In a study by Lee et al. [26], only 15% (out of approximately 948) of patients indicated improved quality of life after completion of platinum-based chemotherapy. Perkowska et al. [5] and Smorąg et al. [27] linked poor quality of life to depression in women in their studies. Kozaka [28], in her review article, clearly emphasised that treatment-related side effects, including physical and emotional burdens, significantly affect women's quality of life.

Plotti et al. (Carboplatin and Paclitaxel) [29], Kim et al. (hyperthermic intraperitoneal chemotherapy—HIPEC) [30], Blagden et al. (carboplatin and paclitaxel) [31], and Penar-Zadarko et al. [32] obtained different results, indicating that chemotherapy does not affect the quality of life in a way that reduces it or keeps it stable [33]. Pergialiotis et al. [34]

indicated that the type of treatment used (in this case, combination therapy with taxanes and platinum) affected quality of life. Also, in Sompolska-Rzechuła [4], women undergoing chemotherapy rated their quality of life positively in the social, functional, emotional, and physical spheres, and adverse symptoms did not affect their well-being negatively.

4.2. Selected Parameters and the Quality of Life of Women with Ovarian Cancer during Chemotherapy

The research has shown that age is one of the factors that strongly determines quality of life. Depending on the number of years and the subsequent study stage, the women felt that their quality of life was affected differently by their functioning, symptoms, or sense of their health. For example, women over 60 were not affected by sexual problems, hormonal/menopausal symptoms, or their body perception. In contrast, higher levels of fatigue, pain, shortness of breath, or gastrointestinal symptoms were reported to affect quality of life. Alternatively, regarding the effect of nausea and vomiting on quality of life, at Stage III of the study, this symptom correlated strongly in 51–60-year-old women. However, Stage IV did not significantly affect this age group, indicating that life stage (age) and related functioning, social roles, and expectations are reflected in the perception of quality of life.

In Nho et al. [15], age was also a factor in reduced quality of life. According to Zhou et al. [35], poor quality of life was also related to age (older age influenced poorer functioning in the physical area, whereas younger age influenced poorer functioning in the mental area). Older people ($\geq$70 years of age), as reported by Walree et al. [36], had a lower sense of the quality of life than younger people (<70 years of age), especially in the domains of general health and in all functional subscales, except for emotional functioning. Panoskaltsis et al. [37] performed a multivariate analysis of the effect of age on the quality of life in women with ovarian cancer undergoing intraperitoneal chemotherapy in hypothermia (HIPEC). Advanced age (>65) was a factor that negatively affected patient survival. In Sompolska-Rzechuła [4], women aged 63–88 had a higher quality of life in terms of social well-being, emotional well-being, functional well-being, and perceived complaints, and women aged 24–63 years had a higher quality of life in terms of physical well-being. In the present study, the severity of the disease had an impact on some quality of life domains, both in the functional areas and the symptoms present, being variable depending on the phase of the study. In our study, the multivariate linear regression model showed that lack of professional activity lowers the quality of life, especially because the other side effects of chemotherapy domain, as well as hair loss in Stage IV of the study.

Chase et al. [18], Friendlander et al. [38], Tachata et al. [19] (disease stage adversely affected the gastrointestinal variable in the patients), and Zhou et al. [35] also observed the impact of the disease stage on quality of life. In contrast, Koole et al. [39], who evaluated the effect of intraperitoneal hyperthermia chemotherapy in Stage III ovarian cancer, showed no negative impact on quality of life. Similarly, Sampolska-Rzechuła et al. [4] found that functional well-being, social well-being, and perceived discomfort were not significantly associated with disease stage.

The research was conducted on the Polish population and should only be related to this population. The authors recommend performing future studies in other national groups and making comparisons, which could provide interesting results and be the subject of interesting discussion.

A significant limitation of our research is the small size of the group. This may limit the ability to conclusively determine the impact of chemotherapy on quality of life. However, it was only possible to recruit the women who met the established criteria during the study period.

The quality of life of the subjects was not assessed by taking into account the scope of the surgery and histologic tumour type. The researchers knew the results of laboratory tests for the examined women, such as the level of haemoglobin, erythrocytes, leukocytes, neurocytes, platelets, and the CA125 antigen. Using multivariate analysis, the article considered these parameters in assessing the quality of life.

The study did not include a comparison group of women without ovarian cancer or women with ovarian cancer who had not received chemotherapy. This may limit the ability to conclusively determine the impact of chemotherapy on quality of life.

This study was partially conducted during the COVID-19 pandemic; however, to maintain the original assumptions, we did not study the impact of COVID-19, which could potentially affect the results.

The innovative value of this study is that the results are paramount and needed in developing treatment and nursing programs to reduce the side effects of chemotherapy, for example, the prevention of nausea and vomiting, appetite enhancement, and coping with hair loss, especially for older and retired women.

5. Conclusions

Deterioration of physical, emotional, cognitive, and social functioning during successive rounds of chemotherapy is associated with the need for improving and intensifying the care associated with cancer treatment.

Gastrointestinal symptoms during treatment require continuous monitoring and evaluation for adjustments to supportive management.

Side effects accompanying treatment for ovarian cancer patients require support from psychologists, dieticians, nurses, and physiotherapists.

The obtained results will help to create a strategy for reducing the severity of chemotherapy side effects, which may improve the quality of life of women with ovarian cancer.

The implications of the above research can be a source of education for patients undergoing chemotherapy, as an indicator of what complications and intensity they can expect at each stage of treatment, additionally taking into account their age. For medical staff (nurses and doctors), quality of life research can support a holistic approach to patients who receive chemotherapy, including preventive action to reduce ailments/complications.

The research was conducted in Poland, only in one city. An interesting prospect would be to extend this study to other centres, including foreign ones, and to conduct comparative studies to see if all patient populations respond the same to chemotherapy using different types of cytostatics.

Supplementary Materials: The following supporting information can be downloaded at: https://www.mdpi.com/article/10.3390/healthcare11182596/s1, Table S1: Women's quality of life according to the QLQ-OV28 in perception of one's own body domain at I stage; Table S2: Women's quality of life according to the QLQ-OV28 in sexuality domain at I stage; Table S3: Women's quality of life according to the QLQ-OV28 in approach to disease/treatment domain at I stage; Table S4: Women's quality of life according to the QLQ-OV28 in gastrointestinal symptoms domain at I stage; Table S5: Women's quality of life according to the QLQ-OV28 in peripheral neuropathy domain at I stage; Table S6: Women's quality of life according to the QLQ-OV28 in hormonal /menopausal symptoms domain at I stage; Table S7: Women's quality of life according to the QLQ-OV28 in other side effects of chemotherapy domain at I stage; Table S8: Women's quality of life according to the QLQ-OV28 in hair loss domain at I stage.

Author Contributions: Conceptualization: G.B. and A.P.; data curation: A.P.; formal analysis: A.P. and G.B.; investigation: A.P.; methodology: A.P. and G.B.; writing—original draft: A.P., G.B. and K.A.K.; writing—review and editing, K.A.K., G.B. and D.F.; supervision: G.B. and D.F. All authors have read and agreed to the published version of the manuscript.

Funding: This research received no external funding.

Institutional Review Board Statement: The study was conducted following the Helsinki Declaration and was approved by the Poznan University of Medical Sciences Ethics Committee, registered under reference numbers 46/16 and 564/16.

Informed Consent Statement: Informed consent was obtained from all subject involved in the study.

Data Availability Statement: Data are available from the authors upon reasonable request.

Conflicts of Interest: The authors declare no conflict of interest.

Abbreviations

ECOG	Eastern Cooperative Oncology Group
EORTC	European Organization for the Research and Treatment of Cancer
EORTC QLQ-C30	European Organization for the Research and Treatment of Cancer Quality of Life Questionnaire—Core 30
EORTC QLQ-OV28	European Organization for the Research and Treatment of Cancer Quality of Life Questionnaire—Ovarian Cancer Module
FIGO	International Federation of Gynaecology and Obstetrics
QLQ-C30	Cancer Quality of Life Questionnaire
QLQ OV28	Ovarian Cancer Quality of Life Questionnaire
QOL	Quality of Life

References

1. Gaona-Luviano, P.; Medina-Gaona, L.A.; Magaña-Pérez, K. Epidemiology of ovarian cancer. *Chin. Clin. Oncol.* **2020**, *9*, 47. [CrossRef] [PubMed]
2. Brett, M.R.; Jennifer, B.P.; Thomas, A.S.; Brett, M.R.; Jennifer, B.P.; Thomas, A.S. Epidemiology of ovarian cancer: A review. *Cancer Biol. Med.* **2017**, *14*, 9–32. [CrossRef] [PubMed]
3. Bray, F.; Ferlay, J.; Soerjomataram, I.; Siegel, R.L.; Torre, L.A.; Jemal, A. Global cancer statistics 2018: GLOBOCAN estimates of incidence and mortality worldwide for 36 cancers in 185 countries. *CA Cancer J. Clin.* **2018**, *68*, 394–424. [CrossRef] [PubMed]
4. Sompolska-Rzechuła, A.; Cymbaluk-Płoska, A.; Chudecka-Głaz, A. Ocena jakości życia kobiet z chorobą nowotworową leczonych metodą chemioterapii. *Pr. Nauk. Uniw. Ekon. We Wrocławiu* **2017**, *483*, 152–612.
5. Perkowska, E.; Terlikowski, S.; Terlikowski, R.; Moczydłowska, A.; Ziemczyk, B. Quality of life for women treated for ovarian cancer. *Pieleg. Chir. Angiol/Surg. Vasc. Nurs.* **2020**, *1*, 25–30.
6. Leppert, W.; Woroń, J. Nudności i wymioty u chorych na nowotwory—Zalecenia postępowania terapeutycznego. *Gastroenterol. Klin.* **2016**, *8*, 85–98.
7. Płużański, A. Nudności i wymioty towarzyszące wysokoemetogennej chemioterapii—Analiza klinicznej praktyki. *Nowotw. J. Oncol.* **2015**, *65*, 122–127. [CrossRef]
8. Jabłońska, I.; Drabik, U. Charakterystyka aspektów jakości życia pacjentów z rakiem odbytnicy. *Probl. Pieleg.* **2009**, *17*, 144–151.
9. Nagańska, E. Powikłania neurologiczne po chemioterapii. *Neurol. Dyplomie* **2019**, *4*, 47–53.
10. Megari, K. Quality of life in chronic disease patients. *Health Psychol. Res.* **2013**, *1*, e27. [CrossRef]
11. Bączyk, G.; Formanowicz, D.; Gmerek, Ł.; Krokowicz, P. Health-related quality of life assessment among patients with inflammatory bowel diseases after surgery—Review. *Gastroenterol. Rev.* **2017**, *12*, 6–16. [CrossRef] [PubMed]
12. Bhat, G.; Karakasis, K.; Oza, A.M. Measuring Quality of Life in Ovarian Cancer Clinical Trials—Can We Improve Objectivity and Cross Trial Comparisons? *Cancers* **2020**, *12*, 3296. [CrossRef] [PubMed]
13. Zalewski, K.; Misiek, M.; Góźdź, S.; Bidziński, M. Nowy system klasyfikacji zaawansowania nowotworów jajnika, jajowodu i otrzewnej—Stan na 2014 rok. *Onkol. Prakt. Klin.* **2015**, *11*, 129–134.
14. Campbell, R.; Costa, D.S.J.; Stocklera, M.; Lee, Y.C.; Ledermann, J.A.; Berton, D.; Sehouli, J.; Roncolato, F.T.; Connell, R.O.; Okamoto, A.; et al. Measure of Ovarian Symptoms and Treatment concerns (MOST) indexes and their associations with health-related quality of life in recurrent ovarian cancer. *Gynecol. Oncol.* **2022**, *166*, 254–262. [CrossRef]
15. Nho, J.H.; Kim, S.R.; Nam, J.H. Symptom clustering and quality of life in patients with ovarian cancer undergoing chemotherapy. *Eur. J. Oncol. Nurs.* **2017**, *30*, 8–14. [CrossRef]
16. Hwang, K.H.; Cho, O.H.; Yoo, Y.S. Symptom clusters of ovarian cancer patients undergoing chemotherapy, and their emotional status and quality of life. *Eur. J. Oncol. Nurs.* **2016**, *21*, 215–222. [CrossRef]
17. Shirali, E.; Yarandi, F.; Ghaemi, M.; Montazeri, A. Quality of Life in Patients with Gynecological Cancers: A Web-Based Study. *Asian Pac. J. Cancer Prev.* **2020**, *21*, 1969–1975. [CrossRef]
18. Chase, D.M.; Marín, M.R.; Backes, F.; Han, S.; Graybill, W.; Mirza, M.R.; Pothuri, B.; Mangili, G.; O'Malley, D.M.; Berton, D.; et al. Impact of disease progression on health-related quality of life of advanced ovarian cancer patients—Pooled analysis from the PRIMA trial. *Gynecol. Oncol.* **2022**, *166*, 494–502. [CrossRef]
19. Techata, A.; Muangmool, T.; Wongpakaran, N.; Charoenkwan, K. Effect of cancer stage on health-related quality of life of patients with epithelial ovarian cancer. *J. Obstet. Gynaecol.* **2022**, *42*, 139–145. [CrossRef]
20. Słoniewski, R.; Dąbrowska-Bender, M.; Religioni, U.; Fronczak, A.; Staniszewska, A.; Duda-Zalewska, A.; Milewska, M.; Kędzierska, M.; Matkowski, R.A.; Dykowska, G.; et al. A Comparative Analysis of Quality of Life in Women Diagnosed with Breast and Ovarian Cancer. *Int. J. Environ. Res. Public Health* **2022**, *19*, 6705. [CrossRef]

21. Lee, J.-J.; Longcoy, L.-T.H.; Tai, C.-Y. Symptom Distress and Quality of Life in Women With Newly Diagnosed Ovarian Cancer Undergoing Chemotherapy: A Longitudinal Approach. *Clin. J. Oncol. Nurs.* **2022**, *26*, 643–650. [PubMed]
22. Sarkar, S.; Sahoo, P.K.; Pal, R.; Tanumy, M.; Mahata, S.; Chatterjee, P.; Vernekar, M.; Mandal, S.; Bera, T.; Nasare, V.D. Assessment of quality of life among advanced ovarian cancer patients in a tertiary care hospital in India. *Support. Care Cancer* **2022**, *30*, 3371–3378. [CrossRef] [PubMed]
23. Śniadecki, M.; Ostrowski, A.; Liro, M.; Wydra, D.G. Chemioterapia dootrzewnowa w raku jajnika. *Nowotw. J. Oncol.* **2013**, *63*, 311–319. [CrossRef]
24. Bhugwandass, C.S.; Pijnenborg, J.M.A.; Pijlman, B.; Ezendam, N.P.M. Effect of chemotherapy on health-related quality of life among early-stage ovarian cancer survivors: A study from the population-based PROFILES registry. *Curr. Oncol.* **2016**, *23*, 556–562. [CrossRef] [PubMed]
25. Perkowska, E.; Terlikowski, S.; Terlikowski, R.; Moczydłowska, A.; Markowska, T.; Marcinowicz, L. Evaluation of the quality of life of ovarian cancer patients in the context of selected quantitative variables such as body mass, number of miscarriages and time from diagnosis. *Fam. Med. Prim. Care Rev.* **2019**, *21*, 355–359.
26. Lee, C.Y.; King, M.T.; O'Connell, R.L.; Lanceley, A.; Joly, F.; Hilpert, F.; Davis, A.; Roncolato, F.T.; Okamoto, A.; Bryce, J.; et al. Symptom burden and quality of life with chemotherapy for recurrent ovarian cancer: The Gynecologic Cancer InterGroup-Symptom Benefit Study. *Int. J. Gynecol. Cancer* **2022**, *32*, 761–768. [CrossRef]
27. Smorąg, K.; Jeżowska–Smorąg, I.; Florkowski, A.; Zboralski, K.; Macander, M.; Gądek, I.; Wilk, B.; Wierzbiński, P. Jakość życia i depresyjność u kobiet z rozpoznaniem raka trzonu macicy i raka jajnika–analiza porównawcza. *Folia Medica Lodz.* **2015**, *42*, 123–143.
28. Kozaka, J. Jakość życia chorych na raka jajnika. *Psychoonkologia* **2014**, *2*, 66–72.
29. Plotti, F.; Scaletta, G.; Aloisi, A.; Luvero, D.; Capriglione, S.; Miranda, A.; Montera, R.; De Cicco Nardone, C.; Terranova, C.; Angioli, R. Quality of Life in Platinum-Sensitive Recurrent Ovarian Cancer: Chemotherapy Versus Surgery Plus Chemotherapy. *Ann. Surg. Oncol.* **2015**, *22*, 2387–2394. [CrossRef]
30. Kim, J.H.; Lee, D.-E.; Lee, Y.; Ha, H.I.; Chang, Y.J.; Chang, S.-J.; Park, S.-Y.; Lim, M.C. Quality of life outcomes from the randomised trial of hyperthermic intraperitoneal chemotherapy following cytoreductive surgery for primary ovarian cancer (KOV-HIPEC-01). *J. Gynecol. Oncol.* **2022**, *33*, e54. [CrossRef]
31. Blagden, S.P.; Cook, A.D.; Poole, C.; Howells, L.; McNeish, I.A.; Dean, A.; Kim, J.W.; O'Donnell, D.M.; Hook, J.; James, E.C.; et al. Weekly platinum-based chemotherapy versus 3-weekly platinum-based chemotherapy for newly diagnosed ovarian cancer (ICON8): Quality-of-life results of a phase 3, randomised, controlled trial. *Lancet Oncol.* **2020**, *21*, 969–977. [CrossRef]
32. Penar-Zadarko, B.; Binkowska-Bury, M.; Wolan, M.; Gawelko, J.; Urbański, K. Longitudinal assessment of quality of life in ovarian cancer patients. *Eur. J. Oncol. Nurs.* **2013**, *17*, 381–385. [CrossRef] [PubMed]
33. Oza, A.M.; Matulonis, U.A.; Malander, S.; Hudgens, S.; Sehouli, J.; del Campo, J.M.; Berton-Rigaud, D.; Banerjee, S.; Scambia, G.; Berek, J.S.; et al. Quality of life in patients with recurrent ovarian cancer treated with niraparib versus placebo (ENGOT-OV16/NOVA): Results from a double-blind, phase 3, randomised controlled trial. *Lancet Oncol.* **2018**, *19*, 1117–1125. [CrossRef] [PubMed]
34. Pergialiotis, V.; Sotiropoulou, I.M.; Liatsou, E.; Liontos, M.; Frountzas, M.; Thomakos, N.; Rodolakis, A.; Haidopoulos, D. Quality of life of ovarian cancer patients treated with combined platinum taxane chemotherapy: A systematic review of the literature. *Support. Care Cancer* **2022**, *30*, 7147–7157. [CrossRef] [PubMed]
35. Zhou, Y.; Irwin, M.L.; Ferrucci, L.M.; McCorkle, R.; Ercolano, E.A.; Li, F.; Stein, K.; Cartmel, B. Health-related quality of life in ovarian cancer survivors: Results from the American Cancer Society's Study of Cancer Survivors—I. *Gynecol. Oncol.* **2016**, *14*, 543–549. [CrossRef] [PubMed]
36. van Walree, I.C.; Hamaker, M.; van de Poll-Franse, L.V.; Vos, M.C.; Boll, D.; van Huis-Tanja, L.H.; Ezendam, N.P.M. Older ovarian cancer survivors report lower long-term health-related quality of life than younger survivors: A study from the population-based profiles registry. *Gynecol. Oncol.* **2019**, *153*, 391–398. [CrossRef]
37. Panoskaltsis, T.; Papadimitriou, C.; Pallas, N.; Karamveri, C.; Kyziridis, D.; Hristakis, C.; Kiriakopoulos, V.; Kalakonas, A.; Vaikos, D.; Tzavara, C.; et al. Prognostic Value of En-Block Radical Bowel Resection in Advanced Ovarian Cancer Surgery With HIPEC. *Cancer Control.* **2023**, *30*, 1–13. [CrossRef]
38. Friedlander, M.; Rau, J.; Lee, C.K.; Meier, W.; Lesoin, A.; Kim, J.-W.; Poveda, A.; Buck, M.; Scambia, G.; Shimada, M.; et al. Quality of life in patients with advanced epithelial ovarian cancer (EOC) randomised to maintenance pazopanib or placebo after first-line chemotherapy in the AGO-OVAR 16 trial. Measuring what matters-patient-centered end points in trials of maintenance therapy. *Ann. Oncol.* **2018**, *29*, 737–743.
39. Koole, S.N.; Kieffera, J.M.; Sikorska, K.; Schagen van Leeuwen, J.H.; Schreuder, H.W.R.; Hermans, R.H.; de Hingh, I.; van der Velden, J.; Arts, H.; van Ham, M.; et al. Health-related quality of life after interval cytoreductive surgery with or without hyperthermic intraperitoneal chemotherapy (HIPEC) in patients with stage III ovarian cancer. *Eur. J. Surg. Oncol.* **2021**, *47*, 101–107. [CrossRef]

healthcare

MDPI

Review

Emotional Dysregulation in Anorexia Nervosa: Scoping Review of Psychological Treatments

Enrica Cogodi [1], Jessica Ranieri [1,2], Alessandra Martelli [3] and Dina Di Giacomo [2,*]

1 Postgraduate in Clinical Psychology, University of L'Aquila, 67100 L'Aquila, Italy; enrica.cogodi@graduate.univaq.it (E.C.); jessica.ranieri@univaq.it (J.R.)
2 Life, Health and Environmental Sciences Department, University of L'Aquila, 67100 L'Aquila, Italy
3 Faculty of Biosciences and Agri-Food and Environmental Technologies, University of Teramo, 64100 Teramo, Italy; alessandra.martelli@unite.it
* Correspondence: dina.digiacomo@univaq.it

Abstract: Eating disorders are complex psychiatric disorders characterized by compensatory and restrictive behavior and a preoccupation with one's body. Eating and purging behaviors are considered dysfunctional emotional regulation strategies. Therefore, psychological treatment is essential. The most common psychological interventions are dialectical behavior therapy (DBT), cognitive–behavioral therapy (CBT), family therapy (FBT), multi-family group therapy (MFTG) and mentalization-based treatment (MBT). The aim of this study was to summarize the current evidence on the impact of psychological treatments on emotional regulation difficulties and psychological symptoms in patients with eating disorders, especially anorexia nervosa. A search was conducted on PubMed and Web of Science using the terms "anorexia nervosa" and "emotion dysregulation". Of the 278 initial articles, we included 15 publications. The results indicate that the acquisition of coping strategies, through DBT, leads to an improvement in anxiety and alexithymia. DBT, CBT and MBT lead to a reduction in the use of dysfunctional emotional regulation strategies too. Eating disorders involve both physical and mental health; therefore, it is desirable for future research to focus on the mutual synergy between the mental and physical components by evaluating various factors, such as biomarkers and the most appropriate therapeutic approach, with respect to the treatment setting.

Keywords: emotion dysregulation; eating disorders; anorexia nervosa; psychological treatment; BMI

1. Introduction

Eating disorders (ED) are complex psychiatric disorders characterized by unhealthy exercise, a preoccupation with body weight, restrictive eating behaviors and compensatory behaviors. They are associated with compromised interpersonal functioning, poor quality of life, clinical and psychiatric comorbidity and high levels of mortality [1]. Usually, eating disorders occur at any age, but they are more frequent in early to mid-adolescence, especially among females [2].

According to the DSM-5 classification [3], the main EDs are anorexia nervosa (AN), bulimia nervosa (BN) and binge eating disorder (BED). BN is characterized by binge eating followed by purging behaviors such as vomiting or the use of laxatives and body concerns, which promote the maintenance of a normal body weight, while BED is characterized by recurrent episodes of binge eating (≥1/week for a minimum of 3 months) that promote the onset of obesity [4]. Meanwhile, AN is characterized by a refusal to maintain a healthy body weight, an intense fear of gaining weight, body image distortion and weight control behaviors such as excessive exercise and self-induced vomiting [5].

Regarding AN, two subtypes exist: the restricting subtype of anorexia (AN-R) and the binge–purge subtype of anorexia (AN-BP). The latter is characterized by binge eating or purging behaviors, such as self-induced vomiting or the use of laxatives, whereas the restricting subtype of anorexia nervosa is characterized by strict limitations in the amounts and types of food consumed [6].

According to Haynos and Fruzzetti's model [7], some of the typical behaviors of patients with anorexia, such as binge eating, caloric restriction or purging, can be considered as maladaptive strategies to regulate aversive emotional states in social and emotional conflict. Therefore, AN can be described as a maladaptive emotion regulation strategy that attenuates psychological distress [8,9]. In fact, some authors have noted that patients with AN showed more negative emotions prior to and more positive emotions after restrictive eating, and exercise was associated with a decrease in negative affect after but not prior to physical activity. These findings indicate that a low-calorie diet and excessive exercise might be used as an emotional regulation strategy [8,10].

According to the multidimensional model proposed by Gratz and Roemer [11], emotional dysregulation is characterized by (a) difficulties in the awareness and understanding of emotions, (b) difficulties in the acceptance of emotions, (c) difficulties in controlling impulsive behavior and engaging in goal-directed behavior when experiencing negative emotions and (d) a lack of functional and appropriate emotional regulation strategies to modulate emotional responses in order to fulfil personal goals and situational demands.

Some evidence shows that individuals with anorexia nervosa have higher levels of alexithymia [12], deficits in emotional awareness and emotional clarity [13], difficulties in forming mental representations of emotions [14], problems in recognizing, expressing and understanding emotions [8], a lower ability to regulate emotions and fewer emotional regulation strategies to use when they are upset [15], more difficulties in regulating positive affective states [16], maladaptive beliefs about experiencing emotions that lead to the non-acceptance of emotional experiences [17], negative body self-image [1], difficulties in empathy [18] and interoceptive deficits [19].

In patients with ED, interoceptive deficits refer to difficulties in the identification of hunger signals and satiety and confusion between these body sensations and emotions [19]. Some common traits among individuals with AN, such as social isolation, cognitive rigidity, reward insensitivity, needs for symmetry and perfectionism, appear to be related to emotional overcontrol and they favor the maintenance of an eating psychopathology [12]. A lack of adaptive emotional regulation strategies, such as problem-solving skill difficulties, avoidance, suppression and rumination, was linked to a greater eating psychopathology [12].

Santos and Haynos [16] found that the greater non-acceptance of positive emotions was associated with greater anxiety and depression in AN and less restriction was linked to impulsivity in response to positive emotions. It has been hypothesized that anxiety could be associated with a fear of food and the subsequent avoidance and restriction of food in these patients.

Some studies have found no association between body mass index (BMI) and difficulties in emotional regulation for individuals with AN, while other studies have reported an association between emotional regulation deficits and underweight patients with AN compared to those in recovery. Other studies have found that BMI was positively associated with emotional regulation difficulties, the avoidance of affect and distress intolerance, and an improvement in emotional regulation deficits was associated with weight gain, independently of psychological treatment [20]. Further, it is hypothesized that patients with AN-BP have greater emotion regulation difficulties compared to patients with AN-R, but only in the emotional impulsivity area [21]. Other studies have investigated the differences between AN-R and AN-BP [1,8,12,16,21]. In AN-R, emotional regulation difficulties tend to be characterized by emotional overcontrol as a lack of emotion expression and emotional inhibition, while, in AN-BP, emotional regulation difficulties tend to be characterized by impulsivity and difficulties in inhibiting behavior when experiencing negative emotions [12].

Racine and Wildes [17] demonstrated that BMI was unrelated to emotional dysregulation, but depressive symptoms influenced changes in emotional regulation difficulties and AN symptoms. Further, depressive and alexithymic symptoms were associated with deficits in emotional regulation strategies in adolescents with anorexia, and alexithymia may be a negative prognostic factor for AN, independently of depressive symptoms and disease severity.

The role of emotional dysregulation in ED maintenance has received increased attention in both research and treatment. The most commonly investigated treatments in ED are dialectical behavior therapy (DBT), cognitive–behavioral therapy (CBT) and family-based treatment (FBT), followed by multifamily therapy group (MFTG) and mentalization-based treatment (MBT).

DBT is based on biosocial theory, according to which biological vulnerability and a poor environmental context cause difficulties in emotional regulation [22]. It aims to help individuals with AN to learn new coping strategies to effectively manage and regulate their emotions [23]. In CBT, the therapist focuses on alliance and motivation. Sessions aim to recognize and modify dysfunctional thoughts related to body image, weight and food. FBT focuses on family relationships and the ways in which parents can help their children to eat; furthermore, another aim of such treatment is to give the patient more responsibility for their own weight restoration [24]. MBT may enhance treatment strategies by adapting interventions to the mental capacities of a patient with ED and to help to maintain a therapeutic relationship and reduce relapse rates [25]. MFTG helps patients and their families to learn and reflect on one another's thoughts, to identify and repair disconnections related to AN [26].

Despite an awareness that emotional dysregulation is a common phenomenon in eating disorders, the knowledge of the efficacy of psychological treatment in reducing emotional regulation deficits is currently poorly investigated. We therefore undertook our study to perform an evidence mapping review regarding the impact of psychological treatment on emotional dysregulation in eating disorder patients, particularly in patients with anorexia. Specifically, the research objectives of this review were to

- summarize the current evidence of the impact of psychological treatment on emotional regulation difficulties and psychological symptoms in eating disorder patients;
- identify gaps in the literature that may require further research;
- identify research questions in terms of the determinants for future implementation actions.

2. Materials and Methods

2.1. Study Design

We conducted an evidence mapping review to analyze the literature focused on emotional dysregulation associated with anorexia nervosa. The framework outlined by the Global Evidence Mapping (GEM) Initiative [27] in their methodological paper on scoping studies was adopted. We performed this review according to the Preferred Reporting Items for Systematic Reviews and Metanalysis (PRISMA)—Extension for Scoping Reviews (PRISMA-R) [28].

2.2. Search Strategy

To identify potentially relevant studies for inclusion, we performed a scoping search of MEDLINE through PubMed and Web of Science in March 2023. The key search terms were "anorexia nervosa" and "emotion dysregulation".

2.3. Inclusion and Exclusion Criteria

To be considered eligible, the titles and abstracts of the retrieved studies had to refer to patients with anorexia nervosa and signs of emotional dysregulation. The range of the search strategy was restricted to the 2013–2023 period. To be included, studies had to (a) be published in the English language; (b) include psychological treatment; (c) include psychological measures. In addition, we excluded all reviews on the topic.

2.4. Article Selection and Data Extraction

To ensure the reliability of the review, the titles and abstracts of the retrieved studies were independently screened by two raters for eligibility. The same two raters also evaluated the full texts for inclusion that were retrieved by online databases and the faculty interlibrary service. Any disagreement between the raters was successfully resolved by discussion until a consensus was reached. The following data were extracted from each paper: (a) general information—authors, publication year, country and involved institution (e.g., university, medical center); (b) study characteristics—study design, sample size, target sample, range age; (c) biomarkers, comorbidity, psychological measures used and psychological treatment; (d) data related to the research question of the review—ED treatment program, a summary of outcomes.

2.5. Data Synthesis

The general information, the study characteristics and the psychological measures used and the data related to the research question of the review were descriptively synthesized. To explore the presence and the impact of emotional dysregulation in young adult patients with anorexia nervosa, the results were summarized referring to ED treatment program outcomes.

3. Procedure

3.1. Search Results

The literature search of the PubMed, Web of Science and Scopus electronic databases provided a total of 278 publications. After removing 44 duplicates, 234 references were identified for screening. Based on the inclusion/exclusion criteria, two reviewers screened all titles and abstracts for eligibility and successfully resolved disagreements by consensus. The full texts of the remaining 73 papers with potential for inclusion were examined comprehensively.

Out of a total of 73 articles assessed for eligibility, 58 were excluded and the reasons for exclusion were reported. Figure 1 shows all details of the study search and selection process. Finally, 15 studies were included.

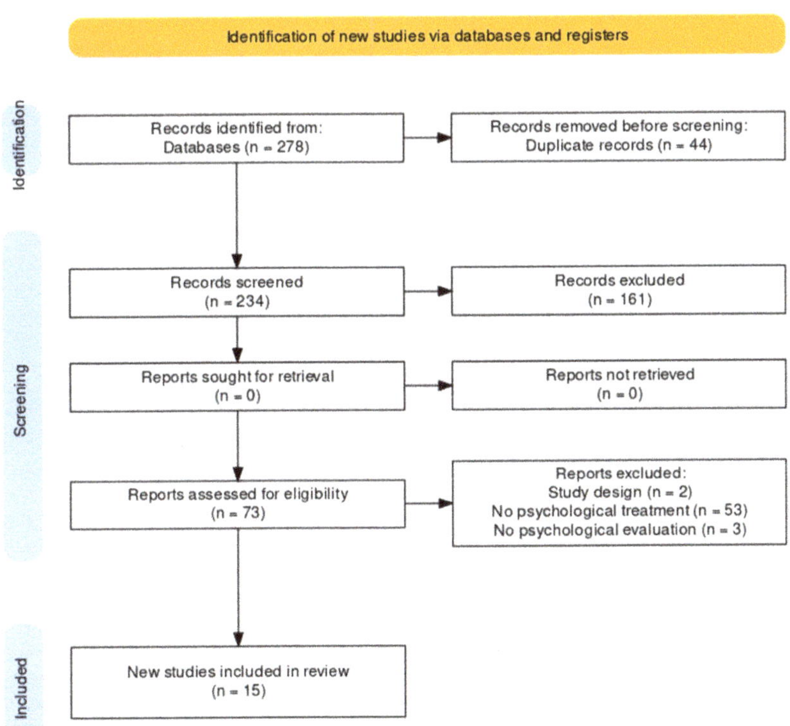

Figure 1. PRISMA flowchart of the study selection process for the review.

3.2. Characteristics of the Included Studies

In Tables 1–3 the main characteristics of the included studies are summarized. We identified the following study characteristics: (a) study design, (b) authors, (c) eating disorders, (d) target sample, (e) sample size, (f) types of treatment, (g) duration of treatment and (h) number of dropouts.

Table 1. Main characteristics of the included studies with DBT.

Study Design	Authors	ED Patients	Target Sample	Sample Size	Type of Treatment	Duration of Treatment	N Dropouts
Observational study	Preyde et al., 2016 [19]	AN-R; AN-BP; BN; EDNOS	YO; AD	$n = 104$	DBT	Not specified	28
	Brown et al., 2019 [29]	AN-R; AN-BP; BN; BED; OSFED	YO; AD	$n = 135$	DBT	97.07 ± 53.16 days	65
	O'Mara et al., 2021 [30]	AN; BN; EDNOS	YO; AD	$n = 54$	DBT	11.3 ± 6.1 weeks	Not specified
Case Series Analysis	Federici et al., 2013 [31]	AN-P; AN-R; EDNOS	YO; AD	$n = 7$	DBT	6 months	Not specified
Quasi-experimental	Reilly et al., 2022 [23]	AN-BP; BN; OSFED	YO; AD	$n = 62$	DBT + pharmacological treatment	Not specified	1

Legend: AN-R = Anorexia Nervosa, Restricting Type; AN-BP = Anorexia Nervosa, Binge–Purging Type; BN = Bulimia Nervosa; EDNOS = Eating Disorder Not Otherwise Specified; BED = Binge Eating Disorder; OSFED = Other Specified Feeding and Eating Disorder; AN = Anorexia Nervosa; AN-P = Anorexia Nervosa, Purging Type; YO = Young; AD = Adult; DBT = Dialectical Behavior Therapy.

Table 2. Main characteristics of the included studies with mixed treatments.

Study Design	Authors	ED Patients	Target Sample	Sample Size	Type of Treatment	Duration of Treatment	N Dropouts
Pilot RCT/RCT	Steinglass et al., 2018 [32]	AN	YO; AD	$n = 22$	SPT; REaCH	1 months	1
	Neyman-Carlsson et al., 2019 [24]	AN	YO; AD	$n = 78$	CBT; FBT	18 months	4
	Petersson et al., 2022 [33]	AN; BN; BED; OSFED	YO; AD	$n = 46$	CBT; affect school	8 weeks	16
Observational study	Rowsell et al., 2016 [12]	AN	YO; AD	$n = 108$	CBT; DBT; interpersonal therapy	14.4 ± 7.1 weeks	52
	Bodell et al., 2022 [34]	AN; BN; BED; PD; ARFID	CH; YO; AD	$n = 265$	CBT; FBT	26 - 750 days	130
	Martin et al., 2022 [35]	AN; BN; BED; OSFED	CH; YO; AD	$n = 127$	FBT; CBT; DBT	Not specified	High rates
	Reilly et al., 2022 [36]	AN-R; AN-BP; BN; OSFED	CH; YO; AD	$n = 1276$	DBT; couples/FBT	83.27 ± 53.32 days	293
Case Series Report	Caslini et al., 2015 [37]	AN-R; BN; EDNOS	YO; AD	$n = 8$	Cognitive restructuring techniques; supportive psychotherapy	One year	Not specified

Legend: AN = Anorexia Nervosa; BN = Bulimia Nervosa; BED = Binge Eating Disorder; OSFED = Other Specified Feeding and Eating Disorder; PD = Purging Disorder; ARFID = Avoidant/Restrictive Food Intake Disorder; AN-R = Anorexia Nervosa, Restricting Type; AN-BP = Anorexia Nervosa, Binge–Purging Type; EDNOS = Eating Disorder Not Otherwise Specified; CH = Child; YO = Young; AD = Adult; SPT = Standard Supportive Psychotherapy; REaCH = Regulating Emotions and Changing Habits; CBT = Cognitive–Behavioral Therapy; FBT = Family-Based Treatment; DBT = Dialectical Behavior Therapy; Couples/FBT = Family-Based Treatment and Adjunctive Couples Therapy.

Table 3. Main characteristics of the included studies with other treatments.

Study Design	Authors	ED Patients	Target Sample	Sample Size	Type of Treatment	Duration of Treatment	N Dropouts
Pilot study	Tantillo et al., 2019 [26]	AN; OSFED	YO; AD	$n = 10$	MFTG	26 weeks	Not specified
Observational study	Zeeck et al., 2021 [25]	AN; BN; OSFED; CG	YO; AD	$n = 38$	MBT	2 years	5

Legend: AN = Anorexia Nervosa; OSFED = Other Specified Feeding and Eating Disorder; BN = Bulimia Nervosa; CG = Control Group; YO = Young; AD = Adult; MFTG = Multifamily Therapy Group; MBT = Mentalization-Based Treatment.

All studies focused on patients with eating disorders and difficulties in emotion regulation. Regarding ED patients, the included studies involved patients with several conditions, including anorexia nervosa (AN), bulimia nervosa (BN), binge eating disorder (BED), eating disorders not otherwise specified (EDNOS), other specified feeding and eating disorders (OSFED), avoidant/restrictive food intake disorder (ARFID) and purging disorder (PD).

3.3. *Sources of Articles*

Figure 2 summarizes general information about the subject areas of the included studies. All papers were published in peer-reviewed journals from 2013 to 2023. Concerning the publication year, we noted a growing and emerging interest in the last ten years, showing a general intention to better understand the association between eating disorders and difficulties in emotional regulation; in fact, only one article, dated 2013, was found (6.7%), whereas five articles ware found dated 2022 (33%). We observed that almost all of the first authors' institutions were universities (n = 13; 86%), highlighting the greater interest of academic staff rather than clinical staff.

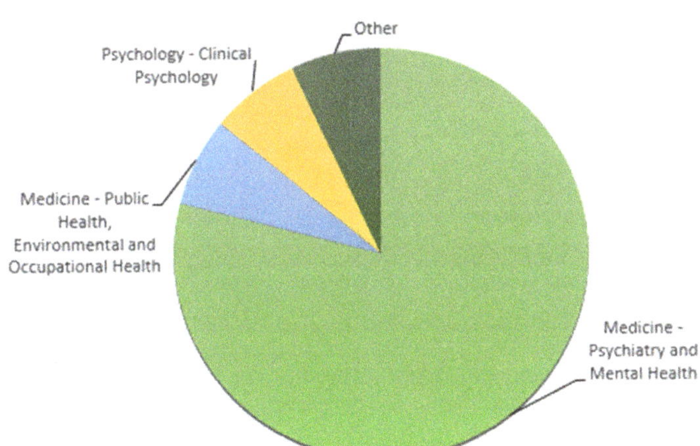

Figure 2. Subject areas of the included studies.

4. Results

The 15 selected studies differed in their study design and methods and included research carried out using quantitative and qualitative designs.

Tables 1–3 report the details of the studies with, respectively, DBT, mixed treatment and other treatments. Tables 4 and 5 report a summary of the included studies, respectively, with and without biomarkers. Table 6 reports the details of the measures and outcomes of the included studies. We describe the following features from each included paper: (a) authors; (b) biomarkers; (c) psychological measures; (d) comorbidities; (e) symptoms; (f) ED treatment program; and (g) outcomes. All papers focused on difficulties in emotional regulation and the use of strategies to regulate emotions in young adults with eating disorders, while the outcomes referred to psychological measures (e.g., anxiety, depression, emotional dysregulation, etc.) and the efficacy of the psychological treatment (e.g., dialectical behavior therapy, family-based therapy, cognitive–behavioral therapy, etc.).

Table 4. Summary of included studies with biomarkers.

Authors	Bio Markers	Psychological Measures	Comorbidities	Symptoms
Federici et al., 2013 [31]	BMI; potassium; sodium; Qtc intervals	EDE-Q; DSHI	MDD; PTSD; ADHD; OCD; BPD; PD NOS; ANX NOS	ED symptoms; self-injurious behaviors
Caslini et al., 2015 [37]	BMI	EDI 2; DES; TAS-20	Obsessive Disorder; Histrionic Disorder; Borderline Disorder; Avoidant Disorder; Obsessive/Schizoid Disorder	ED symptoms; dissociative experiences; alexithymia
Rowsell et al., 2016 [12]	BMI	EDE-Q; DERS; BSI	Not Specified	ED psychopathology; emotional dysregulation; ANX; DEP
Steinglass et al., 2018 [32]	BMI	EDA-5; SCID-I; SRHI; EDE-Q; BDI; STAI-T; DERS; questionnaire to measure, at the beginning, the expectations of treatment and, at the end, treatment satisfaction post-treatment	Not Specified	DEP; ANX; ED severity; habit strength; emotional dysregulation
Brown et al., 2019 [29]	BMI	DBT-WCCL DSS; EDE-Q; BDI-II; DERS	Mood Disorder; Anxiety Disorder; Alcohol Use Disorder; Substance Use Disorder	DEP; severity of ED symptoms; emotional dysregulation; frequency of DBT skills
Neyman-Carlsson et al., 2019 [24]	BMI	EDI-3; RAB-R	Not Specified	ED symptoms; psychological traits
Tantillo et al., 2019 [26]	BMI	LEA; LAERS; MINI; EDE	Mood Disorder; Panic Disorder; Generalized Anxiety; PTSD	ED examination; acknowledge emotions; emotional regulation strategies
Zeeck et al., 2021 [25]	BMI	EDE; EDI-2; SCID-5; GSI; SCL-90-R; BFKE; IIP-K; DERS; CTQ; RFQ	Depression; Anxiety Disorder; OCD; PTSD; Somatoform Disorder; Dysthymia	Eating psychopathology; attachment; general psychopathology; interpersonal problems; emotional regulation; traumatization
Bodell et al., 2022 [34]	BMI	EDE-Q; LOCES-brief; CIA; DERS; ERS; CES-D	Not Specified	DEP; ED severity; loss of control; ED-related impairment; emotional regulation and reactivity
Martin et al., 2022 [35]	BMI	EDE-Q; AAQ-II	Not Specified	ED behaviors and cognitions; psychological inflexibility; experiential avoidance
Petersson et al., 2022 [33]	BMI	EDE-Q; DERS-36; TAS-20	Not Specified	ED cognitions and behaviors; emotional dysregulation; alexithymia

Legend: BMI = Body Mass Index; EDE-Q = Eating Disorder Examination Questionnaire; DSHI = Deliberate Self-Harm Inventory; MDD = Major Depressive Disorder; PTSD = Posttraumatic Stress Disorder; ADHD = Attention Deficit/Hyperactivity Disorder; OCD = Obsessive Compulsive Disorder; BPD = Borderline Personality Disorder; PD NOS = Personality Disorder Not Otherwise Specified; ANX NOS = Anxiety Disorder Not Otherwise Specified; ED Symptoms = Eating Disorder Symptoms; EDI-2 = Eating Disorders Inventory-2; DES = Dissociative Experiences Scale; TAS-20 = Toronto Alexithymia Scale-20; DERS = Difficulties in Emotion Regulation Scale; BSI = Brief Symptom Inventory; ANX = Anxiety; DEP = Depression; EDA-5 = Eating Disorder Assessment for DMS-5; SCID-I = Structured Clinical Interview for DMS-IV Axis I Disorders; SRHI = Self-Report Habit Index; BDI = Beck Depression Inventory; STAI-T = Spielberg State Trait Anxiety Inventory—Trait Version; DBT-WCCL DSS = DBT Ways of Coping Checklist—DBT Skills Subscale; DBT = Dialectical Behavior Therapy; EDI-3 = Eating Disorder Inventory-3; RAB-R = Rating of Anorexia and Bulimia Interview—Revised Version; LEA = Lack of Emotional Awareness; LAERS = Limited Access to Emotion Regulation Strategies; MINI = Mini-International Neuropsychiatric Interview; EDE = Eating Disorder Examination; SCID-5 = Structured Clinical Interview for DMS-5; GSI = Global Severity Index; SCL-90-R = Symptom Check-List; BFKE = Bielefelder Fragebogen zu Klientenerwartungen; IIP-K = Inventory of Interpersonal Problems; CTQ = Childhood Trauma Questionnaire; RFQ = Reflective Functioning Questionnaire; LOCES-Brief = Loss of Control Over Eating Scale-Brief; CIA = Clinical Impairment Assessment; ERS = Emotion Reactivity Scale; CES-D = Center for Epidemiologic Studies Depression Scale; AAQ-II = Acceptance and Action Questionnaire-II; DERS-36 = Difficulties in Emotion Regulation Scale-36.

Table 5. Summary of included studies without biomarkers.

Authors	Biomarkers	Psychological Measures	Comorbidities	Symptoms
Preyde et al., 2016 [19]	-	EDI-3; RAB-R	Not Specified	Emotional dysregulation; interoceptive deficits; ED risk
O'Mara et al., 2021 [30]	-	BAI; NMR	Not Specified	ANX; negative mood regulation expectancies
Reilly et al., 2022 [23]	-	BEST; UPPS-P; ERS; EDE-Q; WCCL; DBT skills use questionnaire	Major Depressive Disorder; Social Anxiety Disorder; PTSD	BPD symptoms; emotional reactivity; bulimic symptoms; negative urgency
Reilly et al., 2022 [36]	-	EDE-Q; TAS-20; BDI-II	Not Specified	DEP; alexithymia; ED cognitions and behaviors

Legend: EDI-3 = Eating Disorder Inventory-3; BAI = Beck Anxiety Inventory; NMR = Generalized Expectancy for Negative Mood Regulation Scale; BEST = Borderline Evaluation of Severity Over Time; UPPS-P = UPPS-P Negative Urgency Scale; ERS = Emotional Reactivity Scale; EDE-Q = Eating Disorders Examination—Questionnaire; WCCL = Ways of Coping Checklist; TAS-20 = Toronto Alexithymia Scale-20; BDI-II = Beck Depression Inventory-II; PTSD = Posttraumatic Stress Disorder; BPD = Borderline Personality Disorder; ANX = Anxiety; DEP = Depression; ED = Eating Disorder.

Table 6. Features of psychological treatment protocols in AN.

	Authors	Psychological Treatment	Program Target	Protocol Treatment	Statistical Analyses	Outcomes
Study with biomarkers and psychological treatment	Federici et al., 2013 [31]	MED-DBT	Emotional regulation	Group and individual sessions	No	Reduction in suicidal/self-injurious behavior, ED symptoms
	Caslini et al., 2015 [37]	Psychotherapy	Cognitive restructuring; emotional literacy and regulation	Weekly session	Wilcoxon test	Reduction in dissociative symptoms, impulse regulation and improved body satisfaction
	Rowsell et al., 2016 [12]	Cognitive behavioral interventions; interpersonal therapy; DBT skills training	Emotional regulation	Hybrid inpatient/day treatment	Independent samples *t*-tests; ANOVA; MANOVA; Mixed MANOVA	AN-BP improved more than AN-R in inhibiting impulsive behaviors
	Steinglass et al., 2018 [32]	REaCH SPT	Cue awareness; emotional regulation psychoeducation; goal setting;	Twelve 45-min sessions three times per week	Pearson correlations; ANCOVA	REaCH was associated with reduction in eating disorder psychopathology and habit strength of dietary behaviors and physical activity
	Brown et al., 2019 [29]	DBT	Mindfulness	5 h weekly group sessions	ANOVA; separate linear regression; RWA	Increased use of DBT skills; ED, depressive and emotional dysregulation symptoms
	Neyman-Carlsson et al., 2019 [24]	CBT FBT	Identification and modification of patient's dysfunctional thoughts and behaviors Developing functional family relations	60 1 h weekly sessions Forty 90 min sessions	*t*-tests; ANOVA; multiple and stepwise regression	In the CBT group, a lower degree of emotional dysregulation predicted a positive change in BMI. In the FBT group, an impaired ability to understand and respond to emotions predicted an increase in weight
	Tantillo et al., 2019 [26]	R4R	Development of emotional and relational processing skills	16 sessions of 90 min each	Within-patient standardized	R4R is an MFTG
	Zeeck et al., 2021 [25]	MBT	Reflective functioning; emotional regulation; interpersonal problems	Individual weekly session; one group session; a session with the family or partner	*t*-tests; multiple regression analysis; hierarchical stepwise regressions	Improvement in eating pathology, general psychopathology
	Bodell et al., 2022 [34]	CBT; FBT	Not detailed	Not detailed	ANCOVA; longitudinal multilevel models	Higher emotional reactivity was associated with loss of control, eating severity, ED severity and ED-related impairment

Table 6. *Cont.*

	Authors	Psychological Treatment	Program Target	Protocol Treatment	Statistical Analyses	Outcomes
Study with biomarkers and psychological treatment	Martin et al., 2022 [35]	CBT; FBT; DBT	Behavioral change	Not detailed	Pearson correlations; mediation model	Improvements in unhealthy exercise at month 2
	Petersson et al., 2022 [33]	Affect school treatment + CBT	Psychoeducation about a specific affect	Eight daytime 2 h group sessions	Pearson test; Spearman rank	The AS group reported a reduction in alexithymia, an improvement in eating disorder cognitions
Study without biomarkers and psychological treatment	Preyde et al., 2016 [19]	DBT	Emotional dysregulation	Not detailed	*t*-tests; bivariate linear regression	Improvement in the eating disorder and affective problems composite (APC)
	O'Mara et al., 2021 [30]	DBT	Mindfulness	Twice weekly sessions; group activities	Paired sample *t*-tests	Improvement in anxiety and a reduction in expectancies for negative mood dysregulation
	Reilly et al., 2022 [23]	DBT or DBT + lamotrigine	Emotional regulation	6 h a day for 5–6 days a week; skills group sessions	MLMs	Reduction in emotional reactivity, negative urgency and symptoms of borderline personality disorder
	Reilly et al., 2022 [36]	DBT	Not detailed	Individual therapy; biweekly skills groups	Two piece-wise multilevel models	Reduction in alexithymia
		FBT/couples therapy	Not detailed	Weekly sessions 10 h of treatment/day, 6 days a week		

Legend: MED-DBT = Multidiagnostic Eating Disorder Dialectical Behavior Therapy; ED = Eating Disorders; PTSD = Posttraumatic Stress Disorder; ANOVA = Analysis of Variance; MANOVA = Multivariate Analysis of Variance; AN-R = Anorexia Nervosa, Restricting Type; AN-BP = Anorexia Nervosa, Binge–Purging Type; DERS = Difficulties in Emotion Regulation Scale; REaCH = Regulating Emotions and Changing Habits; SPT = Supportive Psychotherapy; ANCOVA = Analysis of Covariance; DBT = Dialectical Behavior Therapy; RCI = Reliable Change Index; RWA = Relative Weights Analyses; ED = Eating Disorder; CBT = Cognitive–Behavioral Therapy; BMI = Body Mass Index; R4R = Reconnecting for Recovery; MFTG = Multifamily Therapy Group; AN = Anorexia Nervosa; MBT = Mentalization-Based Treatment; FBT = Family-Based Treatment; REML = Restricted Maximum Likelihood; IOP = Intensive Outpatient Program; PHP = Partial Hospitalization Treatment; MLMs: Multilevel Models.

As summarized in Table 4, the treatments mostly used in the studies with biomarkers were dialectical behavior therapy (DBT) and cognitive–behavioral therapy (CBT), followed by family-based treatment (FBT) and multifamily therapy interventions. Applying DBT, new coping skills such as mindfulness, distress tolerance, emotional regulation and interpersonal effectiveness were taught to help patients to regulate their emotions. The results showed a reduction in the use of dysfunctional emotional regulation strategies in AN and EDNOS patients, determined by the typical symptoms of the eating disorder. In fact, treatment was associated with an improvement in the adaptive expression of one's emotions, a greater assumption of responsibility in decision-making and a reduction in self-harm and suicidal behavior [31]. The early acquisition of these skills (at one month) predicted a greater improvement in the ED pathology and depressive and emotional dysregulation symptoms at discharge [29]. Furthermore, the acquisition of cognitive and behavioral restructuring strategies produced a pre–post treatment improvement with respect to dissociative symptomatology, impulse regulation and body satisfaction in AN and BN patients [37].

Difficulties with emotion regulation were mostly treated during a mixed cognitive–behavioral, dialectical behavioral and interpersonal treatment in a sample of patients with AN who were admitted to a specialized intensive hospital-based treatment program. Patients with binge–purge anorexia nervosa (AN-BP), rather than the restricting subtype of anorexia nervosa (AN-R), reported greater difficulties with emotional regulation overall, particularly with refraining from impulsive behaviors when experiencing negative emotions. During the treatment, AN-BP patients achieved more pronounced improvements in impulse control compared to AN-R patients. With regard to emotional dysregulation, improvements produced by treatment significantly predicted changes in eating psychopathology over time, regardless of the impact due to increased body weight. The improvements found with respect to emotional clarity and involvement in goal-directed behavior in the presence of an altered emotional state corresponded to 36% of the improvements in eating psychopathology [12].

The behavioral intervention defined as Regulating Emotions and Changing Habits (REaCH) was focused on the creation of new behavioral routines and the elimination of maladaptive habits. This intervention was associated with a greater reduction in eating psychopathology and the severity of eating and physical activity habits, compared to supportive therapy alone, at the end of treatment in AN patients [32].

Neyman-Carlsson et al. [24] compared two types of psychological treatment: FBT and CBT. They showed that in the group of patients with anorexia who received family-based therapy (FBT), an impaired understanding of other people's emotions predicted an increase in body weight; then, bulimic symptoms and emotional dysregulation were predictors of an increased number of diagnostic symptoms. However, in the group of patients undergoing CBT, a low level of emotional dysregulation and greater interoceptive deficits were able to predict changes in BMI.

The multifamily intervention called "Reconnecting for Recovery" (R4R) demonstrated its effectiveness in terms of improving eating psychopathology and emotion recognition in individuals with AN. These benefits were significant at the 6-month follow-up but not at the end of treatment. These findings demonstrate that changes in the ability to monitor, evaluate and modify emotional experiences take time [26].

Overall, AN, BN and BED patients undergoing DBT, FBT or CBT demonstrated an improvement in emotional reactivity compared to the control group [34] and a reduction in unhealthy physical exercise at two months from psychological treatment. Unhealthy exercise was prevalent among individuals with anorexia nervosa, as unhealthy exercise and restrictive eating may be used to avoid unpleasant and dysfunctional emotions. Increased emotional reactivity at two months was mediated by an improvement in emotion management, particularly in emotional avoidance, at one month after treatment. This effect was stronger for individuals with AN than other ED diagnoses [35]. Moreover, high emotional reactivity was associated with a greater reduction in overall eating symptoms and loss of control related to the severity of the symptomatology. However, emotional reactivity was not associated with binge eating or impairment-related changes in eating disorders [34].

Petersson et al. [33] compared the effectiveness of a psychological treatment called "affect school treatment". Parallel to the intervention, the AS group and the control group received treatment as usual, which included individual psychotherapy (CBT). The "affect school treatment" included psychoeducation sessions on specific affective states like joy, fear, interest/startle, shame, anger, disgust and worry, followed by deep reflection. The last session focused on stress and pain education and their prevention. The AS group, rather than the CBT group, showed an improvement in alexithymic symptoms at the 6-month follow-up and a greater improvement in emotional regulation difficulties, eating-disorder-related thinking styles and behavior at the 6- and 12-month follow-ups.

AN patients undergoing mentalization-based therapy (MBT) showed an improvement in the general psychopathology of the eating disorder at discharge, both in terms of a reduction in bulimic symptoms and with respect to an improvement in BMI. Furthermore, the reduction in emotional regulation difficulties was evident both at discharge and at the 3-month follow-up. During the follow-up period, the reduction in general psychopathology was maintained, while there was a slight increase in eating pathology. Patients did not report an improvement in interpersonal function over the course of treatment but did so in the time period after discharge. The study found a strong association between the "Uncertainty" subscale of the Reflective Functioning Questionnaire (RFQ) and emotional dysregulation, bulimic symptoms and general psychopathology [25].

In the evaluation of the effectiveness of psychological treatment with respect to the emotional and psychological components assessed in the studies in which biomarkers were not recorded (Table 5), significant improvements in emotional regulation difficulties, anxiety, interoceptive deficits, binge eating and alexithymia emerged at the end of dialectical behavior therapy. Alexithymia manifested the cognitive symptoms of the eating disorder as rumination; therefore, an impairment in the ability to identify emotions appears to be correlated with the greater severity of the eating disorder [19,33].

Reilly et al. (2022) compared the effect of a combined intervention (psychological and pharmacological treatment) to that of psychological treatment alone [23]. The results showed that those who received both the psychological intervention and a mood stabilizer (lamotrigine) had a greater reduction in emotional and behavioral regulation difficulties than the control group, as well as in borderline personality disorder symptoms. Moreover, after lamotrigine administration, the patients showed the greater utilization of the skills acquired during dialectical behavior therapy.

Our review highlights the lack of attention in clinical practice given to clinical and psychosocial index measurement in the short and long term that are indicative of the eating disorder severity and quality of life. Moreover, future research could be oriented toward evaluating psychological treatments' efficacy in psychoeducation about the impact of emotional regulation strategies on eating disorder management. Moreover, most of the studies focused on individual psychological treatment interventions' efficacy, whereas few studies were conducted on group treatment interventions.

5. Discussion

In this review, we analyzed the effectiveness of psychological treatments in managing emotional dysregulation in patients affected by eating disorders. Scientific evidence shows that eating symptoms, restrictive and compensatory, can be defined as dysfunctional emotional regulation strategies. Therefore, psychological treatment is essential.

CBT, DBT and FBT show appreciable levels of effectiveness in reducing eating symptoms associated with emotional difficulties; in particular, patients treated with DBT show increased skills for distress tolerance and more personal responsibility for life decisions [31]. The early acquisition of DBT skills in treatment predicted greater improvements in ED, depressive and emotional dysregulation symptoms [29]. Cognitive ED symptoms were associated with alexithymia symptoms, and this suggests that an impaired ability to identify emotions is related to more severe ED symptoms [36]. In reference to CBT, patients with lower levels of emotional dysregulation strategies, at the end of treatment, exhibited better outcomes [24]. In patients undergoing FBT, bulimic symptoms and difficulties with emotion regulation were predictors of increased diagnostic symptoms [24] and a reduction in alexithymic symptoms [36]. Moreover, for those who followed an MFTG, like R4R, it is highlighted that changes in emotional regulation strategies take time; in fact, the belief that one can access effective emotion regulation strategies was significant at the 6-month follow-up but not at the end of treatment. MBT was associated with an improvement in BMI, bulimic symptoms, interpersonal functioning and psychological quality of life [25]. For mixed treatment, it was found that when experiencing negative emotions, patients with the AN-BP subtype reported greater difficulties with impulse control and emotional regulation than those with the AN-R subtype. Moreover, the AN-BP subtype showed improvements in emotional clarity and engagement in goal-directed behaviors during the treatment, corresponding to improvements in eating disorder psychopathology [12]. Additionally, emotional reactivity was associated with a change in ED symptomatology and a loss of control related to eating severity during treatment, but not with ED-related impairments [34], and emotional avoidance at 1 month mediated the relation between unhealthy exercise at baseline and month 2 [35].

6. Conclusions

Applying a biopsychosocial approach [38] as a strategy to treat individuals who consider health (and illness) as a result of the complex and dynamic interaction of biological (genetic, biochemical, biological, organic), psychological (mood, personality, behavior) and social (cultural, family) factors, future research could develop intervention protocols and techniques that consider the combination of biomarkers and variations in relation to emotional dimensions; the integration of mental and physical health could promote improved well-being. The emerging needs in clinical practice are for a specific theoretical framework and the definition of a treatment setting tailored to the clinical and psychological characteristics of patients with eating disorders.

Author Contributions: Conceptualization, D.D.G.; methodology, E.C.; data curation, J.R. and E.C.; supervision, D.D.G. and A.M.; writing—review and editing, all authors. All authors have read and agreed to the published version of the manuscript.

Funding: This research received no external funding.

Institutional Review Board Statement: Not applicable.

Informed Consent Statement: Not applicable.

Data Availability Statement: No new data were created or analyzed in this study. Data sharing is not applicable to this article.

Conflicts of Interest: The authors declare no conflicts of interest.

References

1. Monell, E.; Clinton, D.; Birgegard, A. Emotion dysregulation and eating disorder outcome: Prediction, change and contribution of self-image. *Psychol. Psychother.-Theory Res. Pract.* **2022**, *95*, 639–655. [CrossRef] [PubMed]
2. Morris, J.; Anderson, S. An update on eating disorders. *Bjpsych Adv.* **2021**, *27*, 9–19. [CrossRef]
3. American Psychiatric Association. *Diagnostic and Statistical Manual of Mental Disorders*, 5th ed.; American Psychiatric Association: Washington, DC, USA, 2013.
4. Malet-Karas, A.; Bernard, D.; Piet, E.; Bertin, E. Disordered eating as a repercussion of sexual assault: A consequence to consider. *Eat. Weight. Disord.-Stud. Anorex. Bulim. Obes.* **2022**, *27*, 2095–2106. [CrossRef] [PubMed]
5. Dalton, B.; Foerde, K.; Bartholdy, S.; McClelland, J.; Kekic, M.; Grycuk, L.; Campbell, I.C.; Schmidt, U.; Steinglass, J.E. The effect of repetitive transcranial magnetic stimulation on food choice-related self-control in patients with severe, enduring anorexia nervosa. *Int. J. Eat. Disord.* **2020**, *53*, 1326–1336. [CrossRef] [PubMed]
6. Zhu, J.; Hay, P.J.; Yang, Y.; Le Grange, D.; Lacey, J.H.; Lujic, S.; Smith, C.; Touyz, S. Specific psychological therapies versus other therapies or no treatment for severe and enduring anorexia nervosa. *Cochrane Database Syst. Rev.* **2023**, *8*, CD011570.
7. Haynos, A.F.; Fruzzetti, A.E. Anorexia nervosa as a disorder of emotion dysregulation: Evidence and treatment implications. *Clin. Psychol. Sci. Pract.* **2011**, *18*, 183–202. [CrossRef]
8. Kolar, D.R.; Neumayr, C.; Roth, M.; Voderholzer, U.; Perthes, K.; Schlegl, S. Testing an emotion regulation model of physical activity in adolescents with anorexia nervosa: A pilot ecological momentary assessment. *Eur. Eat. Disord. Rev.* **2020**, *28*, 170–183. [CrossRef] [PubMed]
9. Merwin, R.M.; Moskovich, A.A.; Wagner, H.R.; Ritschel, L.A.; Craighead, L.W.; Zucker, N.L. Emotion regulation difficulties in anorexia nervosa: Relationship to self-perceived sensory sensitivity. *Cogn. Emot.* **2013**, *27*, 441–452. [CrossRef]
10. Kolar, D.R.; Hammerle, F.; Jenetzky, E.; Huss, M. Smartphone-Enhanced Low-Threshold Intervention for adolescents with Anorexia Nervosa (SELTIAN) waiting for outpatient psychotherapy: Study protocol of a randomised controlled trial. *BMJ Open* **2017**, *7*, e018049. [CrossRef]
11. Gratz, K.L.; Roemer, L. Multidimensional Assessment of Emotion Regulation and Dysregulation: Development, Factor Structure, and Initial Validation of the Difficulties in Emotion Regulation Scale. *J. Psychopathol. Behav. Assess* **2008**, *30*, 315. [CrossRef]
12. Rowsell, M.; MacDonald, D.E.; Carter, J.C. Emotion regulation difficulties in anorexia nervosa: Associations with improvements in eating psychopathology. *J. Eat. Disord.* **2016**, *4*, 12. [CrossRef]
13. Kolar, D.R.; Huss, M.; Preuss, H.M.; Jenetzky, E.; Haynos, A.F.; Bürger, A.; Hammerle, F. Momentary emotion identification in female adolescents with and without anorexia nervosa. *Psychiatry Res.* **2017**, *255*, 394–398. [CrossRef]
14. Monell, E.; Clinton, D.; Birgegard, A. Emotion dysregulation and eating disorders—Associations with diagnostic presentation and key symptoms. *Int. J. Eat. Disord.* **2018**, *51*, 921–930. [CrossRef]
15. van Elburg, A.; Danner, U.N.; Sternheim, L.C.; Lammers, M.; Elzakkers, I. Mental Capacity, Decision-Making and Emotion Dysregulation in Severe Enduring Anorexia Nervosa. *Front. Psychiatry* **2021**, *12*, 545317. [CrossRef]
16. Santos, B.M.; Haynos, A.F. Difficulties with positive emotion regulation in anorexia nervosa. *Eur. Eat. Disord. Rev.* **2023**, *31*, 520–528. [CrossRef]
17. Racine, S.E.; Wildes, J.E. Dynamic Longitudinal Relations Between Emotion Regulation Difficulties and Anorexia Nervosa Symptoms over the Year Following Intensive Treatment. *J. Consult. Clin. Psychol.* **2015**, *83*, 785–795. [CrossRef]
18. Nalbant, K.; Kalayci, B.M.; Akdemir, D.; Akgul, S.; Kanbur, N. Emotion regulation, emotion recognition, and empathy in adolescents with anorexia nervosa. *Eat. Weight. Disord.-Stud. Anorex. Bulim. Obes.* **2019**, *24*, 825–834. [CrossRef]
19. Preyde, M.; Watson, J.; Remers, S.; Stuart, R. Emotional dysregulation, interoceptive deficits, and treatment outcomes in patients with eating disorders. *Soc. Work. Ment. Health* **2016**, *14*, 227–244. [CrossRef]

20. Castro, T.F.; Miller, K.; Araujo, M.X.; Brandao, I.; Torres, S. Emotional processing in recovered anorexia nervosa patients: A 15 year longitudinal study. *Eur. Eat. Disord. Rev.* **2021**, *29*, 955–968. [CrossRef]
21. Haynos, A.F.; Roberto, C.A.; Martinez, M.A.; Attia, E.; Fruzzetti, A.E. Emotion Regulation Difficulties in Anorexia Nervosa Before and After Inpatient Weight Restoration. *Int. J. Eat. Disord.* **2014**, *47*, 888–891. [CrossRef]
22. Rozakou-Soumalia, N.; Dârvariu, Ş.; Sjögren, J.M. Dialectical Behaviour Therapy Improves Emotion Dysregulation Mainly in Binge Eating Disorder and Bulimia Nervosa: A Systematic Review and Meta-Analysis. *J. Pers. Med.* **2021**, *11*, 931. [CrossRef]
23. Reilly, E.E.; Berner, L.A.; Trunko, M.E.; Schwartz, T.; Anderson, L.K.; Krueger, A.; Yu, X.; Chen, J.Y.; Cusack, A.; Nakamura, T.; et al. Evaluating the use of lamotrigine to reduce mood lability and impulsive behaviors in adults with chronic and severe eating disorders. *Eat. Weight. Disord.-Stud. Anorex. Bulim. Obes.* **2022**, *27*, 1775–1785. [CrossRef]
24. Nyman-Carlsson, E.; Birgegard, A.; Engstroem, I.; Gustafsson, S.A.; Nevonen, L. Predictors of outcome among young adult patients with anorexia nervosa in a randomised controlled trial. *Eur. Eat. Disord. Rev.* **2019**, *27*, 76–85. [CrossRef]
25. Zeeck, A.; Endorf, K.; Euler, S.; Schaefer, L.; Lau, I.; Flösser, K.; Geiger, V.; Meier, A.F.; Walcher, P.; Lahmann, C.; et al. Implementation of mentalization-based treatment in a day hospital program for eating disorders-A pilot study. *Eur. Eat. Disord. Rev.* **2021**, *29*, 783–801. [CrossRef]
26. Tantillo, M.; McGraw, J.S.; Lavigne, H.M.; Brasch, J.; Le Grange, D. A pilot study of multifamily therapy group for young adults with anorexia nervosa: Reconnecting for recovery. *Int. J. Eat. Disord.* **2019**, *52*, 950–955. [CrossRef]
27. Bragge, P.; Clavisi, O.; Turner, T.; Tavender, E.; Collie, A.; Gruen, R.L. The Global Evidence Mapping Initiative: Scoping research in broad topic areas. *BMC Med. Res. Methodol.* **2011**, *11*, 92. [CrossRef]
28. Tricco, A.C.; Lillie, E.; Zarin, W.; O'Brien, K.K.; Colquhoun, H.; Levac, D.; Moher, D.; Peters, M.D.; Horsley, T.; Weeks, L.; et al. PRISMA Extension for Scoping Reviews (PRISMA-ScR): Checklist and Explanation. *Ann. Intern. Med.* **2018**, *169*, 467–473. [CrossRef]
29. Brown, T.; Cusack, A.; Anderson, L.; Reilly, E.E.; Berner, L.A.; Wierenga, C.E.; Lavender, J.M.; Kaye, W.H. Early versus Later Improvements in Dialectical Behavior Therapy Skills Use and Treatment Outcome in Eating Disorders. *Cogn. Ther. Res.* **2019**, *43*, 759–768. [CrossRef]
30. O'Mara, S.; VanDine, L.; Tarescavage, A.M.; Ben-Porath, D. Examining DBT Day Treatment in Treating Mood Dysregulation Expectancy and Anxiety in Women Diagnosed with Eating Disorders. *J. Contemp. Psychother.* **2021**, *51*, 15–20. [CrossRef]
31. Federici, A.; Wisniewski, L. An intensive DBT program for patients with multidiagnostic eating disorder presentations: A case series analysis. *Int. J. Eat. Disord.* **2013**, *46*, 322–331. [CrossRef]
32. Steinglass, J.E.; Glasofer, D.R.; Walsh, E.; Guzman, G.; Peterson, C.B.; Walsh, B.T.; Attia, E.; Wonderlich, S.A. Targeting habits in anorexia nervosa: A proof-of-concept randomized trial. *Psychol. Med.* **2018**, *48*, 2584–2591. [CrossRef]
33. Petersson, S.; Arestedt, K.; Birgegard, A. Evaluation of the Affect School as supplementary treatment of Swedish women with eating disorders: A randomized clinical trial. *J. Eat. Disord.* **2022**, *10*, 76. [CrossRef]
34. Bodell, L.P.; Egbert, A.H.; Anaya, C.; Wildes, J.E. Associations between emotion reactivity and eating disorder symptoms in a transdiagnostic treatment-seeking sample. *Int. J. Eat. Disord.* **2022**, *55*, 1390–1396. [CrossRef]
35. Martin, S.J.; Luzier, J.; Saulnier, K.G. Changes in unhealthy exercise in outpatient eating disorder treatment: Examining emotion avoidance mechanisms. *Eat. Weight. Disord.-Stud. Anorex. Bulim. Obes.* **2022**, *27*, 675–682. [CrossRef]
36. Reilly, E.E.; Brown, T.A.; Arunagiri, V.; Kaye, W.H.; Wierenga, C.E. Exploring changes in alexithymia throughout intensive dialectical behavior therapy for eating disorders. *Eur. Eat. Disord. Rev.* **2022**, *30*, 193–205. [CrossRef]
37. Caslini, M.; Rivolta, L.; Zappa, L.E.; Carra, G.; Clerici, M. Psychotherapeutic treatment of eating disorders improve dissociative experiences and impulse regulation but not alexithymia. A case series report. *Riv. Di Psichiatr.* **2015**, *50*, 143–147.
38. Engel, G.L. The Need for a New Medical Model: A Challenge for Biomedicine. *Science* **1977**, *196*, 129–136. [CrossRef]

healthcare

MDPI

Review

Do Atopic Dermatitis and Psoriasis Have an Impact on Cognitive Decline—Latest Research Review

Marcin Kuryłło * and Ewa Mojs

Department of Clinical Psychology, Poznan University of Medical Sciences, 60-812 Poznań, Poland; ewa_mojs@poczta.onet.pl
* Correspondence: marcin@kuryllo.pl

Abstract: Background: Atopic dermatitis and psoriasis are chronic skin diseases that affect the mental health of patients. The relationship between AD and psoriasis and cognitive processes in patients remains unclear. The aim of the review was to answer the question of whether AD and psoriasis have an impact on cognitive decline in patients. Method: A systematic literature search was conducted on PubMed and EBSCO to identify case–control, cross-sectional, or cohort studies that evaluated the association between atopic dermatitis and psoriasis and cognitive impairment. Results: Most of the studies included in the review confirmed cognitive decline in patients with atopic dermatitis and psoriasis. Conclusions: It seems that atopic dermatitis and psoriasis may negatively affect cognitive processes such as working memory, concentration, attention, and speed of motor reactions. Psychological interventions targeting distorted cognitive processing could improve the quality of life of patients with atopic dermatitis and psoriasis.

Keywords: atopic dermatitis; psoriasis; cognitive impairment; cognitive processes

1. Introduction

Atopic dermatitis and psoriasis are common, chronic skin diseases affecting men and women all over the world [1,2]. AD is estimated to affect 15–30% of children and 2–10% of adults [3–5]. AD is characterized by impaired epidermal barrier function, sensitive and dry skin, eczematous lesions that can be localized or disseminated, and intense itching [6]. The prevalence of psoriasis in respective countries ranges from 0.09% to 11.43% [7]. Lesions typically appear as well-defined, erythematous, itchy papules and plaques covered with dry, white, or silvery scales, commonly on the skin of the elbows, knees, lumbosacral region, and scalp. However, they can appear anywhere on the body [6].

Both diseases are associated with an increased risk of comorbidities. Atopic dermatitis may increase the risk of other atopic disorders, including asthma, hay fever, food allergies and eosinophilic oesophagitis [8]. Whereas patients with severe psoriasis face an increased risk of death due to malignant neoplasms, chronic lower respiratory tract infections, diabetes and kidney diseases [9]. Both groups are more susceptible to the risk of dementia, infections and cardiovascular diseases [8,9].

In recent years, there have been many studies on the correlation between psoriasis and AD and mental condition of patients [10–13]. Numerous publications indicate the high prevalence of anxiety and depressive symptoms [14,15], suicidal thoughts [16–19] and alcohol abuse [20,21] among patients with AD and psoriasis.

The association between AD and psoriasis and cognitive processes in patients is still unclear. Cognitive impairment is demonstrated through memory difficulties [22], and difficulties with concentration and decision-making, which translates to the quality of life of the patients. The symptoms range from mild to acute, and the prevalence of cognitive impairment differs depending on the age, level of education and geographical location [23]. Cao S. et al. (2024) emphasized the significant causal association between AD and an increased risk of autism spectrum disorder and also identified bipolar disorder and anorexia nervosa as risk factors for atopic dermatitis [24]. Earlier reports have demonstrated a relationship between AD and psoriasis, and cognitive functions [25–27]. However, the studies were scarce in number. It was only recently, that the interest in this issue has grown, and more publications with study-based findings were published.

2. Method

The review was conducted in accordance with the PRISMA 2020 Statement (Preferred Reporting Items for Systematic Reviews and Meta-Analyses). The PRISMA statement and its extensions are evidence-based recommendations intended to encourage transparent and comprehensive reporting of systematic reviews. The 2020 PRISMA statement replaced the 2009 statement, which was originally developed to help systematic reviewers be transparent about why a review was conducted, what the authors executed, and what they found. PRISMA 2020 includes new reporting guidelines that reflect advances in methods for identifying, selecting, evaluating and synthesizing studies [28] (see Figure 1).

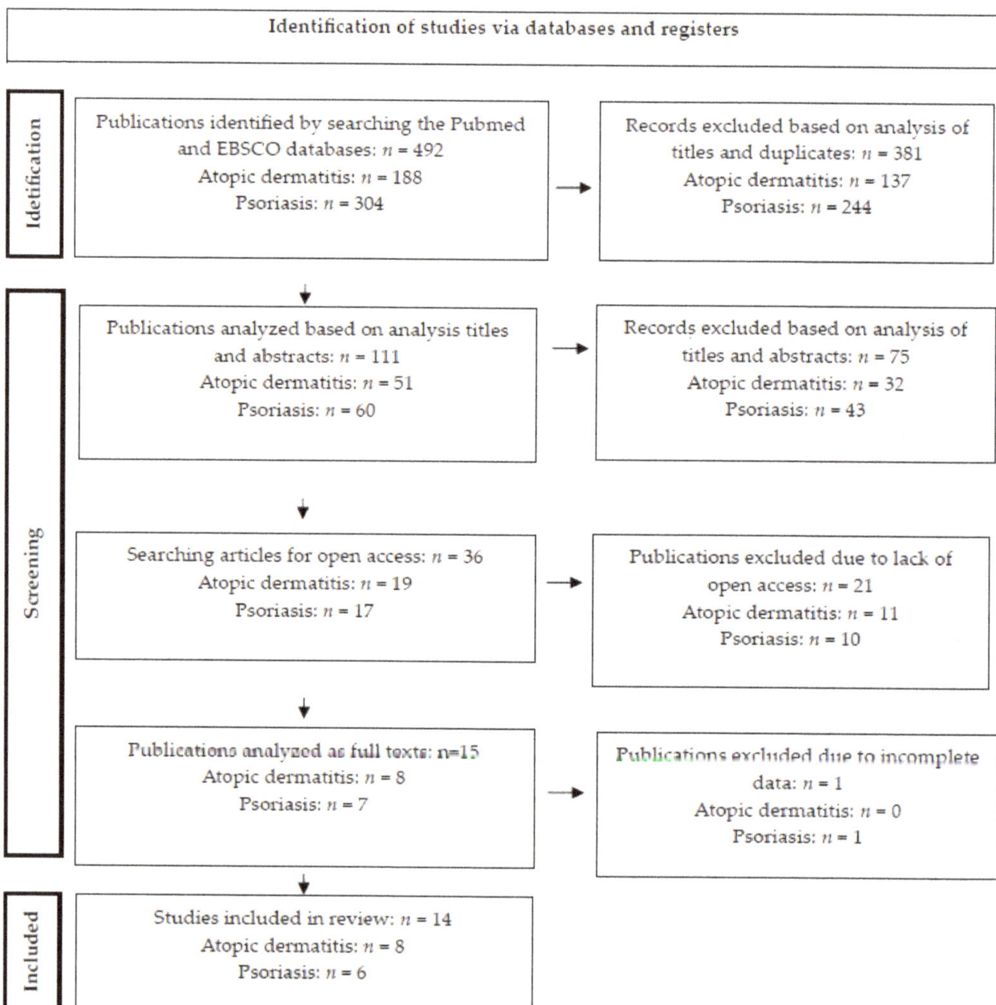

Figure 1. Flow chart of the review process according to PRISMA guidelines.

A systematic review of the scientific literature in PubMed and EBSCO [eBook Open Access (OA) Collection, Academic Search Ultimate, APA PsycInfo, APA PsycArticles, eBook Collection, APA PsycBooks, ERIC, Health Source: Nursing/Academic Edition, Library, Information Science & Technology Abstracts, MEDLINE, Academic Research Source eJournals)] services was performed to identify case–control, cross-sectional or cohort studies where the relationship between atopic dermatitis and psoriasis, and cognitive disorders was assessed. The authors of the review wanted to find an answer to the question whether AD and psoriasis affect the impairment of cognitive functions in patients.

The methodology of the review was formally discussed and agreed within the study group. While searching for the studies, the articles published within the last 6 years (from January 2018 to 18 March 2024) were considered. The searched entries included both the standard headings of medical topics and keywords, such as atopic dermatitis, AD, eczema, psoriasis, plaque psoriasis, cognitive functions, cognitive processes, dementia, memory, attention, thinking, executive functions. The entries were mixed with Boolean operators, and the searched entries were combined and thus it was possible to develop several potential search strategies to find the appropriate results. The included criteria are presented in Table 1.

Table 1. Included criteria according to PECOS.

Population (P)	Exposure (E)	Comparison (C)	Outcome (O)	Study Design (S)
People suffering from psoriasis or atopic dermatitis.	Neuropsychological tests, neuroimaging.	Comparison with a group of healthy people.	Impact on cognitive processes.	Control, prospective, retrospective, longitudinal, observational, cohort or cross-sectional studies.

Source: own study.

Only those studies that included control groups were presented. The review includes articles whose full content is available in open access.

Exclusion criteria: meta-analyses, reviews, systematic reviews, scoping reviews, conference reports, commentaries, theses and non-peer-reviewed publications were excluded from the review.

A computer search for articles was performed in accordance with the identified criteria. First, duplicates were removed from 492 records; then, authors studied the titles. Next, after analyzing the titles and abstracts, the authors excluded 75 articles because they did not comply with the criteria established by the authors. The authors identified 36 potentially relevant articles that clearly presented the premises and research objectives, explaining the purposefulness of sample selection and participant recruitment. Attention was paid to whether appropriate research tools were used, the transparency of research financing sources and open access. The next step was to select open-access articles. The full texts of the selected articles were fully analyzed to avoid the risk of missing potentially important data. Finally, the authors decided to include 14 studies in the presented results. All studies included a control group. The results are presented in Tables 2 and 3:

Table 2. Effects of atopic dermatitis on cognition.

	First Author and Year	Study Design	Aim/Domains Assessed	Study Group	Conclusions
1	Bozsányi S, et al., 2023 [6]	Observational study	Assessment of Frontal Hemispherical Lateralization in Plaque Psoriasis and Atopic Dermatitis.	N = 46 patients with psoriasis, N = 56 patients with AD, N = 29 people without skin diseases, Hungary.	Psychophysiological and psychometric data suggest a shared prevalence of right-hemispheric dominance in both AD and Pso patient groups.
2	Fereidouni M, et al., 2021 [29]	Cross-sectional study	A study of the association of cognitive abilities and emotional function with allergic disorders in young women.	N = 181 female students (N = 54 Allergic Rhino-conjunctivitis, Eczema, Asthma, N = 127 healthy women), between 18 and 27 years of age in Iran.	There was a high prevalence of psychological/psychiatric disorders that included: anxiety, and sleep problems among allergic women. Those with at least one allergy disorder were more likely to have anxiety behavior than healthy individuals (Odds ratio = 1.86; 95% CI: 1.02–3.4), and insomnia symptoms (OR = 2.3; 95% CI: 1.2–4.3).
3	Kim JH, et al., 2023 [30]	Cross-sectional study	Neurodevelopment at 6 years of age in children with atopic dermatitis.	N = 30,557 children with AD, N = 89,452 healthy children, born between 2008 and 2012 in Korea.	AD before age 2 years may be associated with an increased risk of neurodevelopmental dysfunction including gross and fine motor skills in the young childhood period. AD group showed a higher risk of suspected neurodevelopmental dysfunction in the total score (weighted adjusted odds ratio: 1.10; 95% CI: 1.05–1.16], gross motor skills: 1.14; CI 1.04–1.25, and fine motor skills: 1.15; CI 1.06–1.25) than the control group.
4	Kuo HC, et al., 2020 [31]	Observational study	Allergic diseases do not impair the cognitive development of children but do damage the mental health of their caregivers.	N = 109 patients with AD (mean age 6.8 years) N = 82 healthy children (mean age 6.3 years) from Taiwan.	Allergic diseases did not impair the cognitive development of children. Atopic dermatitis did not exhibit an individual effect on children's cognitive scores, ADHD symptoms and severity (SNAP-IV) scores, or caregivers' family APGAR scores.
5	Jackson-Cowan L, et al., 2018 [32]	Cross-sectional study	Childhood atopic dermatitis is associated with cognitive dysfunction: A National Health Interview Survey study from 2008 to 2018.	N = 13,398 children with AD, N = 96,084 children without AD, at ages 2–17 years, USA.	The prevalences of cognitive dysfunction, such as memory impairment (0.87% vs. 0.42%), developmental delays (6.96% vs. 3.87%), and attention deficit (hyperactivity) disorder (10.78% vs. 8.10%) were higher in children with vs. without AD.

Table 2. *Cont.*

	First Author and Year	Study Design	Aim/Domains Assessed	Study Group	Conclusions
6	Magyari A, et al., 2022 [33]	Longitudinal cohort study	Adult atopic eczema and the risk of dementia	*N* = 213,444 patients diagnosed with Atopic eczema, *N* = 1554 223 healthy individuals, aged 60 to 99 years, UK.	Atopic eczema was associated with a small but increased risk of incident dementia. The association increased with the severity of atopic eczema. Participants with atopic eczema had a 27% increased risk of dementia after adjusting for the potential confounders (hazard ratio (HR): 1.27; 95% CI: 1.23–1.30). The magnitude of risk increased with increasing atopic eczema severity.
7	Smirnova J, et al., 2019 [34]	National cohort study	Atopic dermatitis, educational attainment and psychological functioning: a national cohort study.	*N* = 1673 males with AD, *N* = 233,042 males without AD at ages 17–20 years assessed for military conscription in Sweden between 1969 and 1976.	Swedish men with AD did not have lower cognitive function or poorer educational attainment. AD was associated with a greater risk of low stress resilience (adjusted relative risk ratio (RRR) 1.60; 95% confidence interval 1.38 to 1.86). AD was associated with higher cognitive function (b coefficient 0.15; 0.05 to 0.24) and higher educational level (RRR 1.29; 1.13 to 1.47) but adjustment for socioeconomic characteristics of the family of origin attenuated the magnitude of the associations and eliminated statistical significance (b coefficient 0.06; −0.03 to 0.15) and (RRR 1.16; 1.00 to 1.35).
8	Woo YR, et al., 2023 [35]	National cohort study	Increased risk of Dementia in patients with atopic dermatitis.	*N* = 38,391 people with AD, *N* = 2,643,602 people without AD adults $\geq$ 40 years of age, Korean National Health Insurance System (NHIS) database from 2009 to 2016.	The risks of all-cause dementia and Alzheimer's disease were increased in patients with AD. Males with AD had an increased risk of dementia (HR: 1.111; 95% CI: 1.040–1.186) and Alzheimer's disease (HR: 1.099; 95% CI: 1.019–1.184) compared with males without AD.

Source: Own study.

Table 3. Effects of psoriasis on cognition.

	First Author and Year	Study Design	Aim/Domains Assessed	Study Group	Conclusions
1	Deveci E, et al., 2019 [36]	Observational study	Oxidative stress and inflammatory response in patients with psoriasis; is there any relationship between psychiatric comorbidity and cognitive functions?	$N = 37$ patients diagnosed with psoriasis, $N = 37$ healthy volunteers, aged between 18 and 65 years, Turkey.	Psoriasis patients have higher risk factors than healthy controls for cognitive impairment, independent of depression, inflammation and oxidative stress levels. The control group's Öktem Learning (t-test = 3.756, $p < 0.001$); Phonemic Verbal Fluency Test (K-A-S), KAS-K (t = 3.615, $p < 0.001$), KAS-A (t = 3.391, $p < 0.001$), KAS-S (t = 4.441, $p < 0.0001$), scores and completed category number were higher than the patient group (t = 2.082, $p = 0.041$) according to Wisconsin Card Sorting Test. Total recall scores of the control group were higher than patients (U = 503.00, $p < 0.05$) according to Mann–Whitney U test.
2	Kim M, et al., 2020 [37]	National cohort study	Increased risk of Alzheimer's disease in patients with psoriasis	$N = 535{,}927$ patients diagnosed with psoriasis, $N = 2{,}679{,}635$ healthy subjects, aged 40–64 years, Korea.	In a multivariable-adjusted model, patients with psoriasis showed a significantly increased risk of Alzheimer's disease (hazard ratio: 1.09; 95% CI: 1.07–1.12, $p < 0.0001$) compared to controls without psoriasis. Among patients with psoriasis, the risk of Alzheimer's disease was significantly increased in psoriasis patients not receiving systemic therapy compared to those receiving systemic therapy (hazard ratio: 1.10; 95% CI, 1.08–1.12 vs. hazard ratio: 0.99; 95% CI: 0.90–1.09, $p < 0.0001$).
3	Kridin K, et al., 2020 [38]	Cross-sectional study	Psoriasis and Dementia	$N = 121{,}801$ patients with psoriasis, $N = 121{,}802$ healthy subjects from Israel, the mean age = 48.9 years.	Psoriasis was associated with a lower prevalence of dementia relative to control subjects. Multivariate analysis adjusting for demographic variables, cardiovascular-related risk factors, and healthcare utilization demonstrated a significant inverse association between psoriasis and dementia in the entire study population (adjusted OR 0.86; 95% CI 0.76–0.96; $p = 0.009$), but not in the subgroup of patients with moderate-to-severe psoriasis (adjusted OR 0.91; 95% CI 0.81–1.02; $p = 0.113$).

Table 3. *Cont.*

	First Author and Year	Study Design	Aim/Domains Assessed	Study Group	Conclusions
4	Marek-Józefowicz L, et al., 2022 [39]	Observational study	Cognitive functions associated with brain imaging markers in patients with psoriasis	*N* = 53 patients with psoriasis, *N* = 36 healthy controls, aged 21–68 years, Poland.	Patients with psoriasis presented worse achievements on all the neuropsychological tests and showed more intense changes on MRI compared to healthy controls. The severity of psoriasis was positively correlated with the intensity of depressive symptoms (R = 0.46, $p = 0.01$) and the time of performance on the Trail Making Test (TMT) part A (R = 0.43, $p = 0.02$). Depressive symptoms were also correlated with performance on the TMT A (R = 0.43, $p = 0.02$).
5	Padma K, et al., 2020 [40]	Cross-sectional study	Cognitive impairment in patients with psoriasis: a clinical study in teaching hospital	*N* = 100 patients with psoriasis, *N* = 100 healthy controls, aged 20–65 years, India.	Patients with psoriasis had cognitive deficits in the domain of attention, concentration and total scores of Standard Mini-Mental Status Examination (SMMSE) and Brief Cognitive Rating Scale (BCRS) for assessing cognitive functions. Study reveals statistical significance between the duration of psoriasis ($p = 0.007$) and cognitive impairment.
6	Zingel R, et al., 2023 [41]	Longitudinal cohort study	Association between psoriasis and dementia.	*N* = 10,583 patients with psoriasis, *N* = 10,583 healthy controls, over 60 years, Germany.	The study found a positive association between psoriasis and all-cause dementia in patients in general practices in Germany. Psoriasis was significantly associated with a dementia risk (HR: 1.24; 95% CI: 1.14–1.35, $p < 0.001$).

Source: Own study.

Due to the fact that the primary studies included in the review were heterogeneous and there were differences in the study groups, methods and measurement tools used, it is impossible to conduct a meta-analysis, so the authors decided to use a narrative approach.

3. Results

3.1. Effects of Atopic Dermatitis on Cognition

Three of the eight studies focused on children. Two of the three studies [30,32] indicated memory disorders, developmental delays and neurodevelopmental problems, including those related to attention and hyperactivity, in children with AD. One other study [31] found no greater cognitive problems in children with atopic dermatitis than in healthy children.

Two of the eight studies [33,35] focused on dementia, and both confirmed a greater risk of developing dementia in people with atopic dermatitis compared to healthy people. The first study [33] showed that the association increased with the severity of atopic eczema. The authors of the second study [35] showed a significant burden of dementia in patients with atopic dermatitis.

One of the eight studies [29] found no significant difference between the atopic dermatitis group and the healthy group in terms of tasks related to cognitive abilities. However, it was shown that people with atopic dermatitis had higher scores on the depression and stress scale.

One of the eight studies [34] did not confirm increased cognitive problems in young men with AD. Swedish males with atopic dermatitis had lower stress tolerance in late adolescence but did not have poorer cognitive function or educational achievement.

One of the eight studies [6] indicated a shared prevalence of right-hemispheric dominance in both atopic dermatitis and psoriasis patients. AD patients with dominant right hemisphere prefrontal activation showed increased markers of inhibition and avoidance, while psoriasis patients showed increased sympathetic nervous system activity.

3.2. Effects of Psoriasis on Cognition

Three of the six studies [36,39,40] confirmed the problems of psoriasis patients associated with worse results in neuropsychological tests and showed more intense changes in MRI compared to the healthy control group and greater problems with concentration and attention.

Three of the six studies [37,38,41] focused on dementia and Alzheimer's disease. Two of three studies [37,41] confirmed a greater risk of developing dementia in people with psoriasis compared to healthy people. One study [38] showed that people with psoriasis have a lower incidence of dementia.

One of the studies included in Table 2 [6] indicated a shared prevalence of right-hemispheric dominance in psoriasis patients.

4. Discussion

Despite advances in understanding the pathophysiology and introducing new treatments for chronic skin conditions, including atopic dermatitis and psoriasis, surviving and treating the disease place a heavy burden on patients, their families and society. The aim of the paper was to present the latest research on the impact of atopic dermatitis and psoriasis on cognitive processes in patients.

Many of the studies published so far have shown that the prevalence of cognitive impairment is higher in people with certain inflammatory skin diseases, including psoriasis and chronic eczema dermatitis [22,23,42,43]. Nine studies included in this review are coherent with those findings [30,32,33,35–37,39–41].

Yi et al. (2024) assessed alterations of intrinsic brain activity and its association with cognitive function in patients with psoriasis. As reported, patients with psoriasis had altered brain activity and connectivity in the key brain areas within the DMN-prefrontal circuit. According to the authors, these brain changes may be the underlying neural correlates for cognitive functioning in patients with psoriasis [44]. The review included a study on the association between the variation in the function of the right and left hemispheres of the brain and the prevalence of atopic dermatitis and psoriasis. Frontal asymmetry is often treated as a predictor or consequence variable regarding motivation, emotional regulation, and psychopathology [6,45]. Each hemisphere of the brain plays a specialized role in cognitive and behavioural processes; therefore, in chronic skin diseases such as psoriasis and atopic dermatitis, the degree of lateralization between the hemispheres may provide insight into the specific links between skin diseases and the psyche. The authors presented data that suggest the dominance of the right hemisphere in both AD and psoriasis patient groups. The study also examined the cognitive and metacognitive abilities of the subjects, but no significant differences were found in these areas between the patients and the control group [6].

Research on the impact of chronic skin diseases in children, including atopic dermatitis and psoriasis, on cognitive processes is inconsistent. Lee et al. (2023) showed that AD was associated with vulnerability in concentrations (aOR: 1.170; CI: 1.093–1.254). The impact of AD on concentrations showed consistent results regardless of sex, exposure to systemic corticosteroids and antihistamines, and age at the diagnosis of AD [46]. A study by Ma EZ (2024) suggested that pediatric AD was generally associated with greater odds of reported difficulties in learning and memory. However, this association was primarily limited to children with neurodevelopmental comorbidities, such as ADHD or learning disabilities [47]. Vittrup et al. (2023) reported that atopic dermatitis, particularly when severe, is associated with lower school performance in childhood and IQ in young men, which can interfere with academic achievements in life [48]. Sockler et al. (2024) did not find any clinically meaningful associations between AD activity and severity and general cognitive function during early childhood and adolescence [49]. The studies included in this review confirm these inconsistencies. Two of the four studies [30,32] indicate greater neurodevelopmental problems in children with AD. One other study [31] found no greater cognitive problems in children with atopic dermatitis than in healthy children.

Similar to studies on the impact of chronic skin diseases on cognitive processes in children, studies on the impact of atopic dermatitis and psoriasis on dementia and Alzheimer's disease are also inconclusive. Two separate teams of researchers Wu CY et al. (2020) and Pezzolo et al. (2021) reported that psoriasis was not found to be a risk factor for dementia [50] and was not associated with preclinical markers or higher dementia risk [51]. While other researchers (Huang KL. et al., 2019) reported a significantly higher risk of dementia (aHR = 1.23; 95% CI: 1.06–1.42) identified in the psoriasis group [52]. Also, Khalaf et al. (2021) confirmed worse cognitive impairment when compared to the controls regardless of the psoriasis severity [53]. Joh et al. (2023) showed that asthma, allergic rhinitis, and atopic dermatitis were significantly associated with increased risk of all-cause dementia and subtypes, with dose-effect relationships with the severity of allergic diseases [54]. Some of the presented research results attempt to answer the question of whether atopic dermatitis and psoriasis influence dementia and Alzheimer's disease [33,35,37,38,41]. The risk of dementia includes genetic factors, aging, environmental factors, certain types of diseases, and unhealthy lifestyles. Psoriasis usually occurs much earlier than dementia; therefore, according to some researchers, there is reason to speculate that psoriasis may also be a risk factor for dementia [55]. A large cross-sectional study from Israel showed an inverse relationship between psoriasis and dementia, patients with psoriasis were less likely to develop dementia than control groups [38].

This review has some limitations. First, only a small number of the interventions presented in this review included randomised controlled trials. Second, although the methodological aspects of experimental design were duly taken into account in the interventions presented, the observations collected here differed in terms of sample size, experimental procedure, approaches, and outcome measures.

Both atopic dermatitis and psoriasis cause a lot of suffering to patients, which is often associated with stress and, as a consequence, mental problems such as depression or anxiety [14,15,56]. Many psychological interventions have been tested for atopic dermatitis and psoriasis [6,57–60] but personalized approaches are lacking due to the potential prevalence of cognitive impairment. Due to the fact that most of the findings of the presented studies indicate the existence of the impact of AD and psoriasis on cognitive functions, it is worth considering the inclusion of psychological interventions in medical treatment conducted by dermatologists. Jen H. et al. (2021) suggested brief cognitive assessments to screen older psoriasis patients with subjective cognitive complaints [61]. Pan TL. et al. (2021) indicated that atopic dermatitis may be an independent risk factor for new-onset dementia and clinicians may monitor the trajectory of neurocognitive function among elderly patients with AD [62].

Overall, this review contributes to the existing literature on the effects of AD and psoriasis on cognition and highlights the importance of further research on this topic.

5. Conclusions

1. Most available studies indicate a negative impact of chronic skin diseases, including atopic dermatitis and psoriasis, on cognitive function in patients;
2. Further research is needed to examine the impact of chronic skin diseases, including atopic dermatitis and psoriasis, on cognitive impairment;
3. The use of psychological interventions targeting distorted cognitive processing in patients with atopic dermatitis and psoriasis could improve their quality of life.

Author Contributions: Conceptualization, M.K. and E.M.; data curation, M.K.; formal analysis, M.K. and E.M.; investigation, M.K.; methodology, M.K. and E.M.; resources, M.K.; writing—original draft, M.K.; writing—review and editing, M.K. and E.M. All authors have read and agreed to the published version of the manuscript.

Funding: This research received no external funding.

Institutional Review Board Statement: Not applicable.

Informed Consent Statement: Not applicable.

Data Availability Statement: The authors confirm that the data supporting the findings of this study are available within the article.

Conflicts of Interest: The authors declare no conflicts of interest.

References

1. Pankowski, D.; Wytrychiewicz-Pankowska, K.; Owczarek, W. Cognitive impairment in psoriasis patients: A systematic review of case–control studies. *J. Neurol.* **2022**, *269*, 6269–6278. [CrossRef] [PubMed]
2. Chen, W.-Y.; Chen, S.-C.; Hsu, S.-Y.; Lin, Y.-A.; Shih, C.-M.; Huang, C.-Y.; Wang, K.-H.; Lee, A.-W. Annoying Psoriasis and Atopic Dermatitis: A Narrative Review. *Int. J. Mol. Sci.* **2022**, *23*, 4898. [CrossRef] [PubMed]
3. Bieber, T. Atopic dermatitis. *Ann. Dermatol.* **2010**, *22*, 125–137. [CrossRef] [PubMed]
4. Chiesa Fuxench, Z.C.; Block, J.K.; Boguniewicz, M.; Boyle, J.; Ong, P.Y. Atopic Dermatitis in America Study: A Cross-Sectional Study Examining the Prevalence and Disease Burden of Atopic Dermatitis in the US Adult Population. *J. Investig. Dermatol.* **2019**, *139*, 583–590. [CrossRef] [PubMed]
5. Tsai, Y.-C.; Tsai, T.-F. Overlapping Features of Psoriasis and Atopic Dermatitis: From Genetics to Immunopathogenesis to Phenotypes. *Int. J. Mol. Sci.* **2022**, *23*, 5518. [CrossRef] [PubMed]
6. Bozsányi, S.; Czurkó, N.; Becske, M.; Kasek, R.; Lázár, B.K.; Boostani, M.; Meznerics, F.A.; Farkas, K.; Varga, N.N.; Gulyás, L.; et al. Assessment of Frontal Hemispherical Lateralization in Plaque Psoriasis and Atopic Dermatitis. *J. Clin. Med.* **2023**, *12*, 4194. [CrossRef] [PubMed]
7. *Global Report on Psoriasis*; World Health Organization: Geneva, Switzerland, 2016.
8. Silverberg, J.I. Comorbidities and the impact of atopic dermatitis. *Ann. Allergy Asthma Immunol.* **2019**, *123*, 144–151. [CrossRef] [PubMed]

9. Abuabara, K.; Azfar, R.S.; Shin, D.B.; Neimann, A.L.; Troxel, A.B.; Gelfand, J.M. Cause-specific mortality in patients with severe psoriasis: A population-based cohort study in the U.K. *Br. J. Dermatol.* **2010**, *163*, 586–592. [CrossRef] [PubMed]
10. Liang, S.E.; Cohen, J.M.; Ho, R.S. Psoriasis and suicidality: A review of the literature. *Dermatol. Ther.* **2019**, *32*, e12771. [CrossRef]
11. Dalgard, F.J.; Gieler, U.; Tomas-Aragones, L.; Lien, L.; Poot, F.; Jemec, G.B.; Misery, L.; Szabo, C.; Linder, D.; Sampogna, F.; et al. The psychological burden of skin diseases: A cross-sectional multicenter study among dermatological out-patients in 13 European countries. *J. Investig. Dermatol.* **2015**, *135*, 984–991. [CrossRef]
12. Silverberg, J.I.; Lei, D.; Yousaf, M.; Janmohamed, S.R.; Vakharia, P.P.; Chopra, R.; Chavda, R.; Gabriel, S.; Patel, K.R.; Singam, V.; et al. Association of atopic dermatitis severity with cognitive function in adults. *J. Am. Acad. Dermatol.* **2020**, *83*, 1349–1359. [CrossRef] [PubMed]
13. Balato, A.; Zink, A.; Babino, G.; Buononato, D.; Kiani, C.; Eyerich, K.; Ziehfreund, S.; Scala, E. The Impact of Psoriasis and Atopic Dermatitis on Quality of Life: A Literature Research on Biomarkers. *Life* **2022**, *12*, 2026. [CrossRef]
14. Leibovici, V.; Canetti, L.; Yahalomi, S.; Cooper-Kazaz, R.; Bonne, O.; Ingber, A.; Bachar, E. Wellbeing, psychopathology and coping strategies in psoriasis compared with atopic dermatitis: A controlled study. *J. Eur. Acad. Dermatol. Venereol.* **2009**, *24*, 897–903.
15. Zaher, H.A.E.M.; Amin, M.E.; Rakhawy, M.Y. Coping with depression and anxiety in patients with psoriasis. *Egypt. J. Psychiatr.* **2010**, *31*, 57–63.
16. Singh, S.; Taylor, C.; Kornmehl, H.; Armstrong, A.W. Psoriasis and suicidality: A systematic review and meta-analysis. *J. Am. Acad. Dermatol.* **2017**, *77*, 425–440.e2. [CrossRef] [PubMed]
17. Pompili, M.; Innamorati, M.; Forte, A.; Erbuto, D.; Lamis, D.A.; Narcisi, A.; Rea, C.; Orsini, D.; D'arino, A.; Arcese, A.; et al. Psychiatric comorbidity and suicidal ideation in psoriasis, melanoma and allergic disorders. *Int. J. Psychiatry Clin. Pract.* **2017**, *21*, 209–214. [CrossRef] [PubMed]
18. Lee, S.; Shin, A. Association of atopic dermatitis with depressive symptoms and suicidal behaviors among adolescents in Korea: The 2013 Korean Youth Risk Behavior Survey. *BMC Psychiatry* **2017**, *17*, 3. [CrossRef] [PubMed]
19. Nicholas, M.N.; Gooderham, M.J. Atopic Dermatitis, Depression, and Suicidality. *J. Cutan. Med. Surg.* **2017**, *21*, 237–242. [CrossRef] [PubMed]
20. Kamiya, K.; Kishimoto, M.; Sugai, J.; Komine, M.; Ohtsuki, M. Risk Factors for the Development of Psoriasis. *Int. J. Mol. Sci.* **2019**, *20*, 4347. [CrossRef]
21. Brenaut, E.; Horreau, C.; Pouplard, C.; Barnetche, T.; Paul, C.; Richard, M.A.; Joly, P.; Matire, M.L.; Aractingi, S.; Aubin, F.; et al. Alcohol consumption and psoriasis: A systematic literature review. *J. Eur. Acad. Dermatol. Venereol.* **2013**, *27*, 30–35. [CrossRef]
22. Damiani, G.; Tacastacas, J.D.; Wuerz, T.; Miller, L.; Fastenau, P.; Bailey, C.; Chawa, M.S.; Argenas, A.; Fiore, M.; Cooper, K.D.; et al. Cognition/Psychological Burden and Resilience in Cutaneous T-Cell Lymphoma and Psoriasis Patients: Real-Life Data and Implications for the Treatment. *BioMed Res. Int.* **2022**, *2022*, 8802469. [CrossRef] [PubMed]
23. Wen, S.; Elias, P.M.; Wakefield, J.S.; Mauro, T.M.; Man, M.Q. The Link between Cutaneous Inflammation and Cognitive Impairment. *J. Eur. Acad. Dermatol. Venereol.* **2022**, *36*, 1705–1712. [CrossRef] [PubMed]
24. Cao, S.; Zhang, Z.; Liu, L.; Li, Y.; Li, W.; Li, Y.; Wu, D. Causal relationships between atopic dermatitis and psychiatric disorders: A bidirectional two-sample Mendelian randomization study. *BMC Psychiatry* **2024**, *24*, 16. [CrossRef] [PubMed]
25. Albińska, P. Psychological aspects of allergic disorders: The difficulties of adult patients with bronchial asthma and atopic dermatitis. *Psychiatr. Psychol. Klin.* **2014**, *14*, 296–303. [CrossRef]
26. Marek, L.; Placek, W.; Borkowska, A. Cognitive impairment and affective temperament in patients with psoriasis. *Przegl. Dermatol.* **2011**, *98*, 483–490.
27. Innamorati, M.; Quinto, R.M.; Lester, D.; Iani, L.; Graceffa, D.; Bonifati, C. Cognitive impairment in patients with psoriasis: A matched case-control study. *J. Psychosom. Res.* **2018**, *105*, 99–105. [CrossRef] [PubMed]
28. Page, M.J.; McKenzie, J.E.; Bossuyt, P.M. The PRISMA 2020 statement: An updated guideline for reporting systematic reviews. *Syst. Rev.* **2021**, *10*, 89. [CrossRef] [PubMed]
29. Fereidouni, M.; Rezapour, H.; Saharkhiz, M.; Mahmoudzadeh, S.; Ayadilord, M.; Askari, M.; Karbasi, S.; Abbaszadeh, A.; Hoseini, Z.S.; Ferns, G.A.; et al. A study of the association of cognitive abilities and emotional function with allergic disorders in young women. *BMC Women Health* **2021**, *21*, 205. [CrossRef] [PubMed]
30. Kim, J.H.; Yi, Y.Y.; Ha, E.K.; Cha, H.R.; Han, M.Y.; Baek, H.S. Neurodevelopment at 6 years of age in children with atopic dermatitis. *Allergol. Int.* **2023**, *72*, 116–127. [CrossRef]
31. Kuo, H.C.; Chang, L.S.; Tsai, Z.Y.; Wang, L.J. Allergic diseases do not impair the cognitive development of children but do damage the mental health of their caregivers. *Sci. Rep.* **2020**, *10*, 13854. [CrossRef]
32. Jackson-Cowan, L.; Cole, E.F.; Silverberg, J.I.; Lawley, L.P. Childhood atopic dermatitis is associated with cognitive dysfunction: A National Health Interview Survey study from 2008 to 2018. *Ann. Allergy Asthma Immunol.* **2021**, *160*, 661–665. [CrossRef] [PubMed]
33. Magyari, A.; Ye, M.; Margolis, D.J.; McCulloch, C.E.; Cummings, S.R.; Yaffe, K.; Langan, S.M.; Abuabara, K. Adult atopic eczema and the risk of dementia: A population-based cohort study. *J. Am. Acad. Dermatol.* **2022**, *87*, 314–322. [CrossRef]
34. Smirnova, J.; Kobyletzki, L.B.; MLindberg, M.; Svensson, A.; Langan, S.M.; Montgomery, S. Atopic dermatitis, educational attainment and psychological functioning: A national cohort study. *Br. J. Dermatol.* **2019**, *180*, 559–564. [CrossRef] [PubMed]
35. Woo, Y.R.; Cho, M.; Han, K.D.; Cho, S.H.; Lee, J.H. Increased Risk of Dementia in Patients with Atopic Dermatitis: A Nationwide Population-Based Cohort Study. *Acta Derm. Venereol.* **2023**, *103*, adv4557. [CrossRef] [PubMed]

36. Deveci, E.; Kocacenk, T.; Şahan, E.; Yılmaz, O.; Öztürk, A.; Kırpınara, I. Oxidative stress and inflammatory response in patients with psoriasis; is there any relationship with psychiatric comorbidity and cognitive functions? *Psychiatry Clin. Psychopharmacol.* **2019**, *29*, 682–695. [CrossRef]
37. Kim, M.; Park, H.E.; Lee, S.H.; Han, K.; Lee, J.H. Increased risk of Alzheimer's disease in patients with psoriasis: A nationwide population-based cohort study. *Sci. Rep.* **2020**, *10*, 6454. [CrossRef] [PubMed]
38. Kridin, K.; Linder, D.; Shalom, G.; Piaserico, S.; Babaev, M.; Freud, T.; Comaneshter, D.; Cohen, A.D. Psoriasis and Dementia: A Cross-sectional Study of 121,801 Patients. *Acta Derm. Venereol.* **2020**, *100*, adv00250. [CrossRef]
39. Marek-Józefowicz, L.; Lemanowicz, A.; Grochocka, M.; Wróblewska, M.; Białczyk, K.; Piec, K.; Kozera, G.M.; Serafin, Z.; Czajkowski, R.; Borkowska, A. Cognitive Functions Associated with Brain Imaging Markers in Patients with Psoriasis. *Int. J. Environ. Res. Public Health* **2022**, *19*, 5687. [CrossRef] [PubMed]
40. Padma, K.; Nanaware, S.S.; Yadiyal, A.; Mathai, P.J. Cognitive impairment in patients with psoriasis: A clinical study in teaching hospital. *J. Family Med. Prim. Care* **2020**, *9*, 4001–4004. [CrossRef]
41. Zingel, R.; Jacob, L.; Smith, L.; Konrad, M.; Kostev, K. Association Between Psoriasis and Dementia: A Retrospective Cohort Study. *J. Alzheimers Dis. Rep.* **2023**, *7*, 41–49. [CrossRef]
42. Gwinnutt, J.M.; Toyoda, T.; Barraclough, M.; Verstappen, S.M.M.; Hornberger, M.; MacGregor, A. Cognitive impairment in the immune-mediated inflammatory diseases compared with age-matched controls: Systematic review and meta-regression. *Semin. Arthritis Rheum.* **2023**, *58*, 152131. [CrossRef] [PubMed]
43. Galili, E.; Barzilai, A.; Shreberk-Hassidim, R.; Merdler, I.; Caspi, T.; Astman, N. Neuropsychiatric comorbidity among adolescents with psoriasis. *Br. J. Dermatol.* **2018**, *178*, 910–916. [CrossRef] [PubMed]
44. Yi, X.; Wang, X.; Fu, Y.; Luo, Y.; Wang, J.; Han, Z.; Kuang, Y.; Chen, X.; Chen, B.T. Altered brain activity and cognitive impairment in patients with psoriasis. *J. Eur. Acad. Dermatol. Venereol.* **2024**, *38*, 557–567. [CrossRef] [PubMed]
45. Reznik, S.J.; Allen, J.J. Frontal asymmetry as a mediator and moderator of emotion: An updated review. *Psychophysiology* **2018**, *55*, e12965. [CrossRef] [PubMed]
46. Lee, E.; Kim, J.H.; Cha, H.R.; Ha, E.H.; Shin, J.; Lee, W.S.; Lee, S.W.; Han, M.Y. Association between atopic dermatitis and school readiness in preschool children. *Pediatr. Allergy Immunol.* **2023**, *34*, e13996. [CrossRef] [PubMed]
47. Ma, E.Z.; Chang, H.R.; Radtke, S.; Wan, J. Symptoms of Cognitive Impairment Among Children with Atopic Dermatitis. *JAMA Dermatol.* **2024**, *6*, e240015. [CrossRef] [PubMed]
48. Vittrup, I.; Andersen, Y.M.F.; Skov, L.; Wu, J.J.; Agner, T.; Thomsen, S.F.; Egeberg, A.; Thyssen, J.P. The association between atopic dermatitis, cognitive function and school performance in children and young adults. *Br. J. Dermatol.* **2023**, *188*, 341–349. [CrossRef] [PubMed]
49. Sockler, P.G.; Hooper, S.R.; Abuabara, K.; Ma, E.Z.; Radtke, S.; Bao, A.; Kim, E.; Musci, R.J.; Kartawira, K.; Wan, J. Atopic dermatitis, cognitive function and psychiatric comorbidities across early childhood and adolescence in a population-based UK birth cohort. *Br. J. Dermatol.* **2024**, *190*, 501–509. [CrossRef] [PubMed]
50. Wu, C.Y.; Hu, H.Y.; Chou, Y.J.; Li, C.P.; Chang, Y.T. Psoriasis is not a risk factor for dementia: A 12-year nationwide population-based cohort study. *Arch. Dermatol. Res.* **2020**, *312*, 657–664. [CrossRef]
51. Pezzolo, E.; Mutlu, U.; Vernooij, M.W.; Dowlatshahi, E.A.; Gisondi, P.; Girolomoni, G.; Nijsten, T.; Ikram, M.A.; Wakkee, M. Psoriasis is not associated with cognition, brain imaging markers, and risk for dementia: The Rotterdam Study. *J. Am. Acad. Dermatol.* **2021**, *85*, 671–680. [CrossRef]
52. Huang, K.L.; Yeh, C.C.; Wu, S.I.; Huang, K.Y.; Yang, Y.H.; Kuo, T.Y.; Liang, H.Y.; Lee, Y.C.; McIntyre, R.S.; Lee, Y.; et al. Risk of Dementia Among Individuals with Psoriasis: A Nationwide Population-Based Cohort Study in Taiwan. *J. Clin. Psychiatry* **2019**, *80*, 18m12462. [CrossRef] [PubMed]
53. Khalaf, O.O.; El-Mesidy, M.S. Cognitive functions assessment in psoriasis patients: A cross-sectional study in university hospital. *Curr. Psychiatry Res. Rev.* **2021**, *17*, 120–126. [CrossRef]
54. Joh, H.K.; Kwon, H.; Son, K.Y.; Yun, J.M.; Cho, S.H.; Han, K.; Park, J.-H.; Cho, B. Allergic Diseases and Risk of Incident Dementia and Alzheimer's Disease. *Ann. Neurol.* **2023**, *93*, 384–397. [CrossRef] [PubMed]
55. Zhao, J.; Li, T.; Wang, J. Association between psoriasis and dementia: A systematic review. *Neurologia* **2021**. *Online ahead of print*. [CrossRef] [PubMed]
56. Cherubin, M.; Tebar, W.R.; Meneghini, V.; Bensenor, I.M. Psoriasis and associated risk factors: A cross-sectional analysis of the Brazilian Longitudinal Study of Adult Health. *Rev. Assoc. Med. Bras.* **2023**, *69*, e20230038. [CrossRef] [PubMed]
57. Offenbächer, M.; Seitlinger, M.; Münch, D.; Schnopp, C.; Darsow, U.; Harfensteller, J.; Schmid-Grendelmeier, P.; Ring, J.; Kohls, N. A pilot study of a mindfulness-based stress reduction programme in patients suffering from atopic dermatitis. *Psych* **2021**, *3*, 663–672. [CrossRef]
58. Linnet, J.; Jemec, G.B. Anxiety level and severity of skin condition predicts outcome of psychotherapy in atopic dermatitis patients. *Int. J. Dermatol.* **2001**, *40*, 632–636. [CrossRef] [PubMed]
59. Waldmann, V. Depth psychology-based psychotherapy of atopic dermatitis. Dermatol. *Psychosom. Dermatol. Psychosom.* **2002**, *3*, 82–86. [CrossRef]
60. Qureshi, A.A.; Awosika, O.; Baruffi, F.; Rengifo-Pardo, M.; Ehrlich, A. Psychological therapies in management of psoriatic skin disease: A systematic review. *Am. J. Clin. Dermatol.* **2019**, *20*, 607–624. [CrossRef]

61. Yen, H.; Chi, C. Is psoriasis associated with dementia or cognitive impairment? A Critically Appraised Topic. *Br. J. Dermatol.* **2021**, *184*, 34–42. [CrossRef]
62. Pan, T.L.; Bai, Y.M.; Cheng, C.M.; Tsai, S.J.; Tsai, C.F.; Su, T.P.; Li, C.T.; Lin, W.C.; Chen, T.J.; Liang, C.S.; et al. Atopic dermatitis and dementia risk: A nationwide longitudinal study. *Ann. Allergy Asthma Immunol.* **2021**, *127*, 200–205. [CrossRef] [PubMed]

MDPI AG
Grosspeteranlage 5
4052 Basel
Switzerland
Tel.: +41 61 683 77 34

Healthcare Editorial Office
E-mail: healthcare@mdpi.com
www.mdpi.com/journal/healthcare

www.ingramcontent.com/pod-product-compliance
Lightning Source LLC
Chambersburg PA
CBHW041949260926
51850CB00019B/2241
9783725863587